Atrial Fibrillation

Editor

HAKAN ORAL

HEART FAILURE CLINICS

www.heartfailure.theclinics.com

Consulting Editors
MANDEEP R. MEHRA
JAVED BUTLER

Founding Editor
JAGAT NARULA

April 2016 • Volume 12 • Number 2

ELSEVIER

1600 John F. Kennedy Boulevard • Suite 1800 • Philadelphia, Pennsylvania, 19103-2899

http://www.theclinics.com

HEART FAILURE CLINICS Volume 12, Number 2
April 2016 ISSN 1551-7136, ISBN-13: 978-0-323-44495-8

Editor: Lauren Boyle
Developmental Editor: Alison Swety

Heart Failure Clinics (ISSN 1551-7136) is published quarterly by Elsevier Inc., 360 Park Avenue South, New York, NY 10010-1710. Months of publication are January, April, July, and October. Business and editorial offices: 1600 John F. Kennedy Boulevard, Suite 1800, Philadelphia, PA 19103-2899. Periodicals postage paid at New York, NY, and additional mailing offices. Subscription prices are USD 240.00 per year for US individuals, USD 431.00 per year for US institutions, USD 100.00 per year for US students and residents, USD 280.00 per year for Canadian individuals, USD 499.00 per year for Canadian institutions, USD 300.00 per year for international individuals, USD 499.00 per year for international institutions, and USD 100.00 per year for Canadian and foreign students/residents. To receive student and resident rate, orders must be accompanied by name of affiliated institution, date of term, and the *signature* of program/residency coordinator on institution letterhead. Orders will be billed at individual rate until proof of status is received. Foreign air speed delivery is included in all *Clinics* subscription prices. All prices are subject to change without notice. **POSTMASTER:** Send address changes to *Heart Failure Clinics*, Elsevier Health Sciences Division, Subscription Customer Service, 3251 Riverport Lane, Maryland Heights, MO 63043. **Customer Service: 1-800-654-2452 (US and Canada). From outside of the US and Canada, call 314-447-8871. Fax: 314-447-8029. For print support, E-mail: JournalsCustomerService-usa@elsevier.com. For online support, E-mail: JournalsOnlineSupport-usa@elsevier.com.**

Reprints. For copies of 100 or more of articles in this publication, please contact the Commercial Reprints Department, Elsevier Inc., 360 Park Avenue South, New York, NY 10010-1710. Tel.: 212-633-3874; Fax: 212-633-3820; E-mail: reprints@elsevier.com.

Heart Failure Clinics is covered in *MEDLINE/PubMed (Index Medicus)*.

Contributors

CONSULTING EDITORS

MANDEEP R. MEHRA, MD, FACC, FACP, FRCP
Heart and Vascular Center, Brigham and Women's Hospital and Harvard Medical School, Boston, Massachusetts

JAVED BUTLER, MD, MPH, MBA
Stony Brook University Heart Institute, Department of Internal Medicine, Stony Brook School of Medicine, Stony Brook University Medical Center, Stony Brook, New York

EDITOR

HAKAN ORAL, MD
Frederick G. L. Huetwell Professor of Cardiovascular Medicine; Professor of Internal Medicine; Director, Cardiac Arrhythmia Service, University of Michigan, Cardiovascular Center, Ann Arbor, Michigan

AUTHORS

JUSTUS M.B. ANUMONWO, PhD
Assistant Professor, Internal Medicine (Cardiovascular Medicine), Department of Internal Medicine, Center for Arrhythmia Research, University of Michigan; Assistant Professor, Department of Molecular and Integrative Physiology, University of Michigan Medical School, Ann Arbor, Michigan

SAMUEL J. ASIRVATHAM, MD, FACC, FHRS
Professor of Medicine and Pediatrics, Division of Cardiovascular Diseases, Department of Internal Medicine; Department of Pediatrics and Adolescent Medicine, Mayo Clinic, Rochester, Minnesota

OMER BERENFELD, PhD
Associate Professor of Internal Medicine and Biomedical Engineering, Center for Arrhythmia Research, University of Michigan, Ann Arbor, Michigan

AMAN CHUGH, MD
Section of Cardiac Electrophysiology, Division of Cardiology, Cardiovascular Center, University of Michigan Hospitals, Ann Arbor, Michigan

THOMAS CHRISTOPHER CRAWFORD, MD
Division of Cardiology, Department of Medicine, University of Michigan, Ann Arbor, Michigan

RALPH J. DAMIANO Jr, MD
Division of Cardiothoracic Surgery, Barnes-Jewish Hospital, Washington University School of Medicine, St Louis, Missouri

EMILE G. DAOUD, MD, FHRS
Section Chief, Electrophysiology Section, Division of Cardiology, Ross Heart Hospital, Wexner Medical Center at The Ohio State University; Professor, Internal Medicine, Wexner Medical Center at The Ohio State University, Columbus, Ohio

CHRISTOPHER V. DeSIMONE, MD, PhD
Division of Cardiovascular Diseases, Department of Internal Medicine, Mayo Clinic, Rochester, Minnesota

PATRICK DILLON, MD
Fellow, Division of Cardiovascular Medicine,
University of Michigan Health System,
Ann Arbor, Michigan

MIKHAIL S. DZESHKA, MD
University of Birmingham Centre for
Cardiovascular Sciences, City Hospital,
Birmingham, United Kingdom; Grodno State
Medical University, Grodno, Belarus

PAUL A. FRIEDMAN, MD, FACC, FHRS
Division of Cardiovascular Diseases,
Department of Internal Medicine, Mayo Clinic,
Rochester, Minnesota

HAMID GHANBARI, MD
Clinical Lecturer, Division of Cardiovascular
Medicine, University of Michigan Health
System, Ann Arbor, Michigan

COLBY HALSEY, MD
Section of Cardiac Electrophysiology, Division
of Cardiology, Cardiovascular Center, University
of Michigan Hospitals, Ann Arbor, Michigan

MATTHEW C. HENN, MD
Division of Cardiothoracic Surgery, Barnes-
Jewish Hospital, Washington University School
of Medicine, St Louis, Missouri

ANDREW B. HUGHEY, MD
Division of Cardiology, Department of
Medicine, University of Michigan, Ann Arbor,
Michigan

JOSÉ JALIFE, MD
Professor of Internal Medicine and The Cyrus
and Jane Farrehi Professor of Cardiovascular
Research; Professor of Molecular and
Integrative Physiology; Director, Center for
Arrhythmia Research; Director, Cardiovascular
Research Center, University of Michigan,
Ann Arbor, Michigan

JÉRÔME KALIFA, MD, PhD
Department of Internal Medicine, Center
for Arrhythmia Research, Ann Arbor,
Michigan

PETER R. KOWEY, MD
Lankenau Institute for Medical Research,
Lankenau Medical Center, Wynnewood,
Pennsylvania; Jefferson Medical College,

Thomas Jefferson University, Philadelphia,
Pennsylvania

RAKESH LATCHAMSETTY, MD
Clinical Lecturer, Department of
Electrophysiology, University of Michigan
Hospital, Ann Arbor, Michigan

CHRISTOPHER P. LAWRANCE, MD
Division of Cardiothoracic Surgery, Barnes-
Jewish Hospital, Washington University School
of Medicine, St Louis, Missouri

GREGORY Y.H. LIP, MD
University of Birmingham Centre for
Cardiovascular Sciences, City Hospital,
Birmingham, United Kingdom

FRED MORADY, MD
Professor, Department of Electrophysiology,
University of Michigan Hospital, Ann Arbor,
Michigan

DILESH PATEL, MD
Electrophysiology Fellow, Electrophysiology
Section, Division of Cardiology, Ross Heart
Hospital, Wexner Medical Center at The Ohio
State University, Columbus, Ohio

WAJEEHA SAEED, MD
Albert Einstein College of Medicine,
Bronx Lebanon Hospital Center, Bronx,
New York

MUHAMMAD RIZWAN SARDAR, MD
Department of Cardiology, Cooper University
Hospital, Camden, New Jersey; Lankenau
Institute for Medical Research, Wynnewood,
Pennsylvania; Jefferson Medical College,
Thomas Jefferson University, Philadelphia,
Pennsylvania

FAISAL F. SYED, BSc (Hons), MBChB, MRCP
Division of Cardiovascular Diseases,
Department of Internal Medicine, Mayo Clinic,
Rochester, Minnesota

MRINAL YADAVA, MD
Division of Cardiology, Department of
Medicine, University of Michigan, Ann Arbor,
Michigan; Department of Medicine,
Michigan State University, East Lansing,
Michigan

Contents

Atrial fibrillation (AF) is the most frequently encountered arrhythmia. Prevalence increases with advancing age and so as its associated comorbidities, like heart failure. Choice of pharmacologic therapy depends on whether the goal of treatment is maintaining sinus rhythm or tolerating AF with adequate control of ventricular rates. Antiarrhythmic therapy and conversion of AF into sinus rhythm comes with the side effect profile, and we should select best antiarrhythmic therapy, individualized to the patient. New antiarrhythmic drugs are being tested in clinical trials. Drugs that target remodeling and inflammation are being tested for their use as prevention of AF or as upstream therapy.

Strategies and technology related to catheter ablation for atrial fibrillation (AF) continue to advance since its inception nearly 20 years ago. Broader selections of patients are now offered ablation with a similar level of procedural outcome and safety standards. It is hoped that improved understanding of the pathophysiologic processes of the initiation and maintenance of AF will refine target selection during ablation and improve long-term procedural efficacy, particularly in patients with persistent and long-standing persistent AF.

Atrial fibrillation is the most common cardiac arrhythmia, and its treatment options include drug therapy or catheter-based or surgical interventions. The surgical treatment of atrial fibrillation has undergone multiple evolutions over the last several decades. The Cox-Maze procedure went on to become the gold standard for the surgical treatment of atrial fibrillation and is currently in its fourth iteration (Cox-Maze IV). This article reviews the indications and preoperative planning for performing a Cox-Maze IV procedure. This article also reviews the literature describing the surgical results for both approaches including comparisons of the Cox-Maze IV to the previous cut-and-sew method.

Atrioventricular junction (AVJ) ablation is an effective therapy in patients with symptomatic atrial fibrillation who are intolerant to or unsuccessfully managed with rhythm control or medical rate control strategies. A drawback is that the procedure mandates a pacing system. Overall, the safety and efficacy of AVJ ablation is high with a majority of the patients reporting significant improvement in symptoms and quality-of-life measures. Risk of sudden cardiac death after device implantation is low, especially with an appropriate postprocedure pacing rate. Mortality benefit with AVJ ablation has been shown in patients with heart failure and cardiac resynchronization therapy devices.

As atrial fibrillation (AF) substantially increases the risk of stroke and other thromboembolic events, most AF patients require appropriate antithrombotic prophylaxis.

Oral anticoagulation (OAC) with either dose-adjusted vitamin K antagonists (VKAs) (eg, warfarin) or non-VKA oral anticoagulants (eg, dabigatran, apixaban, rivaroxaban) can be used for this purpose unless contraindicated. Therefore, risk assessment of stroke and bleeding is an obligatory part of AF management, and risk has to be weighed individually. Antiplatelet drugs (eg, aspirin and clopidogrel) are inferior to OAC, both alone and in combination, with a comparable risk of bleeding events.

Percutaneous left atrial appendage (LAA) closure is being increasingly used as a treatment strategy to prevent stroke in patients with atrial fibrillation (AF) who have contraindications to anticoagulants. Several approaches and devices have been developed in the last few years, each with their own unique set of advantages and disadvantages. In this article, the published studies on surgical and percutaneous approaches to LAA closure are reviewed, focusing on stroke mechanisms in AF, LAA structure and function relevant to stroke prevention, practical differences in procedural approach, and clinical considerations surrounding management.

Atrial fibrillation is the most commonly encountered arrhythmia after cardiac surgery. Although usually self-limiting, it represents an important predictor of increased patient morbidity, mortality, and health care costs. Numerous studies have attempted to determine the underlying mechanisms of postoperative atrial fibrillation (POAF) with varied success. A multifactorial pathophysiology is hypothesized, with inflammation and postoperative β-adrenergic activation recognized as important contributing factors. The management of POAF is complicated by a paucity of data relating to the outcomes of different therapeutic interventions in this population. This article reviews the literature on epidemiology, mechanisms, and risk factors of POAF, with a subsequent focus on the therapeutic interventions and guidelines regarding management.

The mechanisms underlying atrial fibrillation (AF) in humans are poorly understood. In particular, we simply do not understand how atrial AF becomes persistent or permanent. The objective of this brief review is to address the most important factors involved in the mechanism of AF perpetuation, including structural remodeling in the form of fibrosis and electrical remodeling secondary to ion channel expression changes. In addition, I discuss the possibility that both fibrosis and electrical remodeling might be preventable when intervening pharmacologically early enough before the remodeling process reaches a point of no return.

HEART FAILURE CLINICS

THE CLINICS ARE AVAILABLE ONLINE!
Access your subscription at:
www.theclinics.com

Risk Factors and Genetics of Atrial Fibrillation

Justus M.B. Anumonwo, PhD[a,b,*], Jérôme Kalifa, MD, PhD[c]

KEYWORDS

- Atrial Fibrillation • AF • Risk factors • AF genetics • Genetic variants and AF

KEY POINTS

- Atrial fibrillation (AF) is by far the most common sustained tachyarrhythmia.
- Not only is AF frequent but also associated with large incremental costs.
- The magnitude of AF prevalence and its constant increase are felt throughout the world.
- From an epidemiologic point of view, the main challenge in attempting to control AF progression is that the disease is variable in its presentation and in its underlying causes.
- Lone AF is usually the diagnosis when the arrhythmia seems idiopathic.

INTRODUCTION

AF is by far the most common sustained tachyarrhythmia. Lifetime risks for development of AF are approximately 1 in 4 for men and women 40 years of age and older.[1,2] This corresponds to 1% to 2% of the general population.[3] Mostly because of an aging population, the prevalence in the United States alone is expected to rise to 10 to 15 million patients by 2020.[3,4] Not only is this disorder frequent but also associated with large incremental costs. In 2010, it was estimated that the total incremental cost of AF was $8705 per patient, with a national incremental cost of AF as high as $26 billion.[5] And the problem goes well beyond the confines of Western countries. The magnitude of AF prevalence and its constant increase are felt throughout the world, albeit with marked differences in the nature and quality of AF management.[6] From an epidemiologic point-of-view, the main challenge in attempting to control AF progression is that the disease is variable in its presentation and in its underlying causes. Lone AF is usually the diagnosis when the arrhythmia seems idiopathic. Improved knowledge of AF risk factors, however, has facilitated identification of 1 or more risk factors in an ever-larger group of AF patients.[3] Some investigators have gone as far as challenging the mere existence of the lone AF entity,[7] emphasizing the importance of getting up-to-date information on AF risk factors and appreciating how exactly they favor AF maintenance. Recently, a comprehensive compendium has presented a detailed description of AF risk factors (**Fig. 1**).[3] This article presents a simplified review of the AF risk factors, including emerging genetic risks. Each risk factor or clinical entity is presented briefly, together with a possible underlying pathophysiologic mechanism.

AGING

Aging is well accepted as the predominant demographic factor.[3] AF incidence is multiplied by a factor of 15 to 20 between the ages of 35 and 85, whereas in the same time period the prevalence grows from 1% to approximately 15%.[3] The higher relative risk of developing AF in men,[8] however, is

This article originally appeared in Cardiology Clinics, Volume 32, Issue 4, November 2014.
[a] Department of Internal Medicine, Center for Arrhythmia Research, University of Michigan, 2800 Plymouth Road, 026-229N, Ann Arbor, MI 48109, USA; [b] Department of Molecular and Integrative Physiology, University of Michigan Medical School, 1137 East Catherine Street, Ann Arbor, MI 48109, USA; [c] Department of Internal Medicine, Center for Arrhythmia Research, 2800 Plymouth Road, 026-227S, Ann Arbor, MI 48109, USA
* Corresponding author. Department of Internal Medicine, Center for Arrhythmia Research, University of Michigan, 2800 Plymouth Road, 026-229N, Ann Arbor, MI 48109.
E-mail address: anumonwo@umich.edu

Risk Factors

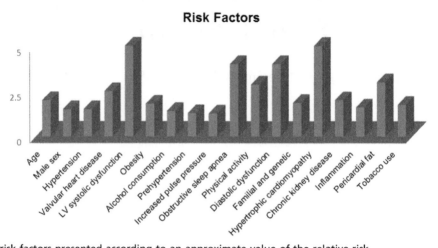

Fig. 1. AF risk factors presented according to an approximate value of the relative risk.

outweighed by increased longevity of women. As a result, women represent half of the overall AF population.[9,10] From a pathophysiologic standpoint, aging is a complex phenomenon. Several of the known aging pathophysiologic processes may contribute to AF development, whereas others remain to be elucidated. Koura and colleagues[11] demonstrated that with aging, the amount of interstitial fibrosis and fatty infiltrates increases, predisposing the atrial muscle to electrical impulse conduction disturbances. These disturbances, such as the so-called zigzag electrical impulse propagation aberrancy, are events that lead to AF initiation and maintenance. At the cellular level, several anomalies may also contribute to age-related AF initiation. For example, atrial myocytes in an aged atrium exhibit a prolonged action potential duration (APD). Also, there is a larger APD heterogeneity across the atrium.[12] Despite this basic understanding, the causes that predominantly link aging and AF are unknown.[13]

HYPERTENSION

Hypertension is a common AF risk factor. Because of the prevalence of hypertension in the general population, it is regarded as the third most common risk factor after age and gender, and it represents the first disease-related risk factor.[14,15] Akin to aging, hypertension is a complex pathophysiologic factor because mechanistic studies are challenging to conduct. Two observations, however, suggest that hypertension per se may be conducive to AF. In spontaneously hypertensive rats, the inducibility of atrial tachycardia was increased, accompanied by a rise in atrial fibrosis.[16] In a sheep model of long-standing elevated blood pressure induced by prenatal corticosteroid exposure

multiple proarrhythmic abnormalities were seen: increased AF stability, reduced conduction velocities, and increased fibrosis with myocyte hypertrophy and myolysis.[17]

HEART FAILURE AND CORONARY ARTERY DISEASE

AF may be caused by any cardiac condition with, however, a predominance of heart failure (HF) and coronary artery disease (CAD).[8,18–22]

HF is a major AF risk factor. HF patients have an approximately 5-fold increased risk of AF onset.[15] The risk of AF increases with the severity of HF clinical symptoms[23] and may relate to the consequences of either systolic or diastolic dysfunction.[24,25] Atrial fibrosis is dramatically increased in the setting of HF, similarly to that in aging and hypertension-related AF. In HF too, the formation of atrial interstitial fibrosis is a strong determinant of the occurrence of AF.[26–28] Specifically, the spatial distribution of atrial fibrosis could be an indicator of AF electrophysiologic mechanisms—reentry or spontaneous focal discharges—and of the exact locations of AF electrical sources. As such, a better knowledge of fibrosis or scar distribution could be an asset in the performance of tailored AF ablation procedures.[29] Finally, HF-related fibrosis formation is one of the main targets of so-called upstream therapies, such as inhibitors of the renin-angiotensin-aldosterone system.[30]

Acute and chronic CAD has emerged as a substantial risk factor of AF onset and perpetuation.[19,31–34] For instance, AF is a well-known complication of acute myocardial infarction,[34] and CAD is a significant risk factor for AF.[4] Although AF after ventricular myocardial infarction might be also triggered by an increase in intra-atrial pressure in the context of acute ventricular dysfunction,[35,36] various works have shown that isolated atrial infarction is common.[37,38] The rate of 17%, reported by Cushing and colleagues[37] in 1942 in the largest study to date, may be the best estimate of its occurrence. These numbers, from postmortem studies, however, suggest that the actual clinical incidence rate might be higher.[39] It was suggested that the pathophysiologic role of atrial ischemia/infarction in AF onset is greatly underestimated.[40,41] Understanding of the patho-physiology linking CAD and AF has benefited from experimental studies. These works have highlighted several atrial ischemia/infarction-related electrophysiologic changes. Spontaneous discharges are significantly more numerous in cells bordering the infarcted region.[42] Atrial ischemia/infarction was also shown to reduce atrial refractory periods,[43] to increase AF induc-ibility and adversely modulate regional electrical impulse propagation,[44] and finally to cause an ac-celeration of atrial drivers.[45] **Fig. 2** is an example of the drastic changes in AF electrical sources nature and frequency after a 90-minute left atrial ischemia episode in an isolated sheep heart.

PERICARDIAL FAT AND OBESITY

Increasingly, clinical investigations report a rela-tionship between obesity and AF risk as well as in the incidence and persistence of AF.[46–51] A sig-nificant portion of the epicardial surface in large mammals is normally covered by adipose tis-sue,[46,47,52] and fat cells (adipocytes) may be involved in myocyte-adipocyte cross talk impor-tant in the normal function of the myocardium.[53,54] Studies in humans and animal models show that obesity significantly increases plasma levels of free fatty acids[55,56] as well as overall visceral and epicardial adiposity.[57,58] With obesity, extensive fatty infiltration results in elevated levels of bio-factors. These biofactors are potentiated by para-crine and vasocrine signaling pathways and overload the myocardium.[59,60] As a result, a dete-rioration of the myocardial function may occur and lead to abnormal impulse initiation mechanisms and myocyte atrophy.[53,54,60,61] In obese patients, it has also been reported that steatosis of the myocardium well correlates with epicardial fat and is an independent contributing factor to myocardial dysfunction. Finally, experimental studies in isolated myocytes show that excess epicardial adiposity, or its biofactors, cause ab-normality in myocardial electrical excitation.[62]

SLEEP APNEA

Obstructive sleep apnea (OSA) has been recently recognized as a major AF risk factor. OSA patients are approximately 4 times more likely to develop AF than non-OSA patients.[3,63] The study of the

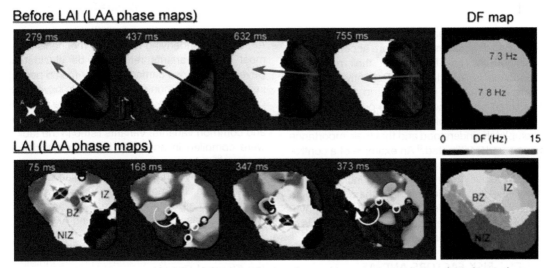

Fig. 2. Optical mapping recordings illustrating the acceleration and increased complexity of AF electrical sources after a 90-minute atrial ischemia (LAI). Four representative movie snapshots before and after LAI during AF and the corresponding dominant frequency (DF) map are shown. AF dynamics were drastically different after LAI. Before LAI, the activity was organized and consistent on a beat-to-beat basis. After LAI, the patterns of activation were changing on a beat-to-beat basis and resulted in complex fibrillatory dynamics: 2 focal discharges within the ischemic zone (IZ) and the border zone (BZ) region at 75 ms evolved into a counterclockwise reentry at 168 ms, which was interrupted by additional IZ-BZ focal discharges at 347 ms to finally give rise to a clockwise rotor. LAA, left atrial appendage; NIZ, non-ischemic zone.

causes linking OSA and AF is complicated by OSA patients often presenting with one or several other AF risk factors.[64] From a practical standpoint, efficacious OSA therapeutic measures, such as positive pressure ventilation, have been shown to decrease AF incidence.[65,66]

ATRIAL DILATATION AND STRETCH

Atrial dilatation and myocardial stretch are well-known risk factors of AF. Several studies have shown that the size of the atrium is a predictor of the occurrence of AF.[20] Stretch is a convenient and measurable way of assessing the risk of AF.[67] From a pathophysiologic point of view, atrial stretch has been shown to lead to a wide range of electrophysiologic changes, including prolongation of late repolarization while early repolarization is shortened, increased excitability, and changes in the nature of AF electrical sources.[68–71] With optical mapping techniques, atrial stretch has been shown to increase the frequency or reentries (rotors) and the spatiotemporal stability of AF waves.[70,71] In patients with HF or mitral valve disease, it is not uncommon to observe restoration of sinus rhythm when the size of the atria diminishes after surgical repair of the valve.[72,73] Moreover, once AF is initiated, the hemodynamic status of the patient worsens because of the loss of atrial contraction,[21] creating a vicious circle that greatly favors AF maintenance.[74]

OTHER RISK FACTORS

Chronic kidney disease, smoking, alcohol, diabetes, and thyroid dysfunction are accepted as independent AF risk factors but their respective importance is still debated. Recently, a review article classified AF risk factors in 3 categories: long established, emerging, and potential, underscoring that many of the AF risk factors remain incompletely understood and that their importance may be underestimated.[3] An example of a controversial risk factor is exercise.[75] Although moderate physical activity may decrease AF incidence,[76] a cumulative life practice of more than 1500 hours is associated with 3-fold AF risk.[3,77,78] Pathophysiologic mechanisms are still unclear, but the role of an increased vagal tone seems to be accepted.[3,79]

GENETIC RISK FACTORS AND AF

Heritability of AF has been suspected as far back as mid-twentieth century, with evidence provided in a study that described familial auricular fibrillation in 3 brothers.[80] Several approaches have been used to determine AF susceptibility genes. Mendelian (monogenic) AF genes have been identified by several approaches, including positional cloning and candidate gene sequencing. Furthermore, whole-exome sequencing (WES) and genome-wide association studies (GWASs) have also significantly contributed to the understanding of AF inheritability. These studies, nevertheless, present a complex picture of the genetic bases of AF, explained in part by the complicated pathophysiology of AF as well as by polygenic inheritance of the identified genes.

Initially a controversial concept, AF heritability in the past decade has increasingly become firmly established by compelling evidence from a variety of studies using various approaches (discussed previously). This is especially the case with lone AF.[81–83] In one such study, evidence for genetic susceptibility to the development of AF was provided by the demonstration that offspring of parents with AF had a significantly increased risk (2–3 fold greater risk), even after controlling for comorbidities.[84] In another recent study examining the risk of an individual in developing lone AF (before age 60), it was reported that family history (of lone AF) is significantly associated with a risk of developing lone AF.[85] In the study, the most significant association was found with first-degree relatives, young age at onset, and multiple affected relatives. In general, there is evidence that lone AF has a greater heritability than AF observed in association with other risk factors.[86]

GENETIC VARIANTS ASSOCIATED WITH AF

There are many genetic variants that predispose to AF, and the underlying molecular mechanisms of most of the variants remain to be elucidated. Several rare (those carried by fewer than 5 people in 1000) and common genetic variants have been compiled in recent reviews[82,87–89] and are summarized in **Tables 1** and **2**, respectively, for the rare and common variants. Variants listed in the tables were compiled in an article by Olesen and colleagues,[88] where a more exhaustive list can be obtained. Many variants encode cardiac ion channels and signaling molecules as well as transcription factors, all of which have been associated with an increase in risk of developing AF.

RARE GENETIC VARIANTS AND AF
Ion Channel Genes

Rare genetic variants (see **Table 1**) are thought to disrupt normal channel properties by causing loss (or gain) in function of affected ion channels. Such variants interfere with channel functionality in the normal cardiac processes of depolarization or repolarization, ultimately leading to the generation

Table 1
Rare genetic variants of ion channel and non–ion channel genes linked to atrial fibrillation

	Gene	Product	Function	Comments
Ion channels	*SCN5A*	α-Subunit	INa channel	GOF; LOF
	SCN1-3B	β-Subunit	INa channel	LOF
	CACNB2	β-Subunit	ICa channel	NI
	CACNA2D4	Aux. subunit	ICa channel	NI
	KCNQ1	α-Subunit	IKs channel	GOF
	KCNE1-5	β-subunit	IKs channel	GOF
	KCND3	α-Subunit	ITO channel	NE; GOF
	KCNH2	α-Subunit	IKr channel	GOF; LOF
	KCNA5	α-Subunit	IKur channel	GOF; LOF
	KCNJ2, 8	α-Subunit	Kir channels	GOF
	ABCC9	Aux. subunit	IKir channel	LOF
	GJA1, 5	α-Subunit	Gap junctions	LOF
Non–ion channels	*GATA4*	Trnscrpt. factor		LOF
	GATA6	Trnscrpt. factor		NI
	GREM2	BMP		Increased inhibition
	LAMNA	Lamin A & C		NI
	NKX2-5	Trnscrpt. factor		NI
	NAPPA	ANP	Natriuretic peptide precursor A	GOF
	NUP155	Nucleoporin		LOF

Abbreviations: ANP, atrial natriuretic peptide; Aux., auxiliary; BMP, bone morphogenic protein; GOF, gain of function; LOF, loss of function; NE, no effect; NI, not investigated; Trnscrpt., transcription.

Adapted from Olesen MS, Nielsen MW, Haunsø S, et al. Atrial fibrillation: the role of common and rare genetic variants. Eur J Hum Genet 2014;22:300–2.

Table 2
Common genetic variants of ion channel and non–ion channel genes linked to atrial fibrillation

Reference SNP ID#	Chromosome	Closest Gene	Comments/SNP Location
rs2200733	4q25	*PITX2*	Paired-like homeodomain transcription factor 2 Upstream
rs2106261	16q22	*ZFHX3*	Zinc finger homeobox 3 Intronic
rs13376333	1q21	*KCNN3*	Ca-activated K channel Intronic
rs3807989	7q31	*CAV1/2*	Caveolin 1/2 Intronic
rs3903239	1q24	*PRRX1*	Homeodomain transcription factor Upstream
rs1152591	14q23	*SYNE2*	Encodes Nesprin 2 Intronic
rs10821415	9q22	*C9orf3*	Open reading frame on chromosome 9 Intronic
rs7164883	15q24	*HCN4*	Pacemaker channel Intronic
rs10824026	10q22	*SYNPO2L*	Encodes a cytoskeletal protein (CHAP) Upstream

Adapted from Olesen MS, Nielsen MW, Haunsø S, et al. Atrial fibrillation: the role of common and rare genetic variants. Eur J Hum Genet 2014;22:298.

of early afterdepolarizations and reentrant electrical excitation. The resultant aberrant excitation processes fit well with the current models proposed for AF initiation mechanisms.[88,90] There are several variants of genes encoding key molecular correlates of the fast voltage-gated sodium channel current (INa); the calcium channel current (ICa); and the slowly (IKs), rapidly (IKr), ultrarapidly (IKur), and transient (ITO) potassium currents as well as the inwardly rectifying (Kir) potassium currents. Thus, *SCN5A* and *SCN1-3B*, the genes that encode respectively α- and β-subunits of the cardiac fast voltage-gated sodium channel, have been linked to AF.[82,91,92] Expression studies demonstrate that the mutations in the identified genes result in changes in properties of encoded channels, such as the kinetics of current inactivation and the total amount of current activated (current density). Using expression data (WES) and predicted function, 2 candidate AF variants that encode the calcium channel subunit (*CACNB2* and *CACNA2D4*, encoding, respectively, β2-subunit and a regulatory subunit of the L-type voltage-gated calcium channel) were identified in 2 separate families.[89] This finding is particularly relevant given that there is ample evidence associating abnormal calcium signaling processes with paroxysmal AF. With the exception of a few cases listed, several of the identified variants of genes encoding voltage-gated potassium channels result primarily in a gain of function of the repolarizing channel currents and, therefore, shorten the APD and the QT interval. Mutations of genes encoding the gap junctional channels (GJA1, GJA5) as well as the auxiliary subunit of the ATP-sensitive inward rectifier channel result in loss of function in the associated channels (see **Table 1**).

Non–Ion Channel Genes

Variants of genes for non–ion channel proteins associated with AF are listed in **Table 1**. As with the case of ion channel genes, precise molecular mechanisms underlying these variants are yet to be fully elucidated. Experimental investigations aimed at understanding the roles of these variants are expected to be complicated, especially considering that some are transcription factors (eg, GATA4/6 and NKX2-5). GATA genes encode cardiac transcription factors and are thought to interact with NKX2-5 genes in processes critical to cardiogenesis (see Olesen and colleagues[88]). Moreover, LAMNA and GREM2 variants have been identified in AF cohort studies, demonstrating abnormalities in cardiac excitation (eg, supra ventricular tachycardia and AF), with evidence in humans as well as in experimental

animal models an effect of variants of the genes on cardiac muscle generation and function. Frame shift and missense mutations in genes encoding atrial natriuretic peptide are associated (cosegregated) with AF.[88,93,94] AF phenotypes have been described with NUP155 mutations in humans and in a murine model,[95] making a strong case for the role of such variants in AF, albeit with precise molecular pathways yet to be established.

COMMON GENETIC VARIANTS AND AF

Since the first description of an association between single nucleotide polymorphisms (SNPs) and AF,[96] GWASs have identified several SNPs as genetic risks associated with AF. In the initial characterization, GWASs were followed by replication studies and demonstrated a strong association between 2 sequence variants on chromosome 4q25 and AF.[96] In the study, an SNP (rs2200733) located (upstream) in proximity of the gene *PITX2* (paired-like homeodomain transcription factor 2, also known as pituitary homeobox 2) was highly associated with AF. Since this observation, several investigations in human and animal models have focused on PITX2c, the dominant isoform of the gene transcript in humans. Not surprisingly, therefore, rs2200733 has been extensively investigated with respect to SNPs and AF. Experimental evidence has been presented for the role of PITX2c in the development of left atrial myocardium, with particular importance for atrial myocytes that reside in the pulmonary vein sleeves.[88,97,98]

Subsequent studies have identified other GWAS loci with SNPs located in regions that are intronic (rs2106261, rs13376333, rs3807989, rs1152591, rs10821415, and rs7164883) or upstream (rs3903239 and rs10824026) of the closest gene (see **Table 2**). In Table 2, the closest genes identified with various SNPs are involved in diverse functions, such as in encoding of transcription factors, cytoskeletal and scaffolding proteins, and ion channels. A significant amount of research effort is focused on mRNA expression of genes within proximity of the location of SNPs, given that they are intronic or upstream of the closest genes. A general contention is that SNPs presumably act as promoters or enhancers of proximate genes.[88]

Finally, it is necessary to briefly address a few other issues regarding the role of rare and common genetic variants in AF. First, there is compelling evidence for a significant overlap between different mutant genes identified in various categories of cardiac arrhythmias. For example, genetic mutations associated with AF are also linked to other cardiac arrhythmias. Thus, AF susceptibility genes identified in the α, β, or subsidiary/accessory subunit of a particular ion channel may also be linked to another cardiac arrhythmias, such as Brugada syndrome and the long QT and short QT syndromes. Consistent with this, a previous report demonstrated the prevalence of early-onset AF in congenital long QT syndrome patients.[99] Second, there is increasing evidence for interactions between rare and common genetic variants in cardiac arrhythmias, including AF.[88] Thus, these variants, by mechanisms yet to be understood, can interact to modify their respective electrophysiologic phenotypes.[100] Third, given various AF susceptibility genes now identified, there has been a contention as to whether genetic testing is warranted in AF.[101,102] All of these are important considerations in any discussion of AF genetics.

In summary, there is a complex picture of the genetic bases of AF, attributable in part to the complicated pathophysiology of AF as well as to complicated inheritance mechanisms of the genes. Thus there is a critical need for up-to-date information on AF risk factors and appreciating how exactly they favor AF maintenance. Furthermore, with regard to genetic variants associated with AF, it is important to have a better understanding of molecular signaling events or mechanisms that ultimately lead to the disruption of normal electrical excitation.

REFERENCES

1. Lloyd-Jones DM, Wang TJ, Leip EP, et al. Lifetime risk for development of atrial fibrillation the framingham heart study. Circulation 2004;110:1042–6.
2. Heeringa J, van der Kuip DA, Hofman A, et al. Prevalence, incidence and lifetime risk of atrial fibrillation: the rotterdam study. Eur Heart J 2006; 27:949–53.
3. Andrade J, Khairy P, Dobrev D, et al. The clinical profile and pathophysiology of atrial fibrillation: relationships among clinical features, epidemiology, and mechanisms. Circ Res 2014;114:1453–68.
4. Miyasaka Y, Barnes ME, Gersh BJ, et al. Secular trends in incidence of atrial fibrillation in olmsted county, minnesota, 1980 to 2000, and implications on the projections for future prevalence. Circulation 2006;114:119.
5. Kim MH, Johnston SS, Chu BC, et al. Estimation of total incremental health care costs in patients with atrial fibrillation in the united states. Circ Cardiovasc Qual Outcomes 2011;4:313–20.
6. Oldgren J, Healey JS, Ezekowitz M, et al. Variations in etiology and management of atrial fibrillation in a prospective registry of 15,400 emergency department patients in 46 countries: the re-ly af registry. Circulation 2014. http://dx.doi.org/10.1161/CIRCULATIONAHA.113.005451.
7. Wyse DG, Van Gelder IC, Ellinor PT, et al. Lone atrial fibrillation: does it exist? A "white paper" of the journal of the American College of Cardiology. J Am Coll Cardiol 2014;63(17):1715–23.
8. Benjamin EJ, Levy D, Vaziri SM, et al. Independent risk factors for atrial fibrillation in a population-based cohort. JAMA 1994;271:840.
9. Feinberg WM, Blackshear JL, Laupacis A, et al. Prevalence, age distribution, and gender of patients with atrial fibrillation. Analysis and implications. Arch Intern Med 1995;155:469–73.
10. Tadros R, Ton AT, Fiset C, et al. Sex differences in cardiac electrophysiology and clinical arrhythmias: epidemiology, therapeutics and mechanisms. Can J Cardiol 2014;30(7):783–92.
11. Koura T, Hara M, Takeuchi S, et al. Anisotropic conduction properties in canine atria analyzed by high-resolution optical mapping preferential direction of conduction block changes from longitudinal to transverse with increasing age. Circulation 2002; 105:2092–8.
12. Anyukhovsky EP, Sosunov EA, Plotnikov A, et al. Cellular electrophysiologic properties of old canine atria provide a substrate for arrhythmogenesis. Cardiovasc Res 2002;54:462–9.
13. Schotten U, Verheule S, Kirchhof P, et al. Pathophysiological mechanisms of atrial fibrillation: a translational appraisal. Physiol Rev 2011;91:265–325.
14. Kannel WB, Abbott RD, Savage DD, et al. Epidemiologic features of chronic atrial fibrillation: the framingham study. N Engl J Med 1982;306:1018–22.
15. Kannel WB, Wolf PA, Benjamin EJ, et al. Prevalence, incidence, prognosis, and predisposing conditions for atrial fibrillation: population-based estimates. Am J Cardiol 1998;82:2N–9N.
16. Choisy SC, Arberry LA, Hancox JC, et al. Increased susceptibility to atrial tachyarrhythmia in spontaneously hypertensive rat hearts. Hypertension 2007; 49:498–505.
17. Kistler PM, Sanders P, Dodic M, et al. Atrial electrical and structural abnormalities in an ovine model of chronic blood pressure elevation after prenatal corticosteroid exposure: implications for development of atrial fibrillation. Eur Heart J 2006;27:3045–56.
18. Roy D, Talajic M, Dubuc M, et al. Atrial fibrillation and congestive heart failure. Curr Opin Cardiol 2009;24:29.
19. Kannel WB, Abbott RD, Savage DD, et al. Coronary heart disease and atrial fibrillation: the framingham study. Am Heart J 1983;106:389–96.
20. Benjamin EJ, Wolf PA, D'Agostino RB, et al. Impact of atrial fibrillation on the risk of death: the framingham heart study. Circulation 1998;98:946–52.

21. Kannel WB, Benjamin EJ. Status of the epidemiology of atrial fibrillation. Med Clin North Am 2008; 92:17–40.

22. Krahn AD, Manfreda J, Tate RB, et al. The natural history of atrial fibrillation: incidence, risk factors, and prognosis in the manitoba follow-up study. Am J Med 1995;98:476–84.

23. Maisel WH, Stevenson LW. Atrial fibrillation in heart failure: epidemiology, pathophysiology, and rationale for therapy. Am J Cardiol 2003;91:2–8.

24. Jais P, Peng JT, Shah DC, et al. Left ventricular diastolic dysfunction in patients with so-called lone atrial fibrillation. J Cardiovasc Electrophysiol 2000;11:623–5.

25. Tsang TS, Gersh BJ, Appleton CP, et al. Left ventricular diastolic dysfunction as a predictor of the first diagnosed nonvalvular atrial fibrillation in 840 elderly men and women. J Am Coll Cardiol 2002; 40:1636–44.

26. Cha TJ, Ehrlich JR, Zhang L, et al. Dissociation between ionic remodeling and ability to sustain atrial fibrillation during recovery from experimental congestive heart failure. Circulation 2004;109: 412–8.

27. Shinagawa K, Shi YF, Tardif JC, et al. Dynamic nature of atrial fibrillation substrate during development and reversal of heart failure in dogs. Circulation 2002;105: 2672–8.

28. Tanaka K, Zlochiver S, Vikstrom KL, et al. Spatial distribution of fibrosis governs fibrillation wave dynamics in the posterior left atrium during heart failure. Circ Res 2007;101:839–47.

29. Trayanova NA. Mathematical approaches to understanding and imaging atrial fibrillation: significance for mechanisms and management. Circ Res 2014; 114:1516–31.

30. Savelieva I, Kakouros N, Kourliouros A, et al. Upstream therapies for management of atrial fibrillation: review of clinical evidence and implications for european society of cardiology guidelines. Part I: primary prevention. Europace 2011;13: 308–28.

31. James TN. Myocardial infarction and atrial arrhythmias. Circulation 1961;24:761–76.

32. Crenshaw M, Brian S, Ward M, et al. Atrial fibrillation in the setting of acute myocardial infarction: the Gusto-I experience. J Am Coll Cardiol 1997; 30:406–13.

33. Wong CK, White HD, Wilcox RG, et al. New atrial fibrillation after acute myocardial infarction independently predicts death: the Gusto-III experience. Am Heart J 2000;140:878–85.

34. Goldberg RJ, Yarzebski J, Lessard D, et al. Recent trends in the incidence rates of and death rates from atrial fibrillation complicating initial acute myocardial infarction: a community-wide perspective. Am Heart J 2002;143:519–27.

35. Tsang T, Barnes ME, Bailey KR, et al. Left atrial volume: important risk marker of incident atrial fibrillation in 1655 older men and women. Mayo Clin Proc 2001;76:467.

36. Moller JE, Hillis GS, Oh JK, et al. Left atrial volume: a powerful predictor of survival after acute myocardial infarction. Circulation 2003;107:2207.

37. Cushing E, Feil H, Stanton E, et al. Infarction of the cardiac auricles (atria): clinical, pathological, and experimental studies. Br Heart J 1942;4:17.

38. Wartman W, Souders J. Localization of myocardial infarcts with respect to the muscle bundles of the heart. Arch Pathol 1950;50:329.

39. Mayuga R, Singer D. Atrial infarction: clinical significance and diagnostic criteria. Practical Cardiol 1985;11:142–60.

40. Bunc M, Starc R, Podbregar M, et al. Conversion of atrial fibrillation into a sinus rhythm by coronary angioplasty in a patient with acute myocardial infarction. Eur J Emerg Med 2001;8:141.

41. Pehkonen E, Honkonen E, Makynen P, et al. Stenosis of the right coronary artery and retrograde cardioplegia predispose patients to atrial fibrillation after coronary artery bypass grafting. Thorac Cardiovasc Surg 1998;46:115–20.

42. Nishida K, Qi XY, Wakili R, et al. Mechanisms of atrial tachyarrhythmias associated with coronary artery occlusion in a chronic canine model. Circulation 2011. http://dx.doi.org/10.1161/CIRCULATIONAHA. 110.972778.

43. Jayachandran JV, Zipes DP, Weksler J, et al. Role of the na+/h+ exchanger in short-term atrial electrophysiological remodeling. Circulation 2000;101: 1861–6.

44. Sinno H, Derakhchan K, Libersan D, et al. Atrial ischemia promotes atrial fibrillation in dogs. Circulation 2003;107:1930–6.

45. Yamazaki M, Avula UM, Bandaru K, et al. Acute regional left atrial ischemia causes acceleration of atrial drivers during atrial fibrillation. Heart Rhythm 2013;10(6):901–9.

46. Al Chekakie MO, Welles CC, Metoyer R, et al. Pericardial fat is independently associated with human atrial fibrillation. J Am Coll Cardiol 2010;56:784–8.

47. Batal O, Schoenhagen P, Shao M, et al. Left atrial epicardial adiposity and atrial fibrillation. Circ Arrhythm Electrophysiol 2010;3:230–6.

48. Abed HS, Wong CX, Brooks AG, et al. Periatrial fat volume is predictive of atrial fibrillation severity. Heart Rhythm 2010;7:S327.

49. Tsao HM, Hu WC, Wu MH, et al. Abundance and distribution of epicardial adipose tissue surrounding the left atrium in patients with atrial fibrillation. Heart Rhythm 2010;7:S327.

50. Shin SY, Yong HS, Lim HE, et al. Total and interatrial epicardial adipose tissues are independently associated with left atrial remodeling in patients with

atrial fibrillation. J Cardiovasc Electrophysiol 2011; 22:647–55.

51. Thanassoulis G, Massaro JM, O'Donnell CJ, et al. Pericardial fat is associated with prevalent atrial fibrillation: the Framingham Heart Study. Circ Arrhythm Electrophysiol 2010;3:345–50.

52. Iacobellis G, Corradi D, Sharma AM. Epicardial adipose tissue: anatomic, biomolecular and clinical relationships with the heart. Nat Clin Pract Cardiovasc Med 2005;2:536–43.

53. Gong D, Yang R, Munir KM, et al. New progress in adipocytokine research. Curr Opin Endocrinol Diabetes Obes 2003;10:115–21.

54. Karmazyn M, Purdham DM, Rajapurohitam V, et al. Signalling mechanisms underlying the metabolic and other effects of adipokines on the heart. Cardiovasc Res 2008;79:279–86.

55. Veiga-Lopez A, Moeller J, Patel D, et al. Developmental programming: impact of prenatal testosterone excess on insulin sensitivity, adiposity, and free fatty acid profile in postpubertal female sheep. Endocrinology 2013;154:1731–42.

56. Kim JY, Park JY, Kim OY, et al. Metabolic profiling of plasma in overweight/obese and lean men using ultra performance liquid chromatography and q-tof mass spectrometry (uplc-q-tof ms). J Proteome Res 2010;9:4368–75.

57. Iacobellis G, Leonetti F. Epicardial adipose tissue and insulin resistance in obese subjects. J Clin Endocrinol Metab 2005;90:6300–2.

58. Silaghi A, Piercecchi-Marti MD, Grino M, et al. Epicardial adipose tissue extent: relationship with age, body fat distribution, and coronaropathy. Obesity (Silver Spring) 2008;16:2424–30.

59. Sacks HS, Fain JN. Human epicardial adipose tissue: a review. Am Heart J 2007;153:907–17.

60. Pantanowitz L. Fat infiltration in the heart. Heart 2001;85:253.

61. Kankaanpaa M, Lehto HR, Parkka JP, et al. Myocardial triglyceride content and epicardial fat mass in human obesity: relationship to left ventricular function and serum free fatty acid levels. J Clin Endocrinol Metab 2006;91:4689–95.

62. Graner M, Siren R, Nyman K, et al. Cardiac steatosis associates with visceral obesity in nondiabetic obese men. J Clin Endocrinol Metab 2013;98:1189–97.

63. Gami AS, Pressman G, Caples SM, et al. Association of atrial fibrillation and obstructive sleep apnea. Circulation 2004;110:364–7.

64. Gami AS, Hodge DO, Herges RM, et al. Obstructive sleep apnea, obesity, and the risk of incident atrial fibrillation. J Am Coll Cardiol 2007;49:565–71.

65. Fein AS, Shvilkin A, Shah D, et al. Treatment of obstructive sleep apnea reduces the risk of atrial fibrillation recurrence after catheter ablation. J Am Coll Cardiol 2013;62:300–5.

66. Ng CY, Liu T, Shehata M, et al. Meta-analysis of obstructive sleep apnea as predictor of atrial fibrillation recurrence after catheter ablation. Am J Cardiol 2011;108:47–51.

67. Vaziri SM, Larson MG, Benjamin EJ, et al. Echocardiographic predictors of nonrheumatic atrial fibrillation. The framingham heart study. Circulation 1994;89: 724–30.

68. Franz MR, Bode F. Acute stretch effects on atrial electrophysiology. In: Khol P, Sachs F, Franz M, editors. Cardiac mechano-electric coupling and arrhythmias. Oxford, UK: Oxford University Press; 2011. p. 168.

69. Franz MR, Bode F. Mechano-electrical feedback underlying arrhythmias: the atrial fibrillation case. Prog Biophys Mol Biol 2003;82:163–74.

70. Kalifa J, Jalife J, Zaitsev AV, et al. Intra-atrial pressure increases rate and organization of waves emanating from the superior pulmonary veins during atrial fibrillation. Circulation 2003; 108:668–71.

71. Yamazaki M, Mironov S, Taravant C, et al. Heterogeneous atrial wall thickness and stretch promote scroll waves anchoring during atrial fibrillation. Cardiovasc Res 2012;94(1):48–57.

72. Keren G, Etzion T, Sherez J, et al. Atrial fibrillation and atrial enlargement in patients with mitral stenosis. Am Heart J 1987;114:1146–55.

73. Haïat R, Scemama A, Halphen C, et al. Spontaneous reduction of late chronic atrial fibrillation after mitral valvuloplasty. Echocardiographic evidence of the restoration of mechanical atrial activity. Arch Mal Coeur Vaiss 1997;90:835–9 [in French].

74. Alpert JS, Petersen P, Godtfredsen J. Atrial fibrillation: natural history, complications, and management. Annu Rev Med 1988;39:41–52.

75. Coumel P. Atrial fibrillation: one more sporting inconvenience? Eur Heart J 2002;23:431–3.

76. Mozaffarian D, Furberg CD, Psaty BM, et al. Physical activity and incidence of atrial fibrillation in older adults the cardiovascular health study. Circulation 2008;118:800–7.

77. Olshansky B, Sullivan R. Increased prevalence of atrial fibrillation in the endurance athlete: potential mechanisms and sport specificity. Phys Sportsmed 2014;42:45–51.

78. Turagam MK, Velagapudi P, Kocheril AG. Atrial fibrillation in athletes. Am J Cardiol 2012;109:296–302.

79. Guasch E, Benito B, Qi X, et al. Atrial fibrillation promotion by endurance exercisedemonstration and mechanistic exploration in an animal model. J Am Coll Cardiol 2013;62:68–77.

80. Wolff L. Familial auricular fibrillation. N Engl J Med 1947.

81. Arnar DO, Thorvaldsson S, Manolio TA, et al. Familial aggregation of atrial fibrillation in iceland. Eur Heart J 2006;27:708–12.

82. Darbar D, Herron KJ, Ballew JD, et al. Familial atrial fibrillation is a genetically heterogeneous disorder. J Am Coll Cardiol 2003;41:2185–92.

83. Ellinor PT, Yoerger DM, Ruskin JN, et al. Familial aggregation in lone atrial fibrillation. Hum Genet 2005;118:179–84.

84. Fox CS, Parise H, D'Agostino RB Sr, et al. Parental atrial fibrillation as a risk factor for atrial fibrillation in offspring. JAMA 2004;291:2851–5.

85. Oyen N, Ranthe MF, Carstensen L, et al. Familial aggregation of lone atrial fibrillation in young persons. J Am Coll Cardiol 2012;60:917–21.

86. Lubitz SA, Ozcan C, Magnani JW, et al. Genetics of atrial fibrillation: implications for future research directions and personalized medicine. Circ Arrhythm Electrophysiol 2010;3:291–9.

87. Olesen MS, Andreasen L, Jabbari J, et al. Very early-onset lone atrial fibrillation patients have a high prevalence of rare variants in genes previously associated with atrial fibrillation. Heart Rhythm 2014;11:246–51.

88. Olesen MS, Nielsen MW, Haunso S, et al. Atrial fibrillation: the role of common and rare genetic variants. Eur J Hum Genet 2014;22:297–306.

89. Weeke P, Parvez B, Blair M, et al. Candidate gene approach to identifying rare genetic variants associated with lone atrial fibrillation. Heart Rhythm 2014;11:46–52.

90. Yang Y, Li J, Lin X, et al. Novel kcna5 loss-of-function mutations responsible for atrial fibrillation. J Hum Genet 2009;54:277–83.

91. Olesen MS, Yuan L, Liang B, et al. High prevalence of long qt syndrome-associated scn5a variants in patients with early-onset lone atrial fibrillation. Circ Cardiovasc Genet 2012;5:450–9.

92. Arnestad M, Crotti L, Rognum TO, et al. Prevalence of long-qt syndrome gene variants in sudden infant death syndrome. Circulation 2007;115:361–7.

93. Hodgson-Zingman DM, Karst ML, Zingman LV, et al. Atrial natriuretic peptide frameshift mutation in familial atrial fibrillation. N Engl J Med 2008; 359:158–65.

94. Abraham RL, Yang T, Blair M, et al. Augmented potassium current is a shared phenotype for two genetic defects associated with familial atrial fibrillation. J Mol Cell Cardiol 2010;48:181–90.

95. Zhang X, Chen S, Yoo S, et al. Mutation in nuclear pore component nup155 leads to atrial fibrillation and early sudden cardiac death. Cell 2008;135: 1017–27.

96. Gudbjartsson DF, Arnar DO, Helgadottir A, et al. Variants conferring risk of atrial fibrillation on chromosome 4q25. Nature 2007;448:353–7.

97. Gage PJ, Suh H, Camper SA. Dosage requirement of pitx2 for development of multiple organs. Development 1999;126:4643–51.

98. Mommersteeg MT, Brown NA, Prall OW, et al. Pitx2c and nkx2-5 are required for the formation and identity of the pulmonary myocardium. Circ Res 2007;101:902–9.

99. Johnson JN, Tester DJ, Perry J, et al. Prevalence of early-onset atrial fibrillation in congenital long qt syndrome. Heart Rhythm 2008;5:704–9.

100. Ritchie MD, Rowan S, Kucera G, et al. Chromosome 4q25 variants are genetic modifiers of rare ion channel mutations associated with familial atrial fibrillation. J Am Coll Cardiol 2012;60: 1173–81.

101. Ackerman MJ, Priori SG, Willems S, et al. HRS/ EHRA expert consensus statement on the state of genetic testing for the channelopathies and cardiomyopathies this document was developed as a partnership between the Heart Rhythm Society (HRS) and the European Heart Rhythm Association (EHRA). Heart Rhythm 2011;8: 1308–39.

102. Everett BM, Cook NR, Conen D, et al. Novel genetic markers improve measures of atrial fibrillation risk prediction. Eur Heart J 2013;34: 2243–51.

Mechanisms of Atrial Fibrillation

Rotors, Ionic Determinants, and Excitation Frequency

Omer Berenfeld, PhD*, José Jalife, MD

KEYWORDS

- Atrial fibrillation • Dominant frequency • Rotors • Remodeling

KEY POINTS

- When a stable, self-sustained rotor forms in the left or right atrium, its high-frequency spinning results in the complex patterns of fibrillatory conduction that characterize atrial fibrillation (AF).
- Although 2 or more rotors can coexist in the atria, the rotor with the highest dominant frequency (DF) predominates and maintains the overall activity.
- In a sheep model of tachypacing-induced AF, the rate of weekly DF increase predicts the time for the transition from paroxysmal to persistent AF.
- The increase in DF during the paroxysmal-to-persistent AF transition is explained by a reduction in the L-type Ca^{2+} current density, which together with an increase in the density of the inward rectifier potassium current, shortens the refractory period to accelerate and stabilize rotors.
- The distribution of DF gradients in patients with paroxysmal AF is different from patients in persistent AF; abolishing DF gradients by radiofrequency ablation of high DF sites predicts freedom of AF.

INTRODUCTION

Atrial fibrillation (AF) is associated with increased morbidity and mortality in patients with cardiovascular disease and its prevalence in the general population continues to increase.[1] However, despite more than 100 years of basic and clinical research, the fundamental mechanisms of AF initiation and maintenance are poorly understood, which has likely contributed to our inability to treat it effectively. A commonly accepted mechanism, the multiple wavelet hypothesis,[2,3] assumes that cardiac fibrillation results from randomly propagating waves with intermittent blockades, annihilation, and re-generation of discrete waves. A more recent variant posits that AF depends on longitudinal/transmural dissociation,[4] with the fibrillatory waves lacking any kind of hierarchical organization. However, multiple theoretic,[5,6] experimental,[7] and clinical[8,9] studies have repeatedly demonstrated that wave propagation during AF is not totally random, but contains deterministic components that depend on self-organized drivers (rotors) that spin at an exceedingly high frequency. The spiraling waves emerging from such rotors give rise to the characteristically complex patterns of fibrillatory conduction as they propagate through the atria. Remarkably, the heterogeneous distribution of ion channels in the atria enables rotors to dwell at specific areas whose structure, electrical properties, and relatively short refractory periods promote rotor attachment.[10] One emergent property of such complex spatiotemporal dynamics was the hierarchical distribution of local

This article originally appeared in Cardiology Clinics, Volume 32, Issue 4, November 2014.
Center for Arrhythmia Research, University of Michigan, 2800 Plymouth Road, Ann Arbor, MI 48109, USA
* Corresponding author. Center for Arrhythmia Research, NCRC Room 026-229S, 2800 Plymouth Road, Ann Arbor, MI 48109.
E-mail address: oberen@umich.edu

heartfailure.theclinics.com

cycle lengths (CLs) that was first reported in early experimental studies by Morillo and colleagues[11] and Harada and colleagues.[12] This was followed by the combined use of phase mapping[13] and dominant frequency (DF) mapping to quantitate the dynamics and the spatial organization of AF activation rates in both atria and by the demonstration that the highest DF corresponded with the location of the rotor that was driving the arrhythmia.[14–17] This article has three major objectives: First, to discuss the electrophysiologic significance of spectral analysis in AF; second, to discuss data that strongly support the hypothesis that remodeling in atrial ionic properties contributes to the transition from paroxysmal to persistent AF (PeAF); and third, to review and discuss clinical data showing a distribution of DFs across the atria during AF and how that distribution may be used to guide ablation procedures.

FREQUENCY-DEPENDENT BREAKDOWN OF WAVE PROPAGATION

To gain insight into the distinct spatial distribution of CLs in the study of Morillo and colleagues,[11] we used spectral analysis of each of the time series recorded at specific locations in both atria to determine their DFs. Most notably, the activation frequencies in certain areas of the left atrium (LA) were always faster than any other region.[15,16] In subsequent studies, we confirmed the hierarchical organization of the DFs.[14] In addition, we demonstrated that such an organization was the result of the exceedingly high frequency at which the spiraling waves emerging from the spinning rotor propagated haphazardly through the heterogeneous atria, undergoing spatially distributed intermittent Wenckebach-like patterns that are typical of fibrillatory conduction.[18,19] In retrospect, this is not too surprising; it is well known that the atria are very heterogeneous in both their anatomic structure and electrophysiologic properties, and waves that propagate at an high frequency in such an environment are likely to encounter obstacles in their path. To illustrate how we investigate the mechanism of fibrillatory conduction, we used a simplified mathematical model of a heterogeneous substrate consisting of a large pectinate muscle connected to a small sheet representing the thin atrial wall (**Fig. 1**).[6] Periodic stimulation was applied to the top free edge of the pectinate bundle (25 mm^2) and the impulse was allowed to propagate downstream to invade the 2-dimensional sheet.[6] The traces on the right show the action potentials (APs) and corresponding power spectra of sites in the bundle and in the sheet. As shown by the top and bottom time series, stimulation at a constant period of 0.119 seconds resulted in a 3:2 propagation pattern across the boundary between the thin bundle and the sheet. This is reflected in the corresponding power spectra as well: Although the source region (the pectinate bundle) displayed a DF of 8.4 Hz, the geometric expansion into the sheet imposed a

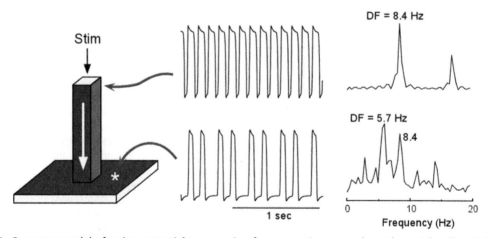

Fig. 1. Computer model of action potential propagation from a pectinate muscle to the atrial wall. A 3-dimensional (60 × 60 × 60 elements) model includes a 1-dimensional bundle attached to a 2-dimensional sheet (*left panel*). Periodic stimulation (*Stim*) was applied at the top edge of the bundle and the impulse was allowed to propagate downward with conduction velocity of ~0.29 m/s and to invade the 2-dimensional sheet. The voltage time series and corresponding power spectra are shown for a site near the stimulation point and a site at the sheet. Comparison between the points indicates a 3:2 pattern of propagation into the sheet with a concomitant spectral transformation and a dominant frequency (DF) shift from 8.4 to 5.7 Hz. (*From* Jalife J, Berenfeld O, Skanes A, et al. Mechanisms of atrial fibrillation: mother rotors or multiple daughter wavelets, or both? J Cardiovasc Electrophysiol 1998;9:S2–12; with permission.)

spectral transformation whereby the DF shifted to 5.7 Hz. The 2 power spectra display additional peaks originating from the combined effect of the sharp AP deflections and the interbeat CL variations. The constant CL at the thin bundle results in a narrow peak at a DF that is the exact inverse of the CL (1/0.119 = 8.4 Hz) with an additional smaller peak at about 16.8 Hz, which is an integer multiple of the DF (ie, a harmonic). The CL of the activity in the sheet, on the other hand, is not constant and can be seen to alternate between short and long values. This in turn gives rise to a more complex profile: Several peaks are seen in the power spectrum, consequent of the combination of various intervals in the time series including not only the long and short CLs, but also their sum and difference. The Fourier algorithm, nevertheless, considers the most stationary combination of the CLs to be the DF at 5.7 Hz, which is the average number of local activations per second,[18,20] corresponding with the 3:2 ratio of the input CL (frequency) of 0.119 sec (8.4 Hz) represented by a smaller peak.

Fig. 2 shows results from an optical mapping experiment in which we used DF analysis in the isolated right atrium (RA) of a sheep heart. In this experiment, the numerical predictions discussed (see **Fig. 1**) are clearly borne out by the complexity of the responses of the RA to high-frequency periodic stimuli. The preparation was subjected to periodic pacing by a bipolar electrode on Bachmann's bundle to simulate activity arriving from a periodic LA source across Bachmann's bundle into the RA.[21] In panel A, stimulation at 5.0 Hz resulted in 1:1 activation of the entire RA and thus the output DF was also 5.0 Hz everywhere on the endocardial (top) and epicardial (bottom) surfaces. However, when pacing at 7.7 Hz, propagation into the RA was no longer 1:1. Instead, a heterogeneous distribution of DF domains was established both in the endocardium and the epicardium, with frequencies ranging between 3.5 and 7.7 Hz. Composite data from 5 experiments are presented in panel B. The DFs measured on the endocardium are plotted as a function of the pacing frequency. Clearly, below 6.7 Hz the response DF showed no dispersion in any of the experiments, which meant that activation was 1:1 everywhere in the RA. Above the "breakdown frequency" of 6.7 Hz, there was a large DF dispersion manifested as multiple domains whose individual frequencies were either equal to or lower than the pacing frequency. In addition, we found that intermittent block patterns occur primarily at branching sites of the pectinate bundles of the atria. Such structurally related blockades led to a significant loss of consistency in the beat-to-beat direction of wave propagation and provided a direct explanation for the difficulty in tracing back the origin of the activation during fibrillatory conduction.[21] We also found that the spatial distribution of AP duration at a low pacing

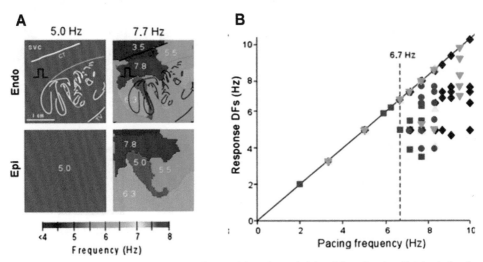

Fig. 2. The "breakdown frequency" in a sheep heart. (*A*) Endocardial (*endo*) and epicardial (*epi*) dominant frequency (DF) maps of same isolated right atrium (RA) preparation paced at 5.0 and 7.7 Hz. Note appearance of heterogeneous DF domains at 7.7 Hz. (*B*) Response DFs versus the pacing rate (n = 5). Each symbol represents one experiment. Pacing Bachmann's bundle at rates below approximately 6.7 Hz results in 1:1 activation. At higher rates, the number of domains increases but the DFs' value decrease. CT, crista terminalis; SVC, superior vena cava. (*From* Berenfeld O, Zaitsev AV, Mironov SF, et al. Frequency-dependent breakdown of wave propagation into fibrillatory conduction across the pectinate muscle network in the isolated sheep right atrium. Circ Res 2002;90:1173–80; with permission.)

rate of 3.3 Hz was different from the distribution of DF domains, which led us to suggest that dispersion of refractoriness at normal frequencies is a poor predictor of the spatial distribution of intermittent block patterns that characterize AF outside the source region.[21]

Relationship Between the Dynamic Patterns of Rotors and DFs

In a set of 5 sheep experiments, we studied patterns of surface wave propagation during PeAF.[22] To establish the patterns of activation underlying the DF_{max} values in the LA, we used phase movies[13] to correlate those with reentries in the posterior LA (PLA) and LA appendage (LAA).[23] In **Fig. 3**A, a dynamic combination of breakthroughs and reentries is seen in the PLA and LAA during AF, with a rotor drifting from the PLA toward the LAA (see Video). As soon as the rotor enters the LAA field of view, the patterns of activation switch from breakthroughs to reentry and the drifting rotor becomes the main source driving the AF. In **Fig. 3**B, concomitant transition in the maximum DF (DF_{max}) values from the PLA to the LAA when

the rotor appears in the field of view of the LAA further confirms the essential role of rotors in this AF model.[22] Further analysis of the DF distribution in our sheep PeAF revealed that, despite a transient back-and-forth drift, the longest sojourn of the rotor was in the PLA, as suggested by the DF map, demonstrating a statistically significant DF gradient from PLA to LAA and RAA (9.1 ± 1.0 vs 7.9 ± 0.7 and 6.9 ± 0.9 Hz, respectively, $P<.05$).

TRANSITION FROM PAROXYSMAL TO PeAF IS REFLECTED BY DF CHANGES

We took advantage of the availability of a sheep model of long-term PeAF to characterize the transition from paroxysmal to PeAF in the frequency domain.[24] Animals were chronically instrumented with a transvenous pacemaker implanted in the RA for intermittent tachypacing (30 seconds) at a rate of 20 Hz whenever the heart was determined to be in sinus rhythm. As expected, with time the paroxysmal AF episodes induced by the tachypacing became progressively longer until becoming at least 7 days, which fit the current clinical definition of PeAF.[25] In 7 animals, the DF of the

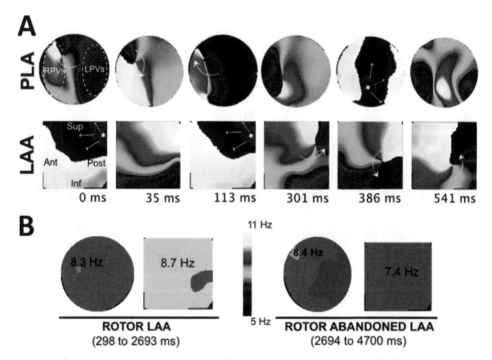

Fig. 3. Patterns of activation in the PLA and LAA of isolated hearts during atrial fibrillation (AF). (*A*) Snapshots from a phase movie show a rotor appearing as a phase singularity point in the field of view of the LAA. The patterns of activation switch from breakthroughs (*asterisks*, 0–113 ms) to a meandering rotor (pivoting around singularity points 301–541 ms). (*B*) The maximum dominant frequency (DF_{max}) is in the LAA when the rotor stays in the field of view and goes back to PLA when the rotor drifts outside the LAA. Ant, anterior; Inf, inferior; LPV, left pulmonary vein; Post, posterior; RPV, right pulmonary vein; Sup, superior. (*Adapted from* Filgueiras-Rama D, Price NF, Martins RP, et al. Long-term frequency gradients during persistent atrial fibrillation in sheep are associated with stable sources in the left atrium. Circ Arrhythm Electrophysiol 2012;5:1160–67; with permission.)

first AF episode recorded from the intracardiac RA lead was relatively slow at 7.5 ± 0.1 Hz (range, 6.5–8.25). Simultaneous DFs from the surface electrocardiograph (ECG) and an implanted loop recorder after QRST subtraction were 7.7 ± 0.2 Hz (range, 6.5–9.25) and 9.0 ± 0.1 Hz (range, 8.9–9.4), respectively. Thus, at the outset there was a significant DF difference between RA and LA (P<.001).[22] Thereafter, DF increased progressively in both atria. At the transition time to PeAF DFs recorded on the RA, surface ECG and LA were higher than during the first episode (P<.001). However, the last DFs recorded after 1 year of uninterrupted PeAF were not different from the transition. Thus, the major increase in DF occurred during the paroxysmal-to-PeAF transition and not during self-sustained PeAF.[24] Additionally, although a significant LA-to-RA frequency gradient was present during the early episodes, this gradient diminished at both the transition (P = .06) and after 12 months of PeAF (P = .1), likely reflecting different remodeling of refractory periods in the two atria. In any given animal, once maximum DF values were achieved, they remained relatively stable even after 1 year of follow-up; there was no difference between maximum DF at transition versus DF at approximately 350 days.[24]

The Rate of DF Increase Predicts the Onset of PeAF

We analyzed several parameters to determine whether or not the time of transition to self-sustained PeAF could be predicted.[24] We first surmised that a critical DF should be reached before self-sustained PeAF developed, but the data did not support this hypothesis. Not only did maximal DF vary among animals, but the rate of DF increase during transition was also highly variable, ranging between 0.003 and 0.15 Hz per day in the RA and between 0.001 and 0.12 Hz per day in the LA. However, sheep that developed uninterrupted PeAF early, also had a steep slope of DF increase with time (dDF/dt), regardless of the DF value during the first episode, whereas those with a delayed onset of PeAF had a shallower DF slope (Fig. 4A). There was a strong inverse nonlinear relationship between time to PeAF onset and dDF/dt regardless of whether DF was determined in the RA, LA, or surface ECG (R^2 = 0.87, 0.92; and 0.71, respectively; see Fig. 4B). The faster the DF increase, the quicker the animal developed self-sustained PeAF. Furthermore, noninvasive measurement of dDF/dt (surface ECG lead I) correlated strongly with RA and LA dDF/dt.[24]

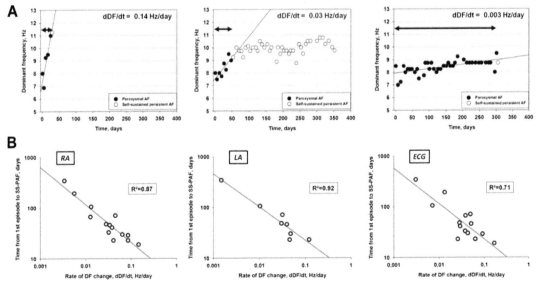

Fig. 4. Rate of increase in dominant frequency (DF) during paroxysmal atrial fibrillation (AF) predicts transition to persistent AF. (*A*) Representative graphs for 3 animals. *Left*, Sheep with the highest slope of DF increase with time (dDF/dt; 0.14 Hz/d; time to transition, 19 days). *Middle*, Intermediate dDF/dt (0.03 Hz/d; time to transition, 46 days). *Right*, Lowest dDF/dt (0.003 Hz/day; time to transition, 346 days). *Left* and *right* from transition group, *middle* from LS-paroxysmal AF group. (*B*) Log–log plots of time from first episode to onset of self-sustained persistent AF versus dDF/dt for the right atrium (RA; intracardiac electrode), left atrium (LA; loop recorder), and electrocardiograph (ECG; surface lead I). Each point represents an animal. The dDF/dt correlated with time to develop self-sustained persistent AF. N = 14 for RA and ECG; N = 8 for LA. (*From* Martins RP, Kaur K, Hwang E, et al. Dominant frequency increase rate predicts transition from paroxysmal to long-term persistent atrial fibrillation. Circulation 2014;129:1472–82; with permission.)

Electrophysiologic Remodeling in Ionic Currents and DF Increase

We conducted computer simulations to address the question of whether differential changes in ion currents could explain DF increase during transition from paroxysmal to the onset of PeAF. We generated APs for control, paroxysmal, and transition AF conditions using the Grandi–Pandit computer model[26] for the human atrial AP (**Fig. 5**A). The membrane ionic current changes were based on our experimental patch-clamp recordings that demonstrated a 65% reduction in the L-type calcium current; a 50% reduction in the sodium inward current; a 75% reduction in the transient outward current; and a 100% increase in the inward rectifier potassium current (I_{K1}).[24] To represent paroxysmal AF, we retained the ionic changes recorded at the end of the transition to PeAF, but reduced the magnitude of L-type calcium current by only 30%, such that the simulated action potential duration

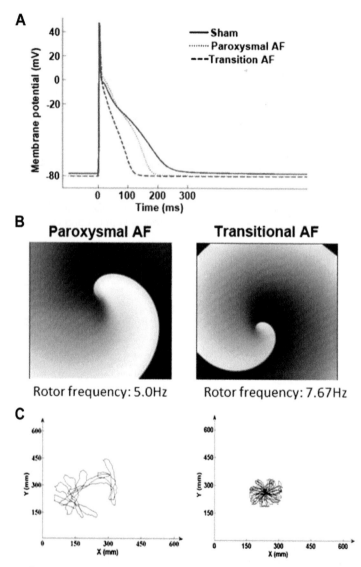

Fig. 5. Simulations predict consequences of ion channel remodeling on rotor frequency. (A) Action potential traces for sham, paroxysmal and transition atrial fibrillation (AF) predicted by experimentally derived ion channel changes. The APD$_{90}$ was abbreviated in both paroxysmal and transition AF compared with sham. Resting membrane potential was hyperpolarized −2 mV. (B) Rotor in paroxysmal (*left*) had lower frequency than transition AF. (C) Rotors in paroxysmal AF meandered considerably and eventually self-terminated on collision with boundary. In transition AF, the rotor was stable, had higher frequency, and persisted throughout the simulation. (*From* Martins RP, Kaur K, Hwang E, et al. Dominant frequency increase rate predicts transition from paroxysmal to long-term persistent atrial fibrillation. Circulation 2014;129:1472–82; with permission.)

at 90% repolarization (APD_{90}) was shortened by 17% in paroxysmal AF, compared with 51% at the transition to PeAF (see **Fig. 5A**).[24]

We conducted simulations on a 2-dimensional sheet model of reentry to investigate whether AP differences between paroxysmal and transition to PeAF would explain the progressive DF increase demonstrated in vivo. Sustained functional reentry (rotor) dynamics showed differential properties. The rotor in paroxysmal AF (see **Fig. 5B**, left) was short lived, and exhibited low rotation frequency (5.0 Hz) and considerable meandering (see **Fig. 5C**, left), eventually self-terminating on collision with boundary edges. In contrast, in the transition to PeAF model, the rotor was stable and persisted throughout the length of the simulation (see **Fig. 5B**, right) with significantly less rotor meander (see **Fig. 5C**, right) and higher DF (7.67 Hz) compared with the transition case. When a reduction in sodium inward current density was not incorporated, the DF increased only

slightly to 8.67 Hz, but the rotor was unstable and eventually stopped.[24]

We also investigated the roles of individual ionic changes in a subset of models where rotors were simulated in 2-dimensional sheets and individual ionic currents were changed compared with controls. The simulation results confirmed that changes in I_{K1} and L-type calcium current are key determinants of rotor acceleration in paroxysmal and transition AF.[24]

TRANSLATION TO PATIENTS: THE HIGH DF SITES AND MAINTENANCE OF AF

AF mapping studies in humans have recognized the presence of temporally and spatially periodic activity[27–29] emanating from the portal vein (PV) region with regularity,[16] suggesting that these structures may have a role in maintaining AF,[17] by harboring either localized short CL reentrant sources and/or focal automatic activity.[30,31] Indeed, in

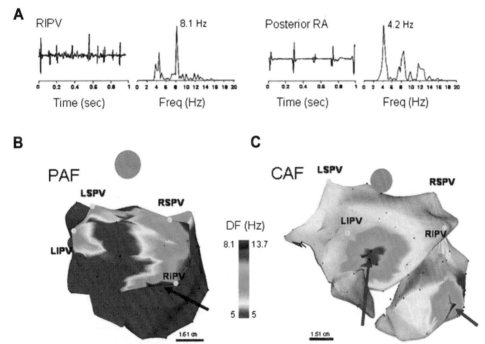

Fig. 6. Dominant frequency (DF) analysis in atrial fibrillation (AF) patients. (*A*) Bipolar electrograms and corresponding power spectra obtained from the RIPV (*left*) and posterior RA in a patient with spontaneous paroxysmal AF. Each site shows distinct DF (8.1 and 4.2 Hz in RIPV and RA, respectively) demonstrating the utility of spectral analysis. (*B*) DF map in a patient with paroxysmal AF (posteroanterior view; 6 hours). Note high DF (HDF) sites in each of the PVs. Ablation sequence in this patient was LSPV, LIPV, RSPV, and RIPV (site of AF termination, *black arrow*); AFCL increased by 10, 25, 9, and 75 ms, respectively, before termination. (*C*) DF map in a patient with permanent AF (24 months). The maximal DF and atrial frequency are higher than the patient in A. In addition, HDF sites are located outside the PVs (*red arrows*). Ablation sequence in this patient was RIPV, RSPV, LSPV, and LIPV; AFCL increased by 5, 2, 0, and 5 ms, respectively. Color bar, DF scale in Hz. CAF, permanent AF; LIPV, left inferior pulmonary vein; LSPV, left superior pulmonary vein; PAF, paroxysmal AF; RIPV, right inferior pulmonary vein; RSPV, right superior pulmonary vein. (*From* Sanders P, Berenfeld O, Hocini M, et al. Spectral analysis identifies sites of high-frequency activity maintaining atrial fibrillation in humans. Circulation 2005;112:789–97; with permission.)

the patient whose DF map is presented in **Fig. 6**B, focal radiofrequency ablation applied to the high DF (HDF) site near the right inferior PV (see **Fig. 6**B, black arrow) effectively terminated AF.[32] A recent study utilizing a morphologically accurate computer model of the atria has demonstrated that the PV region is a preferential site for anchoring rotors.[10,33] In the clinic, paroxysms of short CL activity have been observed in the PVs of patients undergoing AF ablation.[34–36] In addition, sequential ablation of sites showing the shortest CL has been associated with a progressive slowing of AF frequency, culminating in termination in 75% of patients with paroxysmal AF.[37]

DF Mapping in Patients to Guide AF Ablation

Using a blind correlation between atrial DF distribution and ablation, without any attempt at identifying potentially arrhythmogenic sites at the time of the procedure, Sanders and colleagues[32] found that ablation at PVs harboring HDF sites resulted in an increase in the AFCL (≥5 ms) within the coronary sinus (CS) in 89% of cases. The latter was true in patients with either paroxysmal or permanent AF. However, eventual arrhythmia termination occurred during ablation in 15 of 17 patients (88%) with paroxysmal but none with permanent AF (P<.0001). In 13 of the 15 paroxysmal AF patients (87%), arrhythmia termination was associated with ablation at an HDF site; 11 localized to a PV and 2 to the LA roof and the fossa ovalis.

These data, together with other studies by Atienza and colleagues[8,38] and by Lazar and colleagues,[39] clearly indicate that the HDF sites play a role in the maintenance of AF in a significant number of patients. Atienza and colleagues[8] used DF mapping of AF in real-time in drug-refractory paroxysmal and PeAF patients admitted for radiofrequency ablation. After the catheters were in place and sustained AF was induced in paroxysmal AF patients, 3-dimensional reconstruction of the atrial chambers and real-time DF determination were conducted using the CARTO navigation system (Biosense Webster, Diamond Bar, CA, USA) with embedded spectral analysis capabilities. Color-coded DF maps in real time during ongoing AF were superimposed on the atrial shell geometry, displaying low frequencies in red and high frequencies in purple (**Fig. 7**). Once a maximal DF site was identified, ablation started at that site, creating a circumferential set of lesions (see **Fig. 7**). For ethical reasons, because of the observational nature of the study and the a priori unknown outcome of HDF sites ablation, circumferential pulmonary vein isolation was performed in all patients after HDF sites

ablation. The study of Atienza and colleagues[8] demonstrated that the real-time spectral analysis of AF was safe and that it enabled identification and elimination of sources responsible for AF maintenance (see **Fig. 7**). Most important, Atienza and colleagues[8] showed that targeting such sources followed by circumferential PV isolation resulted in long-term sinus rhythm maintenance in 75% of paroxysmal and 50% of PeAF patients. Our study led to the conclusion that radiofrequency ablation leading to the elimination of preexisting DF gradients between the LA and the RA predicts long-term sinus rhythm maintenance in both paroxysmal and PeAF patients.

SUMMARY

The experimental and numerical studies on AF discussed herein were conducted using sheep and simplified computer models, respectively. Obviously, results obtained from animal hearts should be cautiously extrapolated to humans. Similarly, one must be extremely cautious when attempting to generalize the applicability of theoretic concepts derived from numerical experiments. Nevertheless, as discussed, knowledge derived from spectral analysis in the sheep atria may be used to derive important predictions on ionic and structural mechanisms of AF in patients. In general, strong evidence that rotor-like activity is the driving force that maintains human AF in patients is emerging at an accelerating pace.[40,41]

DF mapping in combination with phase mapping, patch clamping, molecular biology, and numerical simulations has contributed to the recognition that inward rectifying K^+ currents play an important role in the dynamics of rotors in both paroxysmal and PeAF.[23,38] This finding has opened the possibility of developing new and effective antiarrhythmic therapies targeting rotor formation or termination.[42,43] For instance, our numerical simulations on AF demonstrate that sustained rotors in the atria depend on the conductance level the inward-rectifiers I_{K1} and the acetylcholine-modulated $I_{K,ACh}$.[10,38,44] $I_{K,ACh}$ activation induces rotor acceleration and stabilization in acute AF.[23,38] However, in PeAF the increase in I_{K1} plays a greater role accelerating and stabilizing rotors.[24] Increasing the degree of rectification of I_{K1} can either slow or abolish rotor activity and AF.[42,43] Hence, one could envision that, in the foreseeable future, development of a new generation of safe and effective antifibrillatory K^+ channel–modifying drugs could lead to protection against AF in patients.

An alternative approach for drug-refractory AF in patients is ablation. However, this approach can

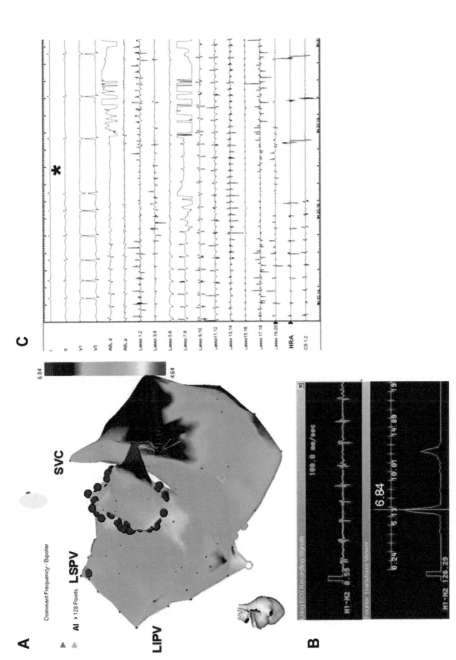

Fig. 7. (A) Real-time atrial dominant frequency (DF) map (posterior view; CARTO system) in a paroxysmal atrial fibrillation (AF) patient. *Purple,* primary maximum DF (DF_max) site on right intermediate pulmonary vein (RIPV). *Red dots,* circumferential ablation line. (*B*) Bipolar recording (*top*) of primary DF_max site and its power spectrum (*bottom*) before ablation. (C) Surface electrocardiograph (ECG) leads and intracardiac lasso catheter electrograms within RIPV; ablation catheter in the encircled area; coronary sinus (CS) and high right atrium (HRA) catheter during isolation of right-sided PVs. Catheters recording outside the encircled area (CS, HRA) show conversion to SR (*asterisk*) whereas the lasso catheter inside RIPV demonstrates ongoing AF. (*From* Atienza F, Almendral J, Jalife J, et al. Real-time dominant frequency mapping and ablation of dominant frequency sites in atrial fibrillation with left-to-right frequency gradients predicts long-term maintenance of sinus rhythm. Heart Rhythm 2009;6:33–40; with permission.)

be challenging in patients with PeAF.[45] In the future, the combined use of time, frequency, and phase domain measures, including electrogram fractionation,[46] principal value decomposition, and DF mapping,[47] should help to elucidate mechanism of impulse propagation and the identification of the drivers and characterization of their dynamics to provide an efficient mean to facilitate patient-specific ablation procedures with well-defined endpoints,[8,48,49] potentially leading to increased efficacy and safety.[50,51]

REFERENCES

1. Chen LY, Shen WK. Epidemiology of atrial fibrillation: a current perspective. Heart Rhythm 2007;4: S1–6.
2. Moe GK. On the multiple wavelet hypothesis of atrial fibrillation. Arch Int Pharmacodyn Ther 1962; 140:183–8.
3. Allessie MA, Lammers WJ, Bonke FI, et al. Experimental evaluation of Moe's wavelet hypothesis of atrial fibrillation. In: Zipes DP, Jalife J, editors. Cardiac electrophysiology and arrhythmias. Orlando (FL): Grune & Stratton; 1985. p. 265–75.
4. de Groot NM, Houben RP, Smeets JL, et al. Electropathological substrate of longstanding persistent atrial fibrillation in patients with structural heart disease: epicardial breakthrough. Circulation 2010; 122:1674–82.
5. Krinskii VI. Excitation propagation in nonhomogenous medium (actions analogous to heart fibrillation). Biofizika 1966;11:676–83.
6. Jalife J, Berenfeld O, Skanes A, et al. Mechanisms of atrial fibrillation: mother rotors or multiple daughter wavelets, or both? J Cardiovasc Electrophysiol 1998;9:S2–12.
7. Allessie MA, Bonke FI, Schopman FJ. Circus movement in rabbit atrial muscle as a mechanism of tachycardia. III. The "leading circle" concept: a new model of circus movement in cardiac tissue without the involvement of an anatomical obstacle. Circ Res 1977;41:9–18.
8. Atienza F, Almendral J, Jalife J, et al. Real-time dominant frequency mapping and ablation of dominant frequency sites in atrial fibrillation with left-to-right frequency gradients predicts long-term maintenance of sinus rhythm. Heart Rhythm 2009;6:33–40.
9. Narayan SM, Krummen DE, Donsky A, et al. Treatment of paroxysmal atrial fibrillation by targeted elimination of stable rotors and focal sources without pulmonary vein isolation: the precise rotor elimination without concomitant pulmonary vein isolation for subsequent elimination of PAF (PRECISE) trial. Heart Rhythm 2013; 10:LBCT4–5.
10. Calvo CJ, Deo M, Zlochiver S, et al. Attraction of rotors to the pulmonary veins in paroxysmal atrial fibrillation: a modeling study. Biophys J 2014;106: 1811–21.
11. Morillo CA, Klein GJ, Jones DL, et al. Chronic rapid atrial pacing: structural, functional, and electro-physiological characteristics of a new model of sustained atrial fibrillation. Circulation 1995;91: 1588–95.
12. Harada A, Sasaki K, Fukushima T, et al. Atrial activation during chronic atrial fibrillation in patients with isolated mitral valve disease. Ann Thorac Surg 1996;61:104–12.
13. Gray RA, Pertsov AM, Jalife J. Spatial and temporal organization during cardiac fibrillation. Nature 1998;392:75–8.
14. Mansour M, Mandapati R, Berenfeld O, et al. Left-to-right gradient of atrial frequencies during acute atrial fibrillation in the isolated sheep heart. Circulation 2001;103:2631–6.
15. Berenfeld O, Mandapati R, Dixit S, et al. Spatially distributed dominant excitation frequencies reveal hidden organization in atrial fibrillation in the langendorff-perfused sheep heart. J Cardiovasc Electrophysiol 2000;11:869–79.
16. Skanes AC, Mandapati R, Berenfeld O, et al. Spatiotemporal periodicity during atrial fibrillation in the isolated sheep heart. Circulation 1998;98: 1236–48.
17. Mandapati R, Skanes A, Chen J, et al. Stable microreentrant sources as a mechanism of atrial fibrillation in the isolated sheep heart. Circulation 2000; 101:194–9.
18. Berenfeld O, Ennis S, Hwang E, et al. Time- and frequency-domain analyses of atrial fibrillation activation rate: the optical mapping reference. Heart Rhythm 2011;8:1758–65.
19. Jalife J. Deja vu in the theories of atrial fibrillation dynamics. Cardiovasc Res 2011;89:766–75.
20. Schuessler RB, Kay MW, Melby SJ, et al. Spatial and temporal stability of the dominant frequency of activation in human atrial fibrillation. J Electrocardiol 2006;39(Suppl 4):S7–12.
21. Berenfeld O, Zaitsev AV, Mironov SF, et al. Frequency-dependent breakdown of wave propagation into fibrillatory conduction across the pectinate muscle network in the isolated sheep right atrium. Circ Res 2002;90:1173–80.
22. Filgueiras-Rama D, Price NF, Martins RP, et al. Long-term frequency gradients during persistent atrial fibrillation in sheep are associated with stable sources in the left atrium. Circulation 2012;5: 1160–7.
23. Sarmast F, Kolli A, Zaitsev A, et al. Cholinergic atrial fibrillation: I-k,i-ach gradients determine unequal left/right atrial frequencies and rotor dynamics. Cardiovasc Res 2003;59:863–73.

24. Martins RP, Kaur K, Hwang E, et al. Dominant frequency increase rate predicts transition from paroxysmal to long-term persistent atrial fibrillation. Circulation 2014;129:1472–82.

25. Calkins H, Kuck KH, Cappato R, et al. 2012 hrs/ehra/ecas expert consensus statement on catheter and surgical ablation of atrial fibrillation: recommendations for patient selection, procedural techniques, patient management and follow-up, definitions, endpoints, and research trial design. Europace 2012; 14:528–606.

26. Grandi E, Pandit SV, Voigt N, et al. Human atrial action potential and Ca2+ model: sinus rhythm and chronic atrial fibrillation. Circ Res 2011;109:1055–66.

27. Wu TJ, Doshi RN, Huang HL, et al. Simultaneous biatrial computerized mapping during permanent atrial fibrillation in patients with organic heart disease. J Cardiovasc Electrophysiol 2002;13: 571–7.

28. Sih HJ, Zipes DP, Berbari EJ, et al. Differences in organization between acute and chronic atrial fibrillation in dogs. J Am Coll Cardiol 2000;36:924–31.

29. Wu TJ, Ong JJ, Chang CM, et al. Pulmonary veins and ligament of Marshall as sources of rapid activations in a canine model of sustained atrial fibrillation. Circulation 2001;103:1157–63.

30. Arora R, Verheule S, Scott L, et al. Arrhythmogenic substrate of the pulmonary veins assessed by high-resolution optical mapping. Circulation 2003; 107:1816–21.

31. Kalifa J, Jalife J, Zaitsev AV, et al. Intra-atrial pressure increases rate and organization of waves emanating from the superior pulmonary veins during atrial fibrillation. Circulation 2003; 108:668–71.

32. Sanders P, Berenfeld O, Hocini M, et al. Spectral analysis identifies sites of high-frequency activity maintaining atrial fibrillation in humans. Circulation 2005;112:789–97.

33. Vigmond EJ, Tsoi V, Kuo S, et al. The effect of vagally induced dispersion of action potential duration on atrial arrhythmogenesis. Heart Rhythm 2004;1:334–44.

34. Kumagai K, Yasuda T, Tojo H, et al. Role of rapid focal activation in the maintenance of atrial fibrillation originating from the pulmonary veins. Pacing Clin Electrophysiol 2000;23:1823–7.

35. O'Donnell D, Furniss SS, Bourke JP. Paroxysmal cycle length shortening in the pulmonary veins during atrial fibrillation correlates with arrhythmogenic triggering foci in sinus rhythm. J Cardiovasc Electrophysiol 2002;13:124–8.

36. Oral H, Ozaydin M, Tada H, et al. Mechanistic significance of intermittent pulmonary vein tachycardia in patients with atrial fibrillation. J Cardiovasc Electrophysiol 2002;13:645–50.

37. Haissaguerre M, Sanders P, Hocini M, et al. Changes in atrial fibrillation cycle length and

38. inducibility during catheter ablation and their relation to outcome. Circulation 2004;109:3007–13.

38. Atienza F, Almendral J, Moreno J, et al. Activation of inward rectifier potassium channels accelerates atrial fibrillation in humans: evidence for a reentrant mechanism. Circulation 2006;114: 2434–42.

39. Lazar S, Dixit S, Callans DJ, et al. Effect of pulmonary vein isolation on the left-to-right atrial dominant frequency gradient in human atrial fibrillation. Heart Rhythm 2006;3:889–95.

40. Narayan SM, Krummen DE, Shivkumar K, et al. Treatment of atrial fibrillation by the ablation of localized sources: confirm (conventional ablation for atrial fibrillation with or without focal impulse and rotor modulation) trial. J Am Coll Cardiol 2012;60:628–36.

41. Rodrigo M, Guillem MS, Climent AM, et al. Body surface localization of left and right atrial high frequency rotors in atrial fibrillation patients: a clinical-computational study. Heart Rhythm 2014. http://dx.doi.org/10.1016/j.hrthm.2014.05.013.

42. Filgueiras-Rama D, Martins RP, Mironov S, et al. Chloroquine terminates stretch-induced atrial fibrillation more effectively than flecainide in the sheep heart. Circulation 2012;5:561–70.

43. Noujaim SF, Stuckey JA, Ponce-Balbuena D, et al. Specific residues of the cytoplasmic domains of cardiac inward rectifier potassium channels are effective antifibrillatory targets. FASEB J 2010; 24(11):4302–12.

44. Pandit SV, Berenfeld O, Anumonwo J, et al. Ionic determinants of functional reentry in a 2-d model of human atrial cells during simulated chronic atrial fibrillation. Biophys J 2005;88(6):3806–21.

45. Oral H, Pappone C, Chugh A, et al. Circumferential pulmonary-vein ablation for chronic atrial fibrillation. N Engl J Med 2006;354:934–41.

46. Nademanee K, McKenzie J, Kosar E, et al. A new approach for catheter ablation of atrial fibrillation: mapping of the electrophysiologic substrate. J Am Coll Cardiol 2004;43:2044–53.

47. Zlochiver S, Yamazaki M, Kalifa J, et al. Rotor meandering contributes to irregularity in electrograms during atrial fibrillation. Heart Rhythm 2008; 5:846–54.

48. Yoshida K, Chugh A, Good E, et al. A critical decrease in dominant frequency and clinical outcome after catheter ablation of persistent atrial fibrillation. Heart Rhythm 2010;7:295–302.

49. Narayan SM, Baykaner T, Clopton P, et al. Ablation of rotor and focal sources reduces late recurrence of atrial fibrillation compared with trigger ablation alone: extended follow-up of the confirm trial (conventional ablation for atrial fibrillation with or without focal impulse and rotor modulation). J Am Coll Cardiol 2014;63:1761–8.

50. Bertaglia E, Zoppo F, Tondo C, et al. Early complications of pulmonary vein catheter ablation for atrial fibrillation: a multicenter prospective registry on procedural safety. Heart Rhythm 2007;4:1265–71.

51. Cappato R, Calkins H, Chen SA, et al. Worldwide survey on the methods, efficacy, and safety of catheter ablation for human atrial fibrillation. Circulation 2005;111:1100–5.

Diagnostic Evaluation and Follow-Up of Patients with Atrial Fibrillation

Patrick Dillon, MD, Hamid Ghanbari, MD*

KEYWORDS

- Atrial fibrillation • Diagnostic evaluation • Follow-up • Risk factors • Symptoms • Quality of life

KEY POINTS

- Atrial fibrillation (AF) is the most common clinically encountered cardiac arrhythmia.
- AF carries significant morbidity and mortality.
- As the prevalence of AF continues to increase, so too will the number of both outpatient and inpatient visits that are either directly or indirectly attributable to the condition.
- Clinicians across many specialties will likely face diagnostic and therapeutic challenges associated with AF more frequently in the coming years and decades.

INTRODUCTION

Atrial fibrillation (AF) is the most common clinically encountered cardiac arrhythmia. The estimated number of patients with AF in the United States is estimated to be between 3 and 6 million.[1] The prevalence of AF is highest in the elderly, and it has been estimated that 4 of 5 patients with AF are 65 years of age or older.[2] Over the next 2 to 3 decades, the incidence is expected to increase to 2.6 million, and the prevalence may increase to more than 12 million.[3]

AF carries with it significant morbidity and mortality. It is an important risk factor for ischemic stroke, and as many as 15% of strokes have been attributed to AF.[4,5] It has also been associated with heart failure, decreased functional status, dementia, lower quality of life, and death.[6–11] As the prevalence of AF continues to increase, so too will the number of both outpatient and inpatient visits that are either directly or indirectly attributable to the condition. Therefore, clinicians across many specialties will likely face diagnostic

and therapeutic challenges associated with AF more frequently in the coming years and decades.

In this review, the diagnostic evaluation and considerations for follow up after the initial diagnosis of AF are discussed. Signs and symptoms, medical history, and physical examination findings useful when evaluating patients at the bedside are highlighted, and diagnostic approaches in varying clinical scenarios are discussed. Important considerations for both short-term and long-term outpatient follow-up are also reviewed.

DIAGNOSTIC EVALUATION
Clinical History

Symptoms
Most patients with AF report symptoms attributable to AF. There are many symptoms related to AF; however, there is significant interindividual and intraindividual variability. The most common symptoms that prompt patients with previously undiagnosed AF to pursue evaluation include palpitations, dyspnea, chest pain, fatigue, and

This article originally appeared in Cardiology Clinics, Volume 32, Issue 4, November 2014.
Disclosures: None.
Division of Cardiovascular Medicine, University of Michigan Health System, 1500 East Medical Center Drive, Ann Arbor, MI 48109, USA
* Corresponding author.
E-mail address: ghhamid@med.umich.edu

Heart Failure Clin 12 (2016) 179–191
http://dx.doi.org/10.1016/j.hfc.2015.08.015
1551-7136/16/$ – see front matter © 2016 Elsevier Inc. All rights reserved.

syncope (**Fig. 1**).[12,13] Palpitations are an unpleasant awareness of the forceful, rapid, or irregular beating of the heart. In a prospective observational study,[12] more than half of patients with AF reported experiencing palpitations. When further subdivided, 79% of patients with paroxysmal and 45% of patients with chronic AF experienced palpitations. The most common precipitating factors were exercise, emotion, postprandial state, and caffeine.

Up to 40% to 50% of patients with AF report dyspnea. The underlying cause of shortness of breath may be difficult to assess, however, because many conditions that cause dyspnea also predispose to AF, like chronic obstructive pulmonary disease (COPD), structural heart disease, and obstructive sleep apnea (OSA).[12,14] Dyspnea related to AF can result in a decline in performance status. The presence of AF, for example, has been shown to be associated with higher New York Heart Association functional class.[15] Furthermore, patients with AF were found to have significantly lower exercise performance compared with similar patients in whom sinus rhythm was restored and maintained.[16]

Chest pain is frequently associated with AF. Fast heart rates, irregular ventricular response, and loss of atrial contraction may lead to a decrease in cardiac output, which contributes to ischemic chest pain in patients with coronary artery disease. Chest pain is seen in patients with AF despite the absence of coronary artery disease, and impaired microvascular flow is a possible explanation.[17,18] Symptoms like lightheadedness and syncope are more likely to be seen in patients with structural heart disease, and although clinically important, they occur less frequently than symptoms described earlier.[19]

Although many patients experience symptoms related to AF, observed frequencies of symptoms may be overestimated, because asymptomatic patients often do not present for evaluation. Several studies have reported that between 10% and 20% of patients with AF are asymptomatic.[12,20–22] One observational study found that patients without symptoms were significantly more likely to be male, carry a diagnosis of diabetes, have a larger left atrial size, have a lower resting heart rate, and have progressed to persistent or permanent AF by the time of AF diagnosis.[22] Furthermore, although CHADS$_2$ and CHA$_2$DS$_2$-VASc scores were similar for symptomatic and asymptomatic patients, asymptomatic patients were less likely to be diagnosed with AF and subsequently treated with anticoagulation. An observational study found that 20% of patients with cryptogenic stroke were given a diagnosis of AF during follow-up after wearing a 30-day event monitor.[23]

Quality of life

Quality of life is significantly reduced in most patients with AF.[24,25] Improvements in symptoms and health-related quality of life (HRQOL) are

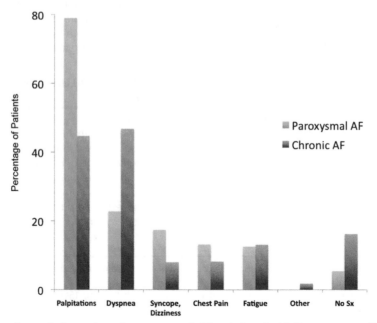

Fig. 1. Frequency of reported symptoms for paroxysmal AF and chronic AF. Sx, symptoms. (*Data from* Levy S, Maarek M, Coumel P, et al. Characterization of different subsets of atrial fibrillation in general practice in France: the ALFA study. The College of French Cardiologists. Circulation 1999;99:3028–35.)

important therapeutic goals in management of patients with AF, along with reducing the risk of stroke, mortality, and cardiovascular morbidity.[19] There have been several global and disease-specific HRQOL measures that have been used in patients with AF. The most commonly used global HRQOL tools in patients with AF are SF-36, SF-12, EuroQOL, and EQ-5D.

The SF-36 is the most widely used generic HRQOL instrument used in patients with AF. It has been validated in many studies evaluating HRQOL in cardiac and noncardiac conditions. It consists of a 36-item questionnaire, which assesses 8 health domains. These domains include general health perception, physical functioning, social functioning, vitality, bodily pain, mental health, and role limitations caused by emotional and physical problems.[26] It also generates psychometrically based physical and mental component summary scores.[26] The SF-12 is a shorter version of SF-36, which uses 12 questions to measure HRQOL.[27] The physical and mental component summary scores from the SF-12 mirror those from the SF-36.[27] The EuroQOL is focused on 5 health domains: mobility, self-care, usual activities, pain/discomfort, and anxiety or depression.[28] It also has the advantage of the EQ-5D method, which can transform raw scores to preference-based utility weights.[29]

The advantage of these global instruments to assess AF-related HRQOL is their long validation track record, generalizability, and large data available from the population with AF. However, these measures, which reflect general health and functioning and scores among patients with AF, are strongly influenced by patient demographics and comorbid conditions.[30] Therefore, these instruments are less sensitive to change, particularly in patients with multiple medical conditions.

The Arrhythmia Symptom Checklist is the most commonly used cardiac questionnaire used in the assessment of HRQOL in patients with AF. It rates the frequency (0–4) and severity (1–3) of 16 symptoms commonly associated with AF.[31] It is easy to use and sensitive to change. However, the symptoms assessed are nonspecific, and it does not assess functional status and patient satisfaction. These factors limit its applicability as a stand-alone HRQOL measure in AF.

More recently, there has been an emphasis on developing several instruments specific to assessment of HRQOL in patients with AF. The Atrial Fibrillation Symptom Score (AFSS) is a 19-item disease-specific measure of quality of life in AF. It includes questions regarding AF-related symptoms, health care use, frequency, overall severity, and duration of symptomatic AF episodes.[16,32,33]

The AF symptom score can be calculated using the AFSS summary score. The AFEQT (Atrial Fibrillation Effect on Quality-of-life) questionnaire is a 20-item instrument designed to assess HRQOL in AF. It assesses 4 health domains: symptoms, activities, treatment concerns, and satisfaction. A summary score is generated based on the first 3 health domains. The responses are shown as a 7-point Likert scale. Patients are asked to indicate the impact of AF on their health status in the previous 4 weeks. The raw scores from each domain are transformed to a 0 to 100 scale, on which a score of 0 indicates the most severe symptoms and score of 100 indicates no limitations.

Assessing symptoms in AF can be challenging, and these instruments are complex and require significant time to complete. This factor has limited their wide clinical adaptation. The Canadian Cardiovascular Society Severity of Atrial Fibrillation (CCS-SAF) scale was created as a concise, symptom-based severity scale intended for routine clinical use in patients with AF.[34] The CCS-SAF scale provides a potentially clinically useful scale for practitioners to assess patient status and to communicate the severity of the functional consequences of the patient's symptoms from AF. It closely approximates patient-reported subjective measures of quality of life in AF and may be practical for clinical use.[32] The Severity of Atrial Fibrillation (SAF) class, derived from CCS-SAF, is imperfectly correlated to generic quality of life measures in the SF-36 and AFSS. This situation presumably occurs because the SAF scale captures, by design, all components of the AF syndrome (including, eg, symptom severity during AF, adverse effects of treatment administered, and the physical and psychological consequences of the disease state), whereas the generic quality of life measures capture only components of the AF illness burden.[32]

Most data focused on assessing HRQOL in patients with AF are derived from intervention studies assessing rate and rhythm control strategies. These studies included patients with highly symptomatic AF with baseline HRQOL scores, which were significantly lower than the general population.[16,25,33,35–37] Studies including less selected patients with AF have also confirmed that most patients with AF have lower HRQOL compared with the general population. In a cross-sectional evaluation of 142 patients (mean age 58 years),[24] patients with AF had significantly worse scores compared with healthy controls. In a cohort of 963 patients included in the FRACTAL (Fibrillation Registry Assessing Costs, Therapies, Adverse Events and Lifestyle) registry,[30] the HRQOL scores were significantly lower than healthy controls.

The baseline comorbid conditions, age, and gender affect HRQOL in patients with AF. This situation is influenced by the use of generic HRQOL instruments, which are affected by age and underlying medical conditions. The severity of heart failure symptoms, chronic pulmonary disease, valvular heart disease, and coronary artery disease has been associated with lower HRQOL in patients with AF.[33,38] Personality traits may also play an important role in perceived HRQOL. Depression, pessimism, and personality traits relating to the response to physical and emotional stressors (anxiety sensitivity and somatization) have been associated with diminished HRQOL in patients with AF.[39,40] Gender plays an important role in HRQOL in patients with AF. Women report a lower HRQOL and greater symptom burden than men.[38,41,42] Older patients report lower symptom burden associated with AF when compared with younger patients.[38] They also tend to have a different symptom pattern, with fatigue and dyspnea being more prominent in the elderly, whereas palpitations are more prominent in younger patients.[38] HRQOL may not be significantly affected in some patients, in particular, the elderly. In a study of 52 patients (mean age 77 years) with chronic AF,[43] there were no observed differences in HRQOL and exercise tolerance compared with age-matched control individuals without AF. Therefore the segment of the population with AF studied influences the impact of AF on HRQOL.

Past medical history

Many conditions predispose to the development of AF, and several risk factors have been established (**Box 1**). Age is an independent risk factor for AF, and every additional decade of life for men and women nearly doubles the risk of developing AF.[2,44] Independent cardiovascular risk factors include hypertension, valve disease, congestive heart failure, and myocardial infarction.[44] A systolic blood pressure higher than 150 mm Hg has been shown to be a statistically significant risk factor for incident AF.[45] As a surrogate of systolic hypertension and aortic stiffness, a widened pulse pressure is a risk for AF, with an adjusted hazard ratio of 1.26 per 20 mm Hg increase in blood pressure.[46]

Although the causal relationship between heart failure and AF is poorly understood, both conditions share common risk factors. The odds ratio of AF for heart failure was 4.5 for men and 5.9 for women in the Framingham Heart Study.[44,47] Increased frequency of AF has been described in the setting of acute coronary syndrome and prevalent myocardial infarction, with an incidence

---

Box 1
Independent risk factors for development of AF

Risk factors for AF

Age

Hypertension

Valvular heart disease

Congestive heart failure

Myocardial infarction

Diabetes mellitus

Obesity (body mass index [calculated as weight in kilograms divided by the square of height in meters] ≥ 30 kg/m^2)

Obstructive sleep apnea

Hyperthyroidism

Cigarette smoking

Heavy ethanol intake

---

between 6% and 21% during acute myocardial infarction.[48] In addition, perhaps the most commonly discussed risk factor is valvular heart disease. Left-sided valvular lesions have been more thoroughly studied than right-sided lesions, and specifically, mitral stenosis and mitral regurgitation. One observational study found that by the time of clinical presentation, 20% of patients with mitral stenosis had already developed AF, and 33% had developed AF by the end of the 10-year follow-up period.[49] Incident AF in degenerative mitral regurgitation caused by flail leaflet was 18% and 48% at 5 and 10 years, respectively, and rates were similar for mitral regurgitation caused by mitral valve prolapse.[50]

AF is a well-recognized manifestation of hyperthyroidism, with a greater than 2-fold increase in risk.[51] In the Canadian Registry for Atrial Fibrillation and Danish National Registry, overt hyperthyroidism was observed in 1% and 8.3% of patients with AF, respectively.[21,52] In addition, patients with subclinical hyperthyroidism as well as patients with thyroid-stimulating hormone levels in the high-normal range have been observed to be at increased risk for AF.[53,54] In contrast, there is not a significant association between AF and hypothyroidism.[55]

Diabetes and metabolic syndrome are independent risk factors for incident AF.[44,56] Accordingly, obesity has been found to predispose to AF, with adjusted hazard ratios of 1.52 and 1.46 for men and women, respectively.[57] In addition, because obesity is a risk factor for OSA, the prevalence of OSA is significantly higher in patients with AF compared with other cardiovascular diseases. It is an independent risk factor for AF in patients younger than 65 years.[58,59] Although these conditions are treatable and even preventable, they continue to increase in incidence and prevalence. Modifiable risk factors like smoking (and resultant COPD) and heavy alcohol use predispose to AF.[60–62]

Medications

A variety of medications have been identified as possible inciting and reversible underlying causes of AF. Generally, the development of AF results from a trigger, whereas the maintenance of AF requires a change in electrophysiologic substrate.[63] The underlying mechanisms of drug-induced AF affect either trigger or substrate and include (1) adrenergic or vagal stimulation, (2) modified atrial conduction, refractoriness, or automaticity, (3) direct cardiotoxicity, (4) coronary vasoconstriction, and (5) electrolyte disturbances.[64]

Adenosine is often used to terminate supraventricular tachycardia (SVT); however, it can induce AF in up to 10% of cases, although this is typically transient, because of the short half-life of adenosine.[65] Other cardiovascular medications that can incite AF include dopamine, dobutamine, and milrinone (by increasing adrenergic stimulation), anticholinergics (by increasing vagal stimulation), and thiazides (by causing electrolyte disturbances). Although digoxin is used for rate control of SVT or AF, toxic levels may lead to the development of atrial tachycardia or even AF.

Although it is difficult to describe a causal relationship between a drug and incident AF, it is important to review medicines when clinically evaluating patients with AF. Although a drug may not necessarily cause AF, it may potentiate tachycardia in the setting of established electrophysiologic substrate for AF. For example, patients with reactive airway disease (a risk factor for AF) may be given β-agonists like albuterol or salmeterol or they may be taking theophylline, a drug that carries increased risk for AF.[66]

PHYSICAL EXAMINATION

All patients with suspected or newly diagnosed AF should receive a complete examination of the cardiovascular system. Initial findings to suggest the presence of AF include an irregular pulse, irregular jugular venous pulsation, and variability in intensity of the first heart sound that occurs with variable ventricular preload. Further observation of the jugular venous pulsation shows an absent a-wave. Although a regular heart rhythm on examination may suggest a sinus rhythm, it is also found in

patients with AF and complete heart block with a junctional or ventricular escape.

Special attention should be given to the presence of murmurs to suggest stenotic or regurgitant lesions, which may contribute to the development of AF. Loss of atrial contraction can lead to hypervolemia and heart failure. Furthermore, decompensation in heart failure status may be the underlying cause of AF. The initial examination to assess for hypervolemia can be important for prognosis, because the presence of increased jugular venous pulsation, peripheral edema, rales, or the presence of a third heart sound were all associated with higher cardiovascular mortality in patients with heart failure and AF.[67]

Diagnostics

An initial clinic visit for evaluation of suspected or documented AF typically includes an electrocardiogram (ECG) and a transthoracic echocardiogram (TTE). ECG may provide evidence of chamber enlargement or hypertrophy or previous myocardial infarction and establish a baseline corrected QT interval if antiarrhythmic medications are a consideration. TTE allows further characterization of valvular heart disease, systolic and diastolic function, chamber hypertrophy, and atrial size. Left atrial dilation suggests underlying electroanatomic remodeling, and identification of left atrial enlargement can guide management. For example, left atrial diameter less than 50 to 55 mm predicts a higher probability of successful catheter ablation of AF.[68] As described earlier, other diagnostics as guided by physical examination should include thyroid function tests, pulmonary function tests, and sleep study.

Advanced imaging modalities may offer more guidance for management decisions in the future. Three-dimensional echocardiography has been suggested to provide a more accurate assessment of left atrial volume when compared with standard two-dimensional echo.[69] If catheter ablation is being considered, cross-sectional imaging with computed tomography or cardiac magnetic resonance (MR) offers detailed information regarding pulmonary vein location and geometry. Furthermore, late gadolinium enhancement MR sequences used to characterize the extent of left atrial fibrosis can predict response to catheter ablation. Mild late gadolinium enhancement, when compared with extensive enhancement, is associated with lower rates of AF recurrence after catheter ablation.[70]

Ambulatory external ECG (AECG) monitoring offers the ability to diagnose clinically suspected paroxysmal AF. Short-term 24-hour to 48-hour continuous monitors have the advantage of documenting AF regardless of patient symptoms but with a trade-off of low sensitivity because of the short duration of observation. Intermittent patient-activated, longer-term recorders increase sensitivity by allowing more time for patients to develop symptoms but fail to document asymptomatic episodes of paroxysmal AF. Newer-generation ambulatory telemetry monitors were developed to overcome limitations of short-term or patient-activated monitors; however, these require storage and review of large amounts of data.

AECG monitoring can also be particularly useful in patients with cryptogenic stroke. Longer-term observation of rhythm in patients with stroke of unclear cause more accurately diagnoses AF. In the EMBRACE trial,[71] patients with cryptogenic stroke or transient ischemic attack were randomly assigned to monitoring with either a 30-day event recorder or with standard 24-hour monitoring. Extended follow-up with 30-day event monitoring significantly improved detection of AF and diagnosed AF in 16% of patients compared with 3% of patients in the standard monitoring group. In another study,[72] longer-term monitoring with an insertable cardiac monitor after cryptogenic stroke diagnosed AF in 12% of patients at 1 year, compared with 2% of patients in the standard monitoring group.

FOLLOW-UP
Anticoagulation

The CHADS$_2$ score has been used for many years to guide anticoagulation therapy to mitigate stroke risk in patients with nonvalvular AF.[73] Guidelines from the European Society of Cardiology (ESC) and more recent guidelines from the American College of Cardiology (ACC), American Heart Association (AHA), and Heart Rhythm Society (HRS) recommend use of the CHA$_2$DS$_2$-VASc score for anticoagulation in nonvalvular AF.[74,75] A CHA$_2$DS$_2$-VASc score of 2 or higher warrants full anticoagulation for patients in whom it is not contraindicated. The ESC guidelines, more so than the ACC/AHA/HRS guidelines, lean toward no anticoagulation, as opposed to aspirin, in patients with CHA$_2$DS$_2$-VASc of zero and toward full anticoagulation, as opposed to aspirin, in patients with CHA$_2$DS$_2$-VASc of 1.

Warfarin, a vitamin K antagonist, interferes with γ-carboxylation of coagulation factors II, VII, IX, and X. Many clinics approach warfarin dosing as a 7-day week total dose divided into smaller daily doses. The international normalized ratio (INR) response should be monitored every 2 to 5 days after initiation of treatment until stable INR levels are documented on stable dosing, after which monitoring is typically performed every 4 weeks. A randomized trial[76] comparing classic clinic-based monthly INR monitoring with home-based weekly point-of-care INR monitoring for patients on warfarin because of mechanical heart valves or AF found no difference in time to first stroke, major bleeding episode, or death between the 2 groups. As user-friendly data-sharing platforms become more available in the health care industry, remote INR monitoring could present an alternative to the clinic-based model of INR monitoring.

Dabigatran, a direct thrombin inhibitor, as well as rivaroxaban and apixaban, activated factor Xa inhibitors, are 3 target-specific oral anticoagulants (TSOA) that have recently been approved by the US Food and Drug Administration for stroke risk mediation in nonvalvular AF.[77–79] The TSOA agents offer alternative anticoagulation treatment to warfarin, with the benefit of fixed dosing regimens and fewer drug-drug interactions. **Tables 1** and **2** compare their pharmacologic and risk profiles. Dabigatran is the most dependent on renal clearance, whereas apixaban is the least dependent. Drug levels increase with decreasing renal function and expose the patient to a higher risk of bleeding. Creatinine clearance calculation is recommended to guide dosing for dabigatran and rivaroxaban, whereas creatinine level is recommended for apixaban dosing. Renal function should be monitored frequently during treatment with TSOAs.

Antiarrhythmic Therapy

Although many studies have shown similar survival rates for rhythm control and rate control strategies,[36,80,81] rhythm control can often be the preferred management choice in patients with severe symptoms. **Fig. 2** and **Table 3** review the use of antiarrhythmic medications in different patient populations. Class IC agents should be avoided in patients with coronary artery disease or heart failure. Dronedarone and sotalol should also be avoided in patients with heart failure.

Amiodarone and ibutilide (available only as intravenous formulation) are commonly used class III agents for patients with recent onset paroxysmal AF in the acute care setting. Both agents have been shown to increase the efficacy of direct-current cardioversion if given before electrical treatment.[82,83]

The class IC agents, flecainide and propafenone, can be used both as a pill-in-the-pocket strategy for intermittent, symptomatic paroxysmal

Table 1
Comparison of warfarin with target-specific oral anticoagulants

	Warfarin	Dabigatran[a]	Rivaroxaban[b]	Apixaban[c]
Target of inhibition	Vitamin K	Thrombin	Factor Xa	Factor Xa
Studied dose (mg)	—	150 twice a day 110 twice a day	20 daily	5 twice a day
Approved dose (mg)	—	150 twice a day 75 twice a day (creatinine clearance 15–30 mL/min)	20 daily 15 daily (creatinine clearance 15–50 mL/min)	5 twice a day 2.5 twice a day
Half-life (h)	40	12–17	5–12	12–15
Peak effect	4–5 d	1–6 h	2–4 h	3–4 h
Renal clearance (%)	None	80	36	27
Excluded creatinine clearance in trial (mL/min)	—	<30	<30	<25
Dialyzable	No	Yes	No	No
Reversal agent	Vitamin K	None	None	None

[a] RE-LY trial.[78]
[b] ROCKET AF trial.[80]
[c] ARISTOTLE trial.[79]

AF or for chronic around-the-clock therapy. A β-blocker or a nondihydropyridine calcium channel blocker should be given at least 30 minutes before class IC agents to prevent rapid 1:1 atrioventricular conduction during atrial flutter.[84] By blocking sodium channels, class IC drugs inhibit cardiac repolarization and prolong the QRS duration. This effect is progressive at faster heart rates. Exercise stress testing immediately after drug initiation can be performed to ensure that QRS duration remains within normal limits.

In patients who are not candidates for class IC drugs or in whom class IC drugs were ineffective, long-term rhythm control can be pursued using class III agents, which include dofetilide, dronedarone, sotalol, and amiodarone. Two studies,

SAFIRE-D (Symptomatic Atrial Fibrillation Investigative Research on Dofetilide)[85] and DIAMOND(Danish Investigation of Arrhythmia and Mortality on Dofetilide),[86] showed maintenance of sinus rhythm using dofetilide in 58% (compared with 25% with placebo) and 79% (compared with 42% with placebo) of patients at 1 year, respectively. Initiation of dofetilide requires inpatient admission for ECG monitoring, because it may prolong the QT interval. It is almost exclusively cleared by the kidneys, and renal function and corrected QT should be monitored at least every 3 months.

Dronedarone is a structural analogue of amiodarone with a more favorable side effect profile. It should not be used in patients with recently

Table 2
Outcomes for target-specific oral anticoagulants compared with warfarin in nonvalvular AF

TSOA	Major Bleeding	Myocardial Infarction	Stroke	Death
Dabigatran 110 mg[a]	0.80 (0.69–0.93) P = .003	1.35 (0.98–1.87) P = .07	0.92 (0.74–1.13) P = .41	0.91 (0.80–1.03) P = .13
Dabigatran 150 mg[a]	0.93 (0.81–1.07) P = .31	1.38 (1.00–1.91) P = .048	0.64 (0.51–0.81) P<.001	0.88 (0.77–1.00) P = .051
Rivaroxaban 20 mg[b]	1.04 (0.90–1.20) P = .58	0.81 (0.63–1.06) P = .12	0.88 (0.74–1.03) P = .12	0.92 (0.82–1.03) P = .15
Apixaban 5 mg[c]	0.68 (0.61–0.75) P<.001	0.88 (0.66–1.17) P = .37	0.79 (0.66–0.95) P = .01	0.89 (0.80–0.998) P = .047

[a] Data from RE-LY trial,[78] results reported as relative risk.
[b] Data from ROCKET AF trial,[80] results reported as hazard ratios.
[c] Data from ARISTOTLE trial,[79] results reported as hazard ratios.

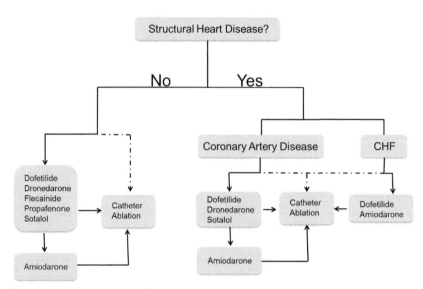

Fig. 2. Use of antiarrhythmic agents in different patient populations. Catheter ablation (*dashed line*) is recommended as a first-line therapy only in patients with paroxysmal AF. CHF, congestive heart failure. (*Data from* Fuster V, Ryden LE, Cannom DS, et al. ACC/AHA/ESC 2006 Guidelines for the Management of Patients with Atrial Fibrillation: a report of the American College of Cardiology/American Heart Association Task Force on Practice Guidelines and the European Society of Cardiology Committee for Practice Guidelines (Writing Committee to Revise the 2001 Guidelines for the Management of Patients With Atrial Fibrillation): developed in collaboration with the European Heart Rhythm Association and the Heart Rhythm Society. Circulation 2006;114:e257–354.)

decompensated heart failure with reduced ejection fraction, because of an observed increase in mortality.[87] When compared with placebo, the use of dronedarone in patients with persistent AF was associated with increased rates of heart failure, stroke, and death from cardiovascular causes. Therefore, its use has been limited to patients with paroxysmal AF.[88]

Sotalol, a β-blocker with class III properties, has been shown to have similar rates of conversion to sinus rhythm when compared with amiodarone but a lower probability of maintaining sinus rhythm.[89] In patients with ischemic heart disease, sotalol has similar efficacy for maintenance of sinus

rhythm when compared with amiodarone. Sotalol should not be used in patients with decreased left ventricular ejection fraction or with left ventricular hypertrophy (wall thickness >1.5 cm). Many experts choose to initiate sotalol therapy in the inpatient setting for ECG and QT interval monitoring.

Although amiodarone can be used in more clinical scenarios compared with the other class III agents, it also carries a significant side effect profile. Adverse effects are common, with prevalence up to 15% in the first year and as high as 50% with long-term use.[90,91] **Table 4** details the HRS recommendations for routine laboratory and diagnostic testing in patients receiving amiodarone.[92]

Table 3
Antiarrhythmic agents used for rhythm control of paroxysmal and persistent AF

Drug	Structurally Normal Heart	Coronary Artery Disease	Heart Failure with Reduced Ejection Fraction	Left Ventricular Hypertrophy
Dofetilide[a]	✔	✔	✔	
Dronedarone	✔	✔		✔
Flecainide[b]	✔			
Propafenone[b]	✔			
Sotalol[a]	✔	✔		
Amiodarone	✔	✔	✔	✔

[a] Use with caution in patients at risk for torsades de pointes.
[b] Should be used with atrioventricular nodal blocking agents.

Table 4
Recommended routine monitoring for patients receiving amiodarone

Test	Timing
Liver function tests	Baseline and every 6 mo
Thyroid function tests	Baseline and every 6 mo
Electrolytes, serum creatinine	Baseline and as indicated
Chest radiograph	Baseline and annually
Pulmonary function tests, with DLco (carbon monoxide diffusion in the lung)	Baseline and for unexplained dyspnea or new chest radiographic findings
Ophthalmologic evaluation	If visual impairment or for symptoms
ECG	Baseline and annually

Radiofrequency Ablation

Radiofrequency catheter ablation (RFA) of AF has evolved as an effective treatment modality to eliminate AF over the last decade. Although antiarrhythmic drugs are often used initially to control AF, RFA can be considered as a first-line treatment in appropriately selected patients. Two randomized controlled trials have compared RFA with antiarrhythmic therapy as first-line rhythm control for patients with paroxysmal AF. In the RAAFT-2 trial,[93] patients randomized to RFA had lower rates of recurrence of AF at 1 and 2 years compared with patients randomized to antiarrhythmic therapy. In the MANTRA-PAF trial,[94] patients randomized to RFA as first-line therapy had lower AF burden at 2 years and had significant increases in physical component of the SF-36 quality of life score. Many cases of recurrent AF after RFA occur in the first 3 to 6 months and do not necessarily exclude long-term success. Several studies have evaluated long-term outcomes after RFA and have described 47% to 56% success in maintenance of sinus rhythm at 5 years after a single RFA.[95–97]

Several observational studies have suggested that RFA may help reduce the risk of stroke in patients with AF.[98,99] In a large study of patients who underwent RFA compared with age-matched and sex-matched controls with and without AF,[100] patients with AF after RFA had a significantly lower risk of stroke compared with selected patients with AF who do not undergo RFA independent of baseline stroke risk score. However, patients

with AF who undergo RFA may represent a healthier population, as suggested by the small risk of mortality and stroke over a long follow-up period. Furthermore, it is possible that subsequent care after ablation may affect outcomes associated with AF. It is unclear whether the reduction in stroke observed in this and other observational studies is related to maintenance of sinus rhythm, anticoagulation, or other procedural and patient-related characteristics. Therefore, management of thromboembolic risk after RFA should be individualized, and clinical risk factors should be carefully considered regardless of whether RFA was performed.

REFERENCES

1. Miyasaka Y, Barnes ME, Gersh BJ, et al. Secular trends in incidence of atrial fibrillation in Olmsted County, Minnesota, 1980 to 2000, and implications on the projections for future prevalence. Circulation 2006;114:119–25.
2. Go AS, Hylek EM, Phillips KA, et al. Prevalence of diagnosed atrial fibrillation in adults: national implications for rhythm management and stroke prevention: the AnTicoagulation and Risk Factors in Atrial Fibrillation (ATRIA) study. JAMA 2001;285:2370–5.
3. Colilla S, Crow A, Petkun W, et al. Estimates of current and future incidence and prevalence of atrial fibrillation in the US adult population. Am J Cardiol 2013;112:1142–7.
4. Risk factors for stroke and efficacy of antithrombotic therapy in atrial fibrillation. Analysis of pooled data from five randomized controlled trials. Arch Intern Med 1994;154:1449–57.
5. Wolf PA, Abbott RD, Kannel WB. Atrial fibrillation as an independent risk factor for stroke: the Framingham study. Stroke 1991;22:983–8.
6. Benjamin EJ, Wolf PA, D'Agostino RB, et al. Impact of atrial fibrillation on the risk of death: the Framingham Heart Study. Circulation 1998;98:946–52.
7. Bunch TJ, Weiss JP, Crandall BG, et al. Atrial fibrillation is independently associated with senile, vascular, and Alzheimer's dementia. Heart Rhythm 2010;7:433–7.
8. Miyasaka Y, Barnes ME, Bailey KR, et al. Mortality trends in patients diagnosed with first atrial fibrillation: a 21-year community-based study. J Am Coll Cardiol 2007;49:986–92.
9. Rienstra M, Lubitz SA, Mahida S, et al. Symptoms and functional status of patients with atrial fibrillation: state of the art and future research opportunities. Circulation 2012;125:2933–43.
10. Thrall G, Lip GY, Carroll D, et al. Depression, anxiety, and quality of life in patients with atrial fibrillation. Chest 2007;132:1259–64.

11. Wang TJ, Larson MG, Levy D, et al. Temporal relations of atrial fibrillation and congestive heart failure and their joint influence on mortality: the Framingham Heart study. Circulation 2003;107:2920–5.

12. Levy S, Maarek M, Coumel P, et al. Characterization of different subsets of atrial fibrillation in general practice in France: the ALFA study. The College of French Cardiologists. Circulation 1999; 99:3028–35.

13. Verma A, Champagne J, Sapp J, et al. Discerning the incidence of symptomatic and asymptomatic episodes of atrial fibrillation before and after catheter ablation (DISCERN AF): a prospective, multicenter study. JAMA Intern Med 2013;173:149–56.

14. Magnani JW, Rienstra M, Lin H, et al. Atrial fibrillation: current knowledge and future directions in epidemiology and genomics. Circulation 2011; 124:1982–93.

15. Chung MK, Shemanski L, Sherman DG, et al. Functional status in rate- versus rhythm-control strategies for atrial fibrillation: results of the Atrial Fibrillation Follow-Up Investigation of Rhythm Management (AFFIRM) Functional Status Substudy. J Am Coll Cardiol 2005;46:1891–9.

16. Singh SN, Tang XC, Singh BN, et al. Quality of life and exercise performance in patients in sinus rhythm versus persistent atrial fibrillation: a Veterans Affairs Cooperative Studies Program Substudy. J Am Coll Cardiol 2006;48:721–30.

17. Brown AM, Sease KL, Robey JL, et al. The risk for acute coronary syndrome associated with atrial fibrillation among ED patients with chest pain syndromes. Am J Emerg Med 2007;25:523–8.

18. Goette A, Bukowska A, Dobrev D, et al. Acute atrial tachyarrhythmia induces angiotensin II type 1 receptor-mediated oxidative stress and microvascular flow abnormalities in the ventricles. Eur Heart J 2009;30:1411–20.

19. Fuster V, Ryden LE, Cannom DS, et al. ACC/AHA/ESC 2006 guidelines for the management of patients with atrial fibrillation: a report of the American College of Cardiology/American Heart Association Task Force on Practice Guidelines and the European Society of Cardiology Committee for Practice Guidelines (Writing Committee to Revise the 2001 Guidelines for the Management of Patients With Atrial Fibrillation): developed in collaboration with the European Heart Rhythm Association and the Heart Rhythm Society. Circulation 2006;114:e257–354.

20. Flaker GC, Belew K, Beckman K, et al. Asymptomatic atrial fibrillation: demographic features and prognostic information from the Atrial Fibrillation Follow-up Investigation of Rhythm Management (AFFIRM) study. Am Heart J 2005;149:657–63.

21. Kerr C, Boone J, Connolly S, et al. Follow-up of atrial fibrillation: the initial experience of the Canadian Registry of Atrial Fibrillation. Eur Heart J 1996;17(Suppl C):48–51.

22. Potpara TS, Polovina MM, Marinkovic JM, et al. A comparison of clinical characteristics and long-term prognosis in asymptomatic and symptomatic patients with first-diagnosed atrial fibrillation: the Belgrade Atrial Fibrillation study. Int J Cardiol 2013;168:4744–9.

23. Elijovich L, Josephson SA, Fung GL, et al. Intermittent atrial fibrillation may account for a large proportion of otherwise cryptogenic stroke: a study of 30-day cardiac event monitors. J Stroke Cerebrovasc Dis 2009;18:185–9.

24. Dorian P, Jung W, Newman D, et al. The impairment of health-related quality of life in patients with intermittent atrial fibrillation: implications for the assessment of investigational therapy. J Am Coll Cardiol 2000;36:1303–9.

25. Hagens VE, Ranchor AV, Van Sonderen E, et al. Effect of rate or rhythm control on quality of life in persistent atrial fibrillation. Results from the Rate Control Versus Electrical Cardioversion (RACE) study. J Am Coll Cardiol 2004;43:241–7.

26. Ware JE. User's manual for the SF-36v2™ health survey. 3rd edition.2009.

27. Ware J Jr, Kosinski M, Keller SD. A 12-item short-form health survey: construction of scales and preliminary tests of reliability and validity. Med Care 1996;34:220–33.

28. EuroQol Group. EuroQol–a new facility for the measurement of health-related quality of life. Health Policy 1990;16:199–208.

29. Rabin R, de Charro F. EQ-5D: a measure of health status from the EuroQol Group. Ann Med 2001;33:337–43.

30. Reynolds MR, Morais E, Zimetbaum P. Impact of hospitalization on health-related quality of life in atrial fibrillation patients in Canada and the United States: results from an observational registry. Am Heart J 2010;160:752–8.

31. Bubien RS, Knotts-Dolson SM, Plumb VJ, et al. Effect of radiofrequency catheter ablation on health-related quality of life and activities of daily living in patients with recurrent arrhythmias. Circulation 1996;94:1585–91.

32. Dorian P, Guerra PG, Kerr CR, et al. Validation of a new simple scale to measure symptoms in atrial fibrillation: the Canadian Cardiovascular Society Severity in Atrial Fibrillation scale. Circ Arrhythm Electrophysiol 2009;2:218–24.

33. Dorian P, Paquette M, Newman D, et al. Quality of life improves with treatment in the Canadian Trial of Atrial Fibrillation. Am Heart J 2002;143:984–90.

34. 2004 Canadian Cardiovascular Society Consensus Conference: atrial fibrillation. Can J Cardiol 2005; 21(Suppl B):9B–73B.

35. Jenkins LS, Brodsky M, Schron E, et al. Quality of life in atrial fibrillation: the Atrial Fibrillation Follow-up Investigation of Rhythm Management (AFFIRM) study. Am Heart J 2005;149:112–20.

36. Carlsson J, Miketic S, Windeler J, et al. Randomized trial of rate-control versus rhythm-control in persistent atrial fibrillation: the Strategies of Treatment of Atrial Fibrillation (STAF) study. J Am Coll Cardiol 2003;41:1690–6.

37. Gronefeld GC, Lilienthal J, Kuck KH, et al. Impact of rate versus rhythm control on quality of life in patients with persistent atrial fibrillation. Results from a prospective randomized study. Eur Heart J 2003;24:1430–6.

38. Reynolds MR, Lavelle T, Essebag V, et al. Influence of age, sex, and atrial fibrillation recurrence on quality of life outcomes in a population of patients with new-onset atrial fibrillation: the Fibrillation Registry Assessing Costs, Therapies, Adverse events and Lifestyle (FRACTAL) study. Am Heart J 2006;152:1097–103.

39. Ong L, Irvine J, Nolan R, et al. Gender differences and quality of life in atrial fibrillation: the mediating role of depression. J Psychosom Res 2006;61:769–74.

40. Ong L, Cribbie R, Harris L, et al. Psychological correlates of quality of life in atrial fibrillation. Qual Life Res 2006;15:1323–33.

41. Paquette M, Roy D, Talajic M, et al. Role of gender and personality on quality-of-life impairment in intermittent atrial fibrillation. Am J Cardiol 2000;86:764–8.

42. Dagres N, Nieuwlaat R, Vardas PE, et al. Gender-related differences in presentation, treatment, and outcome of patients with atrial fibrillation in Europe: a report from the Euro Heart Survey on Atrial Fibrillation. J Am Coll Cardiol 2007;49:572–7.

43. Howes CJ, Reid MC, Brandt C, et al. Exercise tolerance and quality of life in elderly patients with chronic atrial fibrillation. J Cardiovasc Pharmacol Ther 2001;6:23–9.

44. Benjamin EJ, Levy D, Vaziri SM, et al. Independent risk factors for atrial fibrillation in a population-based cohort. The Framingham Heart Study. JAMA 1994;271:840–4.

45. Thomas MC, Dublin S, Kaplan RC, et al. Blood pressure control and risk of incident atrial fibrillation. Am J Hypertens 2008;21:1111–6.

46. Mitchell GF, Vasan RS, Keyes MJ, et al. Pulse pressure and risk of new-onset atrial fibrillation. JAMA 2007;297:709–15.

47. Anter E, Jessup M, Callans DJ. Atrial fibrillation and heart failure: treatment considerations for a dual epidemic. Circulation 2009;119:2516–25.

48. Schmitt J, Duray G, Gersh BJ, et al. Atrial fibrillation in acute myocardial infarction: a systematic review of the incidence, clinical features and prognostic implications. Eur Heart J 2009;30:1038–45.

49. Rowe JC, Bland EF, Sprague HB, et al. The course of mitral stenosis without surgery: ten- and twenty-year perspectives. Ann Intern Med 1960;52:741–9.

50. Grigioni F, Avierinos JF, Ling LH, et al. Atrial fibrillation complicating the course of degenerative mitral regurgitation: determinants and long-term outcome. J Am Coll Cardiol 2002;40:84–92.

51. Sawin CT, Geller A, Wolf PA, et al. Low serum thyrotropin concentrations as a risk factor for atrial fibrillation in older persons. N Engl J Med 1994;331:1249–52.

52. Frost L, Vestergaard P, Mosekilde L. Hyperthyroidism and risk of atrial fibrillation or flutter: a population-based study. Arch Intern Med 2004;164:1675–8.

53. Cappola AR, Fried LP, Arnold AM, et al. Thyroid status, cardiovascular risk, and mortality in older adults. JAMA 2006;295:1033–41.

54. Heeringa J, Hoogendoorn EH, van der Deure WM, et al. High-normal thyroid function and risk of atrial fibrillation: the Rotterdam study. Arch Intern Med 2008;168:2219–24.

55. Kim EJ, Lyass A, Wang N, et al. Relation of hypothyroidism and incident atrial fibrillation (from the Framingham Heart Study). Am Heart J 2014;167:123–6.

56. Watanabe H, Tanabe N, Watanabe T, et al. Metabolic syndrome and risk of development of atrial fibrillation: the Niigata preventive medicine study. Circulation 2008;117:1255–60.

57. Wang TJ, Parise H, Levy D, et al. Obesity and the risk of new-onset atrial fibrillation. JAMA 2004;292:2471–7.

58. Gami AS, Hodge DO, Herges RM, et al. Obstructive sleep apnea, obesity, and the risk of incident atrial fibrillation. J Am Coll Cardiol 2007;49:565–71.

59. Gami AS, Pressman G, Caples SM, et al. Association of atrial fibrillation and obstructive sleep apnea. Circulation 2004;110:364–7.

60. Buch P, Friberg J, Scharling H, et al. Reduced lung function and risk of atrial fibrillation in the Copenhagen City Heart study. Eur Respir J 2003;21:1012–6.

61. Kodama S, Saito K, Tanaka S, et al. Alcohol consumption and risk of atrial fibrillation: a meta-analysis. J Am Coll Cardiol 2011;57:427–36.

62. Mukamal KJ, Tolstrup JS, Friberg J, et al. Alcohol consumption and risk of atrial fibrillation in men and women: the Copenhagen City Heart Study. Circulation 2005;112:1736–42.

63. Iwasaki YK, Nishida K, Kato T, et al. Atrial fibrillation pathophysiology: implications for management. Circulation 2011;124:2264–74.

64. van der Hooft CS, Heeringa J, van Herpen G, et al. Drug-induced atrial fibrillation. J Am Coll Cardiol 2004;44:2117–24.

65. Glatter KA, Cheng J, Dorostkar P, et al. Electrophysiologic effects of adenosine in patients with

supraventricular tachycardia. Circulation 1999;99: 1034–40.

66. Kaakeh Y, Overholser BR, Lopshire JC, et al. Drug-induced atrial fibrillation. Drugs 2012;72: 1617–30.

67. Caldentey G, Khairy P, Roy D, et al. Prognostic value of the physical examination in patients with heart failure and atrial fibrillation: insights from the AF-CHF Trial (Atrial Fibrillation and Chronic Heart Failure). JACC Heart Fail 2014;2:15–23.

68. Oral H, Morady F. How to select patients for atrial fibrillation ablation. Heart Rhythm 2006;3:615–8.

69. Jenkins C, Bricknell K, Marwick TH. Use of real-time three-dimensional echocardiography to measure left atrial volume: comparison with other echocardiographic techniques. J Am Soc Echocardiogr 2005;18:991–7.

70. Oakes RS, Badger TJ, Kholmovski EG, et al. Detection and quantification of left atrial structural remodeling with delayed-enhancement magnetic resonance imaging in patients with atrial fibrillation. Circulation 2009;119:1758–67.

71. Gladstone DJ, Spring M, Dorian P, et al. Atrial fibrillation in patients with cryptogenic stroke. N Engl J Med 2014;370:2467–77.

72. Sanna T, Diener HC, Passman RS, et al. Cryptogenic stroke and underlying atrial fibrillation. N Engl J Med 2014;370:2478–86.

73. Gage BF, Waterman AD, Shannon W, et al. Validation of clinical classification schemes for predicting stroke: results from the National Registry of Atrial Fibrillation. JAMA 2001;285:2864–70.

74. European Heart Rhythm Association, European Association for Cardio-Thoracic Surgery, Camm AJ, et al. Guidelines for the management of atrial fibrillation: the Task Force for the Management of Atrial Fibrillation of the European Society of Cardiology (ESC). Europace 2010;12:1360–420.

75. January CT, Wann LS, Alpert JS, et al. 2014 AHA/ACC/HRS guideline for the management of patients with atrial fibrillation: a report of the American College of Cardiology/American Heart Association Task Force on Practice Guidelines and the Heart Rhythm Society. J Am Coll Cardiol 2014. [Epub ahead of print].

76. Matchar DB, Jacobson A, Dolor R, et al. Effect of home testing of international normalized ratio on clinical events. N Engl J Med 2010;363:1608–20.

77. Connolly SJ, Ezekowitz MD, Yusuf S, et al. Dabigatran versus warfarin in patients with atrial fibrillation. N Engl J Med 2009;361:1139–51.

78. Granger CB, Alexander JH, McMurray JJ, et al. Apixaban versus warfarin in patients with atrial fibrillation. N Engl J Med 2011;365:981–92.

79. Patel MR, Mahaffey KW, Garg J, et al. Rivaroxaban versus warfarin in nonvalvular atrial fibrillation. N Engl J Med 2011;365:883–91.

80. Wyse DG, Waldo AL, DiMarco JP, et al. A comparison of rate control and rhythm control in patients with atrial fibrillation. N Engl J Med 2002;347:1825–33.

81. Van Gelder IC, Hagens VE, Bosker HA, et al. A comparison of rate control and rhythm control in patients with recurrent persistent atrial fibrillation. N Engl J Med 2002;347:1834–40.

82. Capucci A, Villani GQ, Aschieri D, et al. Oral amiodarone increases the efficacy of direct-current cardioversion in restoration of sinus rhythm in patients with chronic atrial fibrillation. Eur Heart J 2000;21: 66–73.

83. Oral H, Souza JJ, Michaud GF, et al. Facilitating transthoracic cardioversion of atrial fibrillation with ibutilide pretreatment. N Engl J Med 1999;340: 1849–54.

84. Alboni P, Botto GL, Baldi N, et al. Outpatient treatment of recent-onset atrial fibrillation with the "pill-in-the-pocket" approach. N Engl J Med 2004;351: 2384–91.

85. Singh S, Zoble RG, Yellen L, et al. Efficacy and safety of oral dofetilide in converting to and maintaining sinus rhythm in patients with chronic atrial fibrillation or atrial flutter: the Symptomatic Atrial Fibrillation Investigative Research on Dofetilide (SAFIRE-D) study. Circulation 2000;102:2385–90.

86. Pedersen OD, Bagger H, Keller N, et al. Efficacy of dofetilide in the treatment of atrial fibrillation-flutter in patients with reduced left ventricular function: a Danish Investigation of Arrhythmia and Mortality on Dofetilide (DIAMOND) substudy. Circulation 2001;104:292–6.

87. Kober L, Torp-Pedersen C, McMurray JJ, et al. Increased mortality after dronedarone therapy for severe heart failure. N Engl J Med 2008;358: 2678–87.

88. Connolly SJ, Camm AJ, Halperin JL, et al. Dronedarone in high-risk permanent atrial fibrillation. N Engl J Med 2011;365:2268–76.

89. Singh BN, Singh SN, Reda DJ, et al. Amiodarone versus sotalol for atrial fibrillation. N Engl J Med 2005;352:1861–72.

90. Jafari-Fesharaki M, Scheinman MM. Adverse effects of amiodarone. Pacing Clin Electrophysiol 1998;21:108–20.

91. Mason JW. Amiodarone. N Engl J Med 1987;316: 455–66.

92. Goldschlager N, Epstein AE, Naccarelli G, et al. Practical guidelines for clinicians who treat patients with amiodarone. Practice Guidelines Subcommittee, North American Society of Pacing and Electrophysiology. Arch Intern Med 2000; 160:1741–8.

93. Morillo CA, Verma A, Connolly SJ, et al. Radiofrequency ablation vs antiarrhythmic drugs as first-line treatment of paroxysmal atrial fibrillation

(RAAFT-2): a randomized trial. JAMA 2014;311: 692–700.

94. Cosedis Nielsen J, Johannessen A, Raatikainen P, et al. Radiofrequency ablation as initial therapy in paroxysmal atrial fibrillation. N Engl J Med 2012; 367:1587–95.

95. Sawhney N, Anousheh R, Chen WC, et al. Five-year outcomes after segmental pulmonary vein isolation for paroxysmal atrial fibrillation. Am J Cardiol 2009; 104:366–72.

96. Ouyang F, Tilz R, Chun J, et al. Long-term results of catheter ablation in paroxysmal atrial fibrillation: lessons from a 5-year follow-up. Circulation 2010; 122:2368–77.

97. Medi C, Sparks PB, Morton JB, et al. Pulmonary vein antral isolation for paroxysmal atrial fibrillation: results from long-term follow-up. J Cardiovasc Electrophysiol 2011;22:137–41.

98. Oral H, Chugh A, Ozaydin M, et al. Risk of thromboembolic events after percutaneous left atrial radiofrequency ablation of atrial fibrillation. Circulation 2006;114:759–65.

99. Bunch TJ, Crandall BG, Weiss JP, et al. Patients treated with catheter ablation for atrial fibrillation have long-term rates of death, stroke, and dementia similar to patients without atrial fibrillation. J Cardiovasc Electrophysiol 2011;22:839–45.

100. Bunch TJ, May HT, Bair TL, et al. Atrial fibrillation ablation patients have long-term stroke rates similar to patients without atrial fibrillation regardless of CHADS2 score. Heart Rhythm 2013;10(9): 1272–7.

Rate Versus Rhythm Control for Atrial Fibrillation

Colby Halsey, MD, Aman Chugh, MD*

KEYWORDS

• Rate • Rhythm • Atrial fibrillation • Heart

KEY POINTS

• Treatment of patients with symptomatic atrial fibrillation (AF) with antiarrhythmic drug therapy in general improves their symptom scores and exercise tolerance; however, large randomized trials have failed to show a mortality benefit with a rhythm-control compared with a rate-control strategy.
• Catheter ablation in patients who have failed or not tolerated medical therapy has been shown to alleviate symptoms and improve quality of life.
• At experienced centers, the risk of a serious procedure-related complication should be low.
• Patients should be alerted to modifiable factors that may decrease the likelihood of unchecked structural remodeling and AF recurrence, such as obesity, sleep apnea, and hypertension.
• Given the increasing incidence of AF, upstream therapies that might prevent AF are urgently needed.

Atrial fibrillation (AF) is a progressive disease that continues to inflict a heavy burden on health care systems and patients. AF portends an increased all-cause mortality, long-term stroke risk, heart failure, and impaired quality of life (QoL).[1–4] Goals of treatment include symptom alleviation, stroke prevention, and identifying modifiable factors that may be contributing to the fibrillatory process, such as obesity, hypertension, and sleep apnea. Medical treatment intended to improve symptoms referable to AF includes rate-controlling medications (rate-control strategy), and antiarrhythmic drugs (AADs) (rhythm-control strategy). Nonpharmacologic options include atrioventricular (AV) junction ablation/permanent pacemaker implantation and catheter ablation to maintain sinus rhythm, respectively. This article reviews the evidence base for the rate-control and rhythm-control strategies and proposes a practical approach in managing patients with AF.

DRUG THERAPY FOR MAINTENANCE OF SINUS RHYTHM

Before discussing trials that have compared rhythm-control and rate-control strategies, a review of the evidence base of each is worthwhile. In the Canadian Trial of Atrial Fibrillation, patients with symptomatic paroxysmal or persistent AF were randomized to amiodarone, sotalol, or propafenone.[1] Rhythm status was ascertained with an electrocardiogram at 3 months, and then every 6 months thereafter. After a mean follow-up of 16 months, 35% of patients who were assigned to amiodarone and 63% of those to either sotalol or propafenone experienced recurrent AF

This article originally appeared in Cardiology Clinics, Volume 32, Issue 4, November 2014.
Supported in part by a grant from the Leducq Transatlantic Network.
Conflict of interest: None.
Section of Cardiac Electrophysiology, Division of Cardiology, Cardiovascular Center, University of Michigan Hospitals, 1500 East Medical Center Drive, SPC 5853, Ann Arbor, MI 48109-5853, USA
* Corresponding author.
E-mail address: achugh@med.umich.edu

Heart Failure Clin 12 (2016) 193–203
http://dx.doi.org/10.1016/j.hfc.2015.08.016
1551-7136/16/$ – see front matter © 2016 Elsevier Inc. All rights reserved.

(P<.001). Drug discontinuation because of adverse effects was noted in 18% of patients randomized to amiodarone versus 11% of those to either sotalol or propafenone (P = .06). In the Sotalol Amiodarone Atrial Fibrillation Efficacy Trial (SAFE-T), patients with persistent AF were randomized to amiodarone, sotalol, or placebo.[2] Rhythm status was assessed with weekly transtelephonic monitoring. The median times to recurrence were 487, 74, and 6 days, respectively. The recurrence rates at 1 year were 48%, 68%, and 87%, respectively. Maintenance of sinus rhythm was associated with an improved QoL and exercise tolerance. Although amiodarone has been shown to be superior in other trials, a high dose of the drug (300 mg per day for the first year after a loading dose) was used in the SAFE-T study. Both study drugs were well tolerated.

Even though amiodarone is probably the most effective antiarrhythmic medication available, its effect is still modest. Further, its potential for end-organ toxicity is also limiting. Class IC agents such as propafenone and flecainide are best avoided in patients with structural disease, such as prior myocardial infarction, heart failure, and significant left ventricular hypertrophy. Given these limitations of both amiodarone and class I drugs, other agents have been introduced that could safely be used in patients with heart disease. The efficacy of dofetilide, a class III antiarrhythmic medication that blocks the delayed rectifier potassium channels (IK$_r$) channel, was tested in more than 1500 patients with systolic heart failure in the Danish Investigations of Arrhythmia and Mortality on Dofetilide Study Group.[3] The investigators noted a lower incidence of AF and hospitalizations in the group randomized to dofetilide. There was no difference in mortality between the dofetilide and placebo groups. However, torsades de pointes was observed in 3.3% of patients randomized to drug therapy. A substudy later revealed that, in a subgroup of 506 patients with atrial arrhythmias at baseline, those randomized to dofetilide were more likely to maintain sinus rhythm at 1 year compared with those randomized to placebo (79% vs 42%; P<.001).[4] There was no effect on mortality but survival was enhanced in those who maintained sinus rhythm.

A major limitation of dofetilide is that it requires in-hospital initiation because it prolongs ventricular repolarization and may cause torsades de pointes. Dose reduction is often required because of QT prolongation (Fig. 1). The potential for drug-drug interaction (eg, with various antibiotics, thiazide diuretics, and verapamil) is also limiting.

Despite its superior efficacy compared with other antiarrhythmics, amiodarone is rarely used as a first-line agent because of the concern of end-organ toxicity. The adverse effects are thought to be related to its iodine content. And thus dronedarone, which is devoid of the iodine moiety, was introduced in hopes of maintaining the efficacy of amiodarone but without its adverse effects on the lungs, liver, and thyroid. In a multicenter clinical trial, 1237 patients with paroxysmal or persistent (after cardioversion) AF

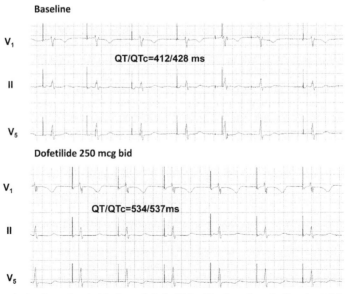

Fig. 1. Prolonged repolarization after initiation of dofetilide. The baseline rhythm is atrial pacing with intrinsic AV nodal conduction. Owing to prolongation of the QT interval and ventricular ectopy (not shown), dofetilide was discontinued and the patient underwent catheter ablation of persistent AF. BID, twice a day.

were randomized in a 2:1 fashion to dronedarone (400 mg twice a day) or placebo. Exclusion criteria included permanent AF, history of bradycardia or torsades de pointes, advanced AV block, severe congestive heart failure (CHF), and renal dysfunction (creatinine>1.7 mg/dL).[5] The median times to AF recurrence were 116 days in the dronedarone group and 53 days in the placebo group (P<.05). At 12 months, AF recurred in 64% of the patients in the dronedarone group and in 75% in the placebo group (P<.001). Although there was some prolongation of the QT interval in the dronedarone group, there were no episodes of torsades de pointes. Further, no evidence of end-organ toxicity related to dronedarone was found.

The ANDROMEDA (Antiarrhythmic Trial with Dronedarone in Moderate to Severe CHF Evaluating Morbidity Decrease) study evaluated the use of dronedarone in patients with systolic left ventricular dysfunction and class III or IV heart failure symptoms. The trial was prematurely terminated because of increased mortality and worsening heart failure in patients randomized to dronedarone.[6] As a result, the package insert now includes a black box warning stating that dronedarone is contraindicated in patients with class IV heart failure symptoms, or in those with class II or III with a recent decompensation. The ATHENA (A Placebo-Controlled, Double-Blind, Parallel Arm Trial to Assess the Efficacy of Dronedarone for the Prevention of Cardiovascular Hospitalization or Death from Any Cause) trial[7] evaluated dronedarone in patients with atrial arrhythmias but without class IV heart failure symptoms. The investigators reported that dronedarone reduced the occurrence of the composite end point of cardiovascular hospitalization or death. The PALLAS (Permanent Atrial Fibrillation Outcome Study Using Dronedarone on Top of Standard Therapy) trial was designed to determine whether dronedarone decreases cardiovascular outcomes in patients with permanent AF. However, the trial was stopped early based on an increased incidence of heart failure, stroke, and death in the study group.[8] A history of permanent AF was also added to a list of contraindications to the drug. Postmarketing experience has revealed rare instances of acute liver injury requiring transplantation attributable to dronedarone. In addition, dronedarone was inferior to amiodarone in suppressing AF.[9]

RATE CONTROL IN AF

Treatment options in controlling the ventricular rate during AF include digoxin, β-blockers, and calcium blockers. Less commonly, amiodarone and dronedarone may be used. In patients in whom the ventricular rate cannot be controlled and in whom sinus rhythm cannot be maintained, AV junction ablation is a reasonable option; this is performed concomitantly with implantation of a permanent pacemaker. This approach is associated with an improvement in QoL, exercise performance, and left ventricular performance.[10] However, in some patients left ventricular function may be worsened by asynchronous right ventricular pacing, an effect that may be ameliorated by addition of a left ventricular lead. AF going unchecked and pacemaker dependence are disadvantages of AV junction ablation.

RATE VERSUS RHYTHM CONTROL

As discussed earlier, both rate-control and rhythm-control interventions have been shown to improve QoL and exercise performance in patients with AF. However, it remained unclear whether one strategy was superior to the other in terms of these parameters and of hard end points such as stroke, heart failure, and death. In 2000, Hohnloser and colleagues[11] published the Pharmacological Intervention in Atrial Fibrillation (PIAF) trial, which randomized 252 patients with symptomatic, persistent AF to rate control with diltiazem versus rhythm control with amiodarone. At the end of the observation period, sinus rhythm was documented in 56% of patients in the amiodarone group versus in 10% in the diltiazem group (P<.001). After a mean follow-up of 12 months, there was no significant difference in the primary end point of QoL. However, exercise performance was improved in the amiodarone group. The investigators also reported a higher rate of hospitalization in the amiodarone group (69% vs 24%). Most of the hospitalizations in the amiodarone group were related to patients requiring electrical cardioversion. The multicenter Strategies of Treatment of Atrial Fibrillation (STAF) trial randomized 200 patients with persistent AF to rate versus rhythm control, allowing for up to 4 cardioversions in the latter.[12] At 36 months, sinus rhythm was maintained in only 23% of patients randomized to rhythm control versus 0% in the rate-control groups. No significant difference was found in the combined primary end point of death, cardiopulmonary resuscitation, cerebrovascular events, and systemic embolism. Again, a higher rate of hospitalizations was observed in patients randomized to rhythm control (P<.001). Of the 19 primary end points that occurred during the study period, 18 occurred during AF and only 1 during sinus rhythm (P = .049). The investigators speculated that improved outcomes would have been observed in the rhythm-control group if sinus rhythm could have been maintained in a higher proportion of patients.

Thereafter, larger studies were conducted that were powered to address the issue of mortality and other hard end points. In 2002, the Atrial Fibrillation Follow-up Investigation of Rhythm Management (AFFIRM) trial, sponsored by the National Heart, Lung and Blood Institute, was published.[13] More than 4000 patients (mean age, 70 years) were randomized to rate versus rhythm control (using AADs and cardioversion) and were followed for a mean of 3.5 years. The prevalence of sinus rhythm in the rhythm-control group was 63% at 5 years. However, rhythm status was assessed only by periodic electrocardiograms in the office setting and long-term ambulatory monitoring was not performed. Mortality rates were 21% versus 24% in the rate-control and rhythm-control groups, respectively (hazard ratio [HR], 1.15; 95% confidence interval, 0.99–1.34; $P = .08$). High crossover rates (15% vs 37.5% in the rate vs rhythm cohorts, respectively) were observed. In addition, QoL was similar in both groups throughout the study. Given the inherent problem using an intention-to-treat analysis in the setting of high crossover rates, the AFFIRM investigators published a follow-up article reporting the on-treatment analysis.[14] In this analysis, the presence of sinus rhythm was associated with a significantly lower risk of death (HR, 0.53). Warfarin use was also associated with decreased mortality. Furthermore, AADs were associated with increased mortality when adjusted for the presence of sinus rhythm, which led the investigators to conclude that, "if an effective therapy for maintenance of sinus rhythm with fewer adverse effects were available, it might be beneficial."[14] Another substudy suggested that AAD use in the AFFIRM study may have been associated with a higher incidence of pulmonary and cancer-related deaths.[15]

In the same issue of the New England Journal of Medicine in which the AFFIRM study was published, the Rate Control versus Electrical Cardioversion (RACE) study also appeared.[16] The investigators randomized 522 patients with persistent recurrent AF (following an initial cardioversion) to rate-control versus rhythm-control strategies. The primary composite end point consisted of death from cardiovascular causes, heart failure, thromboembolic complications, bleeding, implantation of a pacemaker, and severe adverse effects of drugs. After a mean of 2.3 ± 0.6 years of follow-up, sinus rhythm was noted in 39% of the 266 patients in the rhythm-control group, compared with 10% of the 256 patients in the rate-control group. The primary end point occurred in 17% of the patients in the rate-control group and 23% in the rhythm-control group. Thromboembolism was more frequent in the rhythm-control group. Six patients, all in the rhythm-control group, had thromboembolic complications after discontinuation of oral anticoagulant therapy, 5 of whom were in sinus rhythm.

Longitudinal studies have suggested that AF is associated with CHF among other adverse outcomes. The Atrial Fibrillation and Congestive Heart Failure (AF-CHF) study tested the hypothesis that a rhythm-control strategy in patients with heart failure may be associated with improved outcomes.[17] Nearly 1400 patients with left ventricular ejection fraction less than 35%, heart failure, and AF (persistent in more than two-thirds of the patients) were randomized to rhythm-control therapy (primarily with amiodarone) and rate-control therapy. The prevalence of AF in the rhythm-control group, as documented on electrocardiography, was 27% after 4 years of follow-up. However, 58% of patients in the study group experienced AF at some point during the study duration. The prevalence of AF in the rate-control group ranged from 59% to 70% during follow-up. The primary outcome was cardiovascular death, which occurred in 27% of patients randomized to a rhythm-control strategy versus 25% randomized to the rate-control strategy ($P = .59$). As expected, the rate of hospitalizations was higher in the former. The investigators concluded that a rate-control strategy should be pursued in patients with AF and heart failure.

Several large, well-conducted clinical trials failed to show that a sinus rhythm strategy is superior to a rate-control strategy. The former was associated with a trend toward worse outcomes. However, there are several caveats that should be noted. First, most patients (58%) in the AF-CHF trial, for example, who were randomized to a rhythm-control strategy experienced AF at some point during the study period. Also, about 30% to 40% of patients in the rate-control arm were in sinus rhythm during follow-up. Consistent with the results of the AFFIRM study,[13] the absolute difference in the rhythm status between the rhythm-control and rate-control groups was only about 40%. It is thus difficult to argue that a sinus rhythm confers no advantage because sinus rhythm could not consistently be achieved in most cases. Second, the benefits of sinus rhythm may have been neutralized by the harmful effects of AADs. Treatment of AF has been plagued by drug inefficacy, intolerance, and proarrhythmia. Even the newest AAD (ie, dronedarone) has failed to meet expectations, not only in terms of adverse effects but also efficacy. In addition, oral anticoagulation was often discontinued a few weeks after transthoracic cardioversion in these trials. Because AF often recurs despite antiarrhythmic treatment, some patients had thromboembolic complications in the absence of oral anticoagulation, which may have also contributed to adverse outcomes in the rhythm-control arm.

Neither strategy can help reverse the structural remodeling that contributed to development of AF. The cause of these structural abnormalities, which are present even in patients with normal hearts,[18] often cannot be identified. In this sense, AF may merely be a marker, as opposed to the cause, of adverse outcomes. If so, trying to correct the rhythm, in contradistinction to the underlying abnormal atrial substrate, may not yield the desired results.

CATHETER ABLATION VERSUS AAD'S

As the AFFIRM investigators speculated, if sinus rhythm could be achieved reliably and safely, it may be worthwhile. Catheter ablation may fill this void. First described in the late 1990s, catheter ablation of AF has the potential to eliminate AF in most patients with drug-refractory, symptomatic AF. Several trials have been conducted in a variety of settings comparing AAD therapy and catheter ablation. Many of the trials were conducted at a single center and hence are limited by a small sample size. The first such trial was published in 2005 by Wazni and colleagues.[19] Thirty-three and 37 patients were randomized to catheter ablation and AAD therapy, respectively. Most of the patients had paroxysmal as opposed to persistent AF. The ablation protocol consisted of pulmonary vein (PV) isolation (**Figs. 2** and **3**) and the primary end point was symptomatic AF as documented on an event monitor. After 1 year of follow-up, 87% of patients randomized to catheter ablation remained free from symptomatic AF compared with only 37% of patients who received medical therapy (P<.001). Asymptomatic PV stenosis was noted in 2 patients in the ablation arm and there were no other severe complications. Improvement in symptom scores was also noted in the ablation group.

Another randomized study was conducted by Pappone and colleagues[20] in patients with paroxysmal AF. A total of 198 patients were randomized to circumferential PV ablation (CPVA; circular lesions around each PV antrum connected by linear ablation at the posterior LA, and linear ablation at the mitral isthmus, guided by voltage abatement) and medical therapy with antiarrhythmic medications. After 1 year of follow-up, 93% of patients randomized to catheter ablation remained

arrhythmia free compared with 35% of patients in the medical arm. Two complications were noted in the ablation group: one patient with a transient ischemic attack, and another with a small pericardial effusion not requiring drainage. Adverse effects leading to the discontinuation of AADs occurred in nearly 25% of the patients randomized to medical treatment.

Earlier studies comparing catheter ablation and medical therapy primarily included patients with paroxysmal AF. A study published by Oral and colleagues[21] evaluated the impact of catheter ablation, performed at an Italian and American center, in patients with persistent AF. A total of 146 patients were randomized to amiodarone plus 2 cardioversions within the first 3 months alone (control group) or in combination with CPVA (circular lesions around the pulmonary veins, plus linear lesions in the left atrium). Patients were asked to wear an event monitor for at least 5 days of the week for 12 months, and the tracings were interpreted in a blinded fashion. Approximately one-third of the patients in the ablation arm required a repeat procedure for AF or atypical flutter. After 12 months of follow-up, 74% of the patients randomized to CPVA remained in sinus rhythm compared with only 4% of patients in the control group (P<.001). A decrease in the left atrial dimensions and symptom scores were also noted. There were no serious complications.

In the Catheter Ablation Versus Antiarrhythmic Drugs for Atrial Fibrillation (4A) study, investigators randomized 112 patients with paroxysmal AF to either PV isolation (additional ablation allowed at the discretion of the physician) or AAD therapy.[22] After the 12-month follow-up period, catheter ablation was superior to medical therapy in maintaining sinus rhythm (89% vs 23%, respectively; P<.0001). Exercise capacity and QoL were also significantly better in the ablation group. Of the 155 procedures required, 3 severe complications occurred: 2 episodes of cardiac tamponade and 1 case of PV stenosis.

The ThermoCool AF multicenter trial randomized 167 patients with paroxysmal AF in a 2:1 fashion (106 to the ablation arm and 61 to AAD therapy). Similar to the 4A study, PV isolation was required in all patients having ablation and additional ablation was allowed at the discretion of the physician. At the end of the 9-month follow-up, 66% of patients in the ablation group were arrhythmia free compared with only 16% in the AAD group. QoL measures were also higher in the ablation group. The event rates in the ablation and medical arms were 5% (5 of 103) and 9% (5 of 57), respectively.

These randomized studies consistently showed the superiority of catheter ablation versus medical therapy in patients with both paroxysmal and

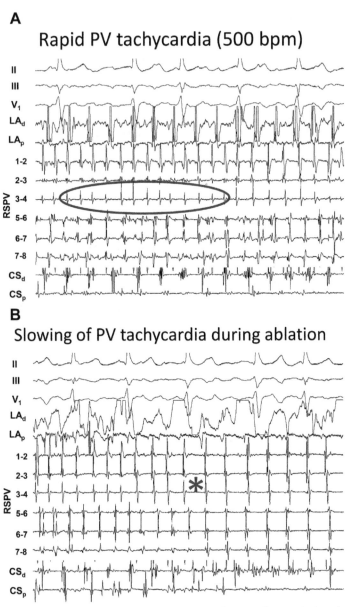

A

Rapid PV tachycardia (500 bpm)

B

Slowing of PV tachycardia during ablation

Fig. 2. (*A*) Rapid PV tachycardia (*red oval*), with a cycle length of 120 milliseconds (500 beats/min) emanating from the right superior PV. See next part. (*B*) With antral ablation around the right-sided PVs, the PV tachycardia is slowed (*asterisk*). See next part. (*C*) With further ablation around the right PV antrum, AF slows further and terminates to normal sinus rhythm (NSR), confirming the mechanistic importance of the PVs in maintaining AF. However, note that the PV is still connected (*black arrow*). See next part. (*D*) A gap was found at the anterior aspect of the circular lesion, where radiofrequency ablation finally eliminates the remaining connection, resulting in PV isolation.

persistent AF (**Table 1**). The risk of serious complications was low. In addition, patients randomized to catheter ablation also had better QoL. As such, catheter ablation in patients with paroxysmal AF who have not responded to AADs[23] is a class I indication.

CATHETER ABLATION AS FIRST-LINE TREATMENT

The early studies comparing catheter ablation with medical therapy recruited patients who had failed treatment with AADs. More recent studies sought

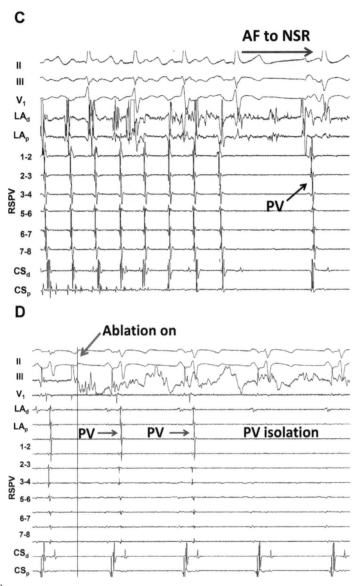

Fig. 2. (*continued*)

to determine whether catheter ablation is superior to medical therapy in AAD-naive patients. The Medical Antiarrhythmic Treatment or Radiofrequency Ablation in Paroxysmal Atrial Fibrillation (MANTRA-PAF) trial (N = 294) assessed catheter ablation as first-line treatment in patients with paroxysmal AF.[24] The ablation protocol involved creation of circular lesions around ipsilateral PVs but did not require documentation of PV isolation. Linear ablation at the roof was also performed. Linear ablations at the mitral and tricuspid isthmi were optional. The primary end points were cumulative and per-visit AF burden as determined via Holter monitoring. Overall, there was no significant difference in the primary end point of cumulative

AF burden (90th percentile of arrhythmia burden, 13% and 19%, respectively; P = .10). At 24 months, AF burden was lower in the ablation group than in the medical group (90th percentile, 9% vs 18%; P = .007), and more patients in the ablation group remained free from AF (85% vs 71%; P = .004). In addition, the physical component, but not the mental component, of the QoL measures was significantly improved in the ablation arm. The total number of adverse events did not differ between the groups (20 patients vs 16 patients; P = .45) but 1 death occurred in the ablation group as a result of a procedure-related cerebral stroke. Cardiac tamponade occurred in 3 patients as a consequence of the ablation procedure.

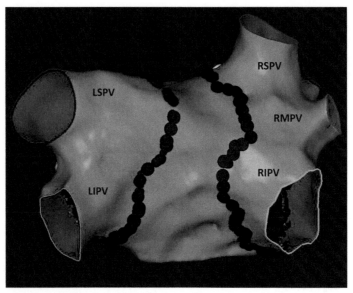

Fig. 3. Three-dimensional map of the posterior left atrium showing the lesion set required for PV isolation. Red tags denote sites at which radiofrequency energy was delivered. LIPV, left inferior PV; LSPV, left superior PV; RIPV, right inferior PV; RMPV, right middle PV; RSPV, right superior PV.

The Radiofrequency Ablation versus Antiarrhythmic Drugs as First-line Treatment of Paroxysmal Atrial Fibrillation (RAAFT-2) investigators randomized 127 drug-naive patients in European and North American centers to radiofrequency ablation versus AADs. In contradistinction to the MANTRA-PAF study, PV isolation was required in all patients having ablation; ablation outside the PVs was performed in about 20% of patients at the discretion of the operator. PV isolation was achieved in 87% of patients and a repeat procedure was performed in 10 patients (15%). Arrhythmia recurrence was noted in 72% of

patients in the AAD group compared with 55% in the ablation group (HR, 0.56; 95% confidence interval, 0.35–0.90; $P = .02$). Similarly, QoL measures were significantly better in the ablation group. Six patients (9%) in the ablation arm experienced complications, including 4 with cardiac tamponade (n = 4), compared with 3 patients (5%) in the AAD group.

Taken together, the trials comparing catheter ablation with drug therapy in AAD-naive patients show either a lack of benefit or a modest reduction in AF recurrence. Also, the risk of serious complications such as perforation/tamponade and stroke

Table 1
Trials comparing ablation and medical therapy for AF

Author, Year	Patients (N)	% Paroxysmal	% Persistent	% Success with AAD	% Success with RFA
Wazni et al,[19] 2005	70	97	3	37	87
Oral et al,[21] 2006	146	0	100	58	74
Jaïs et al,[22] 2008	112	100	0	23	89
Wilber et al,[34] 2010	167	100	0	16	66
Cosedis Nielsen et al,[24] 2012	294	100	0	71	85
Morillo et al,[35] 2014	127	100	0	28	45
Total # of patients	916	468	148	—	—
Average (%)	—	—	—	39	74

Abbreviation: RFA, radiofrequency ablation.
  Data from Refs.[19,21,22,24,34,35]

should be considered. Thus, it is reasonable to consider AADs as part of the initial strategy in the management of patients with symptomatic, paroxysmal AF. The periprocedural risk should also be weighed against the prospect of lifelong treatment with antiarrhythmic medications, especially in young patients. This concern was reflected in the updated AF consensus document. The writing committee concluded that catheter ablation before a trial of medical therapy was reasonable in patients with paroxysmal AF (class IIa indication) provided that it can be performed by an experienced operator.[23]

CATHETER ABLATION OF AF

Despite significant advances in both the understanding of the AF mechanisms and the outcomes of catheter ablation, many challenges remain. At present, paroxysmal AF may be eliminated in about 90% of patients with a low risk of serious complications (1–2%). However, the procedure still involves point-by-point ablation, making for a lengthy and sometimes challenging procedure. Cryoablation offers some advantages, such as that the circumference of the PV may be ablated in a single application, but it is unknown whether long-term outcomes are superior to those of radiofrequency ablation.[25] Multipolar ablation catheters are being investigated to determine their efficacy and safety in patients with both paroxysmal and persistent AF. Another major limitation is the frequency of PV reconnection, which results in the necessity of repeat procedures in about one-third of patients with paroxysmal AF. The PV reconnection rate may be improved by the use of contact force technology. There is also a concern of late attrition over long-term follow-up (>5 years), which may be caused by lack of permanent PV isolation or ongoing remodeling, or both.

Although there is consensus as to the ablation target in patients with paroxysmal AF, the optimal strategy in patients with persistent AF remains elusive. Several approaches have been examined, including PV isolation, ablation of complex/fractionated electrograms, and linear ablation. A PV-only approach is associated with roughly a 40% success rate at best, even with repeat procedures.[26,27] It is reasonable to pursue a more aggressive strategy (ie, more than just PV isolation) in patients with persistent AF given the more extensive atrial remodeling in such patients.[28] When an extensive ablation approach is undertaken in patients with persistent AF, the success may approach 80% to 85%.[29,30] However, these procedures may be lengthy (5 hours or so) and patients frequently require a repeat procedure (about

50%) either for AF or for more organized arrhythmias. The procedure for persistent AF is complex because sources may reside anywhere in the left or even the right atrium. In patients with paroxysmal AF, the target sites (ie, the PVs) may be ablated even during sinus rhythm. Because sources differ from patient to patient in persistent AF and mapping can only be performed during AF, the procedure for persistent AF is much more time consuming. Preliminary studies suggest that AF sources may be localized by sophisticated mapping techniques and that the amount of radiofrequency ablation required may be less than with conventional techniques.[31,32]

SUMMARY

Treatment of patients with symptomatic AF with AAD therapy in general improves their symptom scores and exercise tolerance. However, large randomized trials have failed to show a mortality benefit with a rhythm-control compared with a rate-control strategy. These studies have been marred by modest efficacy of AADs, drug intolerance, and possible adverse effects of medical therapy, which may have neutralized the possible benefits of sinus rhythm. Catheter ablation in patients who have failed or not tolerated medical therapy has been shown to alleviate symptoms and improve QoL.[33] At experienced centers, the risk of a serious procedure-related complication should be low. However, catheter ablation cannot undo the structural remodeling that contributed to the arrhythmia in the first place. Thus, concomitantly with ablation, patients should be alerted to modifiable factors that may decrease the likelihood of unchecked structural remodeling and AF recurrence, such as obesity, sleep apnea, and hypertension. It is also unknown whether AF elimination by catheter ablation improves outcomes such as heart failure, stroke, and death. The ongoing CABANA (Catheter Ablation Versus Antiarrhythmic Drug Therapy for Atrial Fibrillation) trial and others were designed to help answer these important questions. Given the increasing incidence of AF, upstream therapies that might prevent AF are urgently needed.

REFERENCES

1. Roy D, Talajic M, Dorian P, et al. Amiodarone to prevent recurrence of atrial fibrillation. Canadian trial of atrial fibrillation investigators. N Engl J Med 2000; 342:913–20.
2. Singh BN, Singh SN, Reda DJ, et al. Amiodarone versus sotalol for atrial fibrillation. N Engl J Med 2005;352:1861–72.

3. Torp-Pedersen C, Moller M, Bloch-Thomsen PE, et al. Dofetilide in patients with congestive heart failure and left ventricular dysfunction. Danish investigations of arrhythmia and mortality on dofetilide study group. N Engl J Med 1999;341:857–65.

4. Pedersen OD, Bagger H, Keller N, et al. Efficacy of dofetilide in the treatment of atrial fibrillation-flutter in patients with reduced left ventricular function: a Danish Investigations of Arrhythmia and Mortality on Dofetilide (DIAMOND) substudy. Circulation 2001;104:292–6.

5. Singh BN, Connolly SJ, Crijns HJ, et al. Dronedarone for maintenance of sinus rhythm in atrial fibrillation or flutter. N Engl J Med 2007;357:987–99.

6. Kober L, Torp-Pedersen C, McMurray JJ, et al. Increased mortality after dronedarone therapy for severe heart failure. N Engl J Med 2008;358:2678–87.

7. Hohnloser SH, Crijns HJ, van Eickels M, et al. Effect of dronedarone on cardiovascular events in atrial fibrillation. N Engl J Med 2009;360:668–78.

8. Connolly SJ, Camm AJ, Halperin JL, et al. Dronedarone in high-risk permanent atrial fibrillation. N Engl J Med 2011;365:2268–76.

9. Le Heuzey JY, De Ferrari GM, Radzik D, et al. A short-term, randomized, double-blind, parallel-group study to evaluate the efficacy and safety of dronedarone versus amiodarone in patients with persistent atrial fibrillation: the DIONYSOS study. J Cardiovasc Electrophysiol 2010;21:597–605.

10. Brignole M, Gianfranchi L, Menozzi C, et al. Influence of atrioventricular junction radiofrequency ablation in patients with chronic atrial fibrillation and flutter on quality of life and cardiac performance. Am J Cardiol 1994;74:242–6.

11. Hohnloser SH, Kuck KH, Lilienthal J. Rhythm or rate control in atrial fibrillation–Pharmacological Intervention in Atrial Fibrillation (PIAF): a randomised trial. Lancet 2000;356:1789–94.

12. Carlsson J, Miketic S, Windeler J, et al. Randomized trial of rate-control versus rhythm-control in persistent atrial fibrillation: the Strategies of Treatment of Atrial Fibrillation (STAF) study. J Am Coll Cardiol 2003;41:1690–6.

13. Wyse DG, Waldo AL, DiMarco JP, et al. A comparison of rate control and rhythm control in patients with atrial fibrillation. N Engl J Med 2002;347:1825–33.

14. Corley SD, Epstein AE, DiMarco JP, et al. Relationships between sinus rhythm, treatment, and survival in the Atrial Fibrillation Follow-up Investigation of Rhythm Management (AFFIRM) study. Circulation 2004;109:1509–13.

15. Steinberg JS, Sadaniantz A, Kron J, et al. Analysis of cause-specific mortality in the Atrial Fibrillation Follow-up Investigation of Rhythm Management (AFFIRM) study. Circulation 2004;109:1973–80.

16. Van Gelder IC, Hagens VE, Bosker HA, et al. A comparison of rate control and rhythm control in patients with recurrent persistent atrial fibrillation. N Engl J Med 2002;347:1834–40.

17. Roy D, Talajic M, Nattel S, et al. Rhythm control versus rate control for atrial fibrillation and heart failure. N Engl J Med 2008;358:2667–77.

18. Stiles MK, John B, Wong CX, et al. Paroxysmal lone atrial fibrillation is associated with an abnormal atrial substrate: characterizing the "second factor". J Am Coll Cardiol 2009;53:1182–91.

19. Wazni OM, Marrouche NF, Martin DO, et al. Radiofrequency ablation vs antiarrhythmic drugs as first-line treatment of symptomatic atrial fibrillation: a randomized trial. JAMA 2005;293:2634–40.

20. Pappone C, Augello G, Sala S, et al. A randomized trial of circumferential pulmonary vein ablation versus antiarrhythmic drug therapy in paroxysmal atrial fibrillation: the APAF study. J Am Coll Cardiol 2006;48:2340–7.

21. Oral H, Pappone C, Chugh A, et al. Circumferential pulmonary-vein ablation for chronic atrial fibrillation. N Engl J Med 2006;354:934–41.

22. Jaïs P, Cauchemez B, Macle L, et al. Catheter ablation versus antiarrhythmic drugs for atrial fibrillation: the a4 study. Circulation 2008;118:2498–505.

23. January CT, Wann LS, Alpert JS, et al. 2014 AHA/ACC/HRS Guideline for the management of patients with atrial fibrillation: a report of the American College of Cardiology/American Heart Association Task Force on Practice Guidelines and the Heart Rhythm Society. Circulation 2014;129:66–71.

24. Cosedis Nielsen J, Johannessen A, Raatikainen P, et al. Radiofrequency ablation as initial therapy in paroxysmal atrial fibrillation. N Engl J Med 2012;367:1587–95.

25. Packer DL, Kowal RC, Wheelan KR, et al. Cryoballoon ablation of pulmonary veins for paroxysmal atrial fibrillation: first results of the North American Arctic Front (STOP AF) pivotal trial. J Am Coll Cardiol 2013;61:1713–23.

26. Oral H, Knight BP, Tada H, et al. Pulmonary vein isolation for paroxysmal and persistent atrial fibrillation. Circulation 2002;105:1077–81.

27. Tilz RR, Chun KR, Schmidt B, et al. Catheter ablation of long-standing persistent atrial fibrillation: a lesson from circumferential pulmonary vein isolation. J Cardiovasc Electrophysiol 2010;21:1085–93.

28. Yoshida K, Ulfarsson M, Oral H, et al. Left atrial pressure and dominant frequency of atrial fibrillation in humans. Heart Rhythm 2011;8:181–7.

29. Haissaguerre M, Hocini M, Sanders P, et al. Catheter ablation of long-lasting persistent atrial fibrillation: clinical outcome and mechanisms of subsequent arrhythmias. J Cardiovasc Electrophysiol 2005;16:1138–47.

30. Yoshida K, Rabbani AB, Oral H, et al. Left atrial volume and dominant frequency of atrial fibrillation in patients undergoing catheter ablation of persistent

atrial fibrillation. J Interv Card Electrophysiol 2011; 32(2):155–61.

31. Narayan SM, Krummen DE, Shivkumar K, et al. Treatment of atrial fibrillation by the ablation of localized sources: confirm (conventional ablation for atrial fibrillation with or without focal impulse and rotor modulation) trial. J Am Coll Cardiol 2012;60:628–36.

32. Haissaguerre M, Hocini M, Denis A, et al. Driver domains in persistent atrial fibrillation. Circulation 2014; 130(7):530–8.

33. Wokhlu A, Monahan KH, Hodge DO, et al. Long-term quality of life after ablation of atrial fibrillation the impact of recurrence, symptom relief, and placebo effect. J Am Coll Cardiol 2010;55:2308–16.

34. Wilber DJ, Pappone C, Neuzil P, et al. Comparison of antiarrhythmic drug therapy and radiofrequency catheter ablation in patients with paroxysmal atrial fibrillation: a randomized controlled trial. JAMA 2010; 303(4):333–40.

35. Morillo CA, Verma A, Connolly SJ, et al. Radiofrequency ablation vs antiarrhythmic drugs as first-line treatment of paroxysmal atrial fibrillation (RAAFT-2): a randomized trial. JAMA 2014;311(7): 692–700.

Antiarrhythmic Drug Therapy for Atrial Fibrillation

Muhammad Rizwan Sardar, MD[a,b,c,]*,
Wajeeha Saeed, MD[d], Peter R. Kowey, MD[c,e]

KEYWORDS

- Atrial fibrillation • Cardioversion • Antiarrhythmic • Pharmacologic therapy • Rhythm control
- Rate control • Upstream therapy • Prevention

KEY POINTS

- Atrial fibrillation (AF) is a complex disease, requiring better understanding in a multifaceted approach.
- Better research is needed to develop, subclassify, and identify new therapeutic targets, which hold the promise that precise therapies aimed at preventing or reversing AF will be developed.
- Antiarrhythmic therapeutic strategies for AF should be focused on controlling pathophysiologic remodeling, with better prevention and disease-modifying strategies.

Atrial fibrillation (AF) is the most common arrhythmia, and its incidence increases with advanced age. About 1% of patients with AF are younger than 60 years, 12% are between 75 and 85 years, and one-third of patients with AF are older than 80 years.[1–3] It is estimated that there are 3 million AF cases, and prevalence is expected to reach 7 million by 2050.[4,5] Incidence rates of AF vary among different races. Individuals of European descent have lifetime risk of 20% to 25% of developing AF after the 40 years of age.[6] Although risk factors for developing AF are more prevalent in African Americans, their incidence seems to be lower than whites.[7]

AF is associated with a 3-fold to 5-fold increased risk of stroke, and stroke caused by AF has significantly higher mortality and morbidity than without AF. There is a 3-fold increase in the risk of heart failure (HF),[8] 2-fold increased risk of dementia, and higher mortality associated with AF. There are more than 470,000 hospitalizations in the United States with the primary diagnosis of AF, and it is estimated to cause 100,000 deaths per year. AF, besides being one of the leading causes of mortality and morbidity, adds $26 billion to costs in the US health system annually.[9]

Treatment of AF is multifold but revolves around 1 essential consideration: whether or not to attempt to restore sinus rhythm or to treat AF by controlling ventricular rate only. This decision depends on symptom severity, age of the patient, underlying heart disease, and other comorbidities, which may limit therapeutic options.

This article originally appeared in Cardiology Clinics, Volume 32, Issue 4, November 2014.
Disclosures: Fee for Atrial Fibrillation Education Program, North American Center for Continuing Medical Education (M.R. Sardar); no relevant disclosure (W. Saeed); and fee-for-service consultation for Sanofi, Gilead, Otsuka, Servier, ChanRx, Forest, Merck, Cardiome, Xention (P.R. Kowey).
[a] Department of Cardiology, Cooper University Hospital, 3rd Floor Dorrance, One Cooper Plaza, Camden, NJ 08103, USA; [b] Lankenau Institute for Medical Research (LIMR), Wynnewood, PA 19096, USA; [c] Jefferson Medical College, Thomas Jefferson University, Philadelphia, PA 19107, USA; [d] Albert Einstein College of Medicine, Bronx Lebanon Hospital Center, Bronx, NY 10457, USA; [e] Lankenau Institute for Medical Research (LIMR), Lankenau Medical Center, Wynnewood, PA 19096, USA
* Corresponding author. Department of Cardiology, Cooper University Hospital, 3rd Floor Dorrance, One Cooper Plaza, Camden, NJ 08103.
E-mail address: rizwansardar@hotmail.com

AF can be classified as paroxysmal, persistent, and permanent. The term lone AF refers to the finding of AF in patients without obvious structural heart disease. Paroxysmal AF terminates spontaneously or with intervention within 7 days of onset. Persistent AF lasts longer than 7 days, requiring electrical or chemical cardioversion. Long-standing persistent AF is continuous AF for longer than 12 months. Permanent AF describes continuous AF that has failed cardioversion, and the patient and clinician have jointly decided to not pursue restoring or maintaining sinus rhythm. Nonvalvular AF is AF in the absence of rheumatic mitral stenosis, a mechanical or bioprosthetic heart valve, or mitral valve repair.[10]

Symptoms of AF can vary and are individual. They range from fatigue, shortness of breath, palpitations, syncope, hypotension, and HF, with the most common symptom being fatigue. Some of the symptoms may abate with slowing of the heart rate with the use of atrioventricular (AV) nodal blocking agents. Symptom resolution may not be achieved in some patients, who continue to feel fatigued and have exercise intolerance despite adequate heart rate control, which is attributed to the loss of atrial mechanical function. Patients with underlying diastolic dysfunction and left ventricular hypertrophy are particularly sensitive to the loss of AV synchrony. For patients with no deterioration of functional status in AF, rate control may be sufficient. On the other hand, patients with clear functional decline and exacerbation of symptoms may benefit from the rhythm control strategy.

RHYTHM VERSUS RATE CONTROL

Several studies have assessed rhythm versus rate control strategies. The 2 largest trials, AFFIRM (Atrial Fibrillation Follow-up Investigation of Rhythm Management) and RACE (Rate Control Versus Electrical Cardioversion for Persistent Atrial Fibrillation), failed to show any significant benefit in choosing the rhythm control strategy.[11,12] Similar findings were seen in the PIAF (Pharmacological Intervention in Atrial Fibrillation) and STAF (Strategies of Treatment of Atrial Fibrillation) trials.[13,14]

The AFFIRM trial enrolled patients with persistent and paroxysmal AF randomly assigned to rate or rhythm control strategy. There were no significant differences in overall mortality, with a trend toward increase mortality in the rhythm control group. There was also a trend toward more ischemic strokes in rhythm control groups; however, this was mainly in patients who were not adequately anticoagulated.[12]

An AFFIRM substudy analyzing on-treatment analysis[15] showed that the presence of sinus rhythm was associated with a lower risk of mortality, suggesting that adverse effect of antiarrhythmic drugs (AAD) overcomes the potential benefit of sinus rhythm restoration.

The RACE trial[11] randomized only patients with persistent AF, and all patients were anticoagulated irrespective of previous electric cardioversion efforts into rate or rhythm control groups. After a mean follow-up of 2.3 years, the rate control strategy was noninferior to rhythm control for the prevention of death or morbidity. A substudy of the AFFIRM trial[16] looked at exercise tolerance within the rhythm control and rate control strategies for AF and performed serial 6-minute walk tests on 245 patients. There was improvement in walking distance in both groups. Roy and colleagues[17] in 2008 analyzed rhythm versus rate controlled strategy for AF with patients with HF in the AF-CHF trial. This trial enrolled 1376 patients with left ventricular ejection fraction (LVEF) of 35% or less and found no clinically significant differences between the 2 groups in terms of cardiovascular death, all-cause death, stroke, or worsening HF.

Most of the studies evaluating issue of rhythm versus rate control treatment of AF are applicable to patient's age older than 60 years and younger than 80 years but still failed to show mortality benefit with the rhythm control strategy.[11–14,18] This lack of superiority is partly linked to AAD side effects as well as excess stroke risk in patients in whom anticoagulation was discontinued. Although younger (<60 years) and older (>80 years) are not well represented in these studies, the results are still applicable. In the last decade, there has been an increase in the use of rhythm control strategies, which is largely driven by an increase in AF ablations.[19] For younger symptomatic patients with AF without significant underlying heart disease, who are not adequately represented in the earlier studies, restoration of sinus rhythm is still considered a valid approach, because the long-term implications of permanent AF are unknown.

RHYTHM CONTROL

AAD have been available for nearly 100 years and remain a cornerstone in AF therapy.[20] The role of AAD is not only to reduce the arrhythmia burden (frequency and duration of AF) but also to reduce hospitalization associated with AF. Despite the side effects associated with most of the antiarrhythmic pharmacotherapy for AF, AAD are still widely prescribed medications for AF.

Pharmacologic Cardioversion

Chemical cardioversion can be achieved with oral as well as intravenous (IV) AAD. Once the decision to restore sinus rhythm by electric or pharmacologic means is made, duration of AF is an important factor. Patients with duration of AF onset less than 48 hours have a spontaneous conversion rate of 60% in the first 24 hours.[21] Attempting pharmacologic or electrical cardioversion in AF of less than 48 hours duration allows easier restoration of sinus rhythm, increased long-term success rate, and shorter length of stay. Success of sinus rhythm restoration with pharmacologic agents varies by the choice of AAD used; however, average success rate is about 50% in the first 90 minutes from the time of drug administration. The success rate of electrical cardioversion is higher, ranging between 75% and 93%, but requires general anesthesia or conscious sedation and an 8-hour fasting period.[22] Once AF duration is greater than 7 days, pharmacologic cardioversion is less effective, and therefore, electric cardioversion is favored. Both strategies require adequate anticoagulation before cardioversion and for a period of 4 to 6 weeks after. Risk of thromboembolism without anticoagulation is similar with either of the cardioversion strategies.

Decision to Maintain Sinus Rhythm

Reversible causes of AF should be treated before initiating AAD therapy. Multiple studies evaluated short-term and long-term outcomes associated with rate control compared with rhythm control in patients with AF.[11–14,18] Once the decision of rhythm control is made, choice of agent must be individualized, considering side effect profile of the AAD and the potential benefit for a particular patient. Even after successful electrical cardioversion, risk of AF recurrence is high in untreated patients, with relapse rates of 71% to 84% at 1 year. This risk can be reduced by 30% to 50% with the use of AAD.[23]

Available AAD Choices

Over the last 20 to 25 years, AAD have been used for the management and treatment of multiple cardiac arrhythmias. AAD therapy for AF has evolved and involves complex classification, effect on multiple ion channels and adrenergic receptors, with multitude of cardiac and noncardiac side effects.

Most of the AAD used for AF exert their effect as membrane stabilizers or sodium channel blockers and potassium channel blockers. Quinidine and disopyramide have intermediate sodium channel blocking properties and show use dependence, which means the dominant effect of the drug of sodium channel blockade is seen at rapid heart rates. These agents also affect potassium channel (I_{Kr}) at normal or slower heart rates and at lower concentrations, and therefore show reverse use dependence for potassium channel blockade. Propafenone and flecainide have the slowest dissociation from sodium channels, causing more bound drug concentration with a greater degree of slowing conduction at rapid heart rates and, as a result, more use dependence. Potassium channel blockers prolong the action potential duration and refractory period. Sotalol and dofetilide cause reverse use dependence by a potassium channel blocking effect, prolonging repolarization at slower heart rates. Amiodarone and dronedarone affect multiple channels, including sodium, potassium, and calcium.

Many AAD have active metabolites, with pharmacologic action different from the parent compound. Porcainamide, a class IA AAD, blocks sodium channels, but its major metabolite N-acetylprocainamide blocks outward potassium current with little or no effect on sodium channels and behaves like a class III antiarrhythmic agent. Likewise, the class IC agent propafenone is metabolized to 5-hydroxypropafenone, which lacks the β-blocker properties of the parent compound. Therefore, when prescribing, it is prudent to know the active metabolites of AAD.

Quinidine

Quinidine is one of the oldest known AAD and is rarely used for AF, because of its proarrhythmic and noncardiovascular side effects. The effect of quinidine on I_{to} current has generated interest as a potential therapy for Brugada syndrome and idiopathic ventricular fibrillation.[23]

Disopyramide

Disopyramide is a class IA sodium channel blocker with additive anticholinergic, negative ionotropic, and vagolytic properties. Anticholinergic effects led to its recommendation for use in patients with vagally mediated AF.[24] Negative ionotropy makes disopyramide beneficial in treating AF with hypertrophic obstructive cardiomyopathy (HOCM). The same property precludes its use in left ventricular systolic dysfunction.[25] It is rarely used and makes up 1% to 2% of annual AAD prescriptions in the United States.[20]

Flecainide and propafenone

Class IC agents can convert AF into slow atrial flutter, which may conduct 1:1 and can cause hemodynamic compromise. Therefore, it is recommended to coadminister AV nodal blocking agents with class IC agents, although not necessarily in all patients. These agents cause lengthening of the PR segment and prolong the QRS duration up to 25% from baseline. These drugs should be used with caution in patients with underlying conduction delay or bundle branch blocks. Propafenone is metabolized by the liver P-450 system into 2 major active metabolites, 5-hydroxypropafenone and N-depropylpropafenone. The active metabolites are eliminated renally and cannot be cleared by hemodialysis. The dosage of propafenone needs to be reduced in patients with severe hepatic and renal insufficiency. CYP2D6 is genetically absent in 7% of the patients (poor metabolizers) and is inhibited by tricyclic antidepressants, fluoxetine, and quinidine. These drug interactions and genetic poor metabolism can lead to excess drug levels and enhance β-blocker and calcium channel blocker properties of parent propafenone.[26]

These agents are considered for patients in AF without underlying structural heart disease. They both are well tolerated and have a low risk of toxicity. Both flecainide and propafenone are proarrhythmic and have negative ionotropic properties and are therefore contraindicated in patients with left ventricular systolic dysfunction and ischemic heart disease.[27] RAFT (Rythmol Atrial Fibrillation Trial) randomized 523 patients into 3 sustained release propafenone dose groups (225 mg, 325 mg, and 425 mg twice a day, respectively) and followed them for 39 weeks. At the end of the study period, the recurrence rate of AF was 69% in the placebo group, higher than all tested doses of propafenone (52% in 225 mg, 42% in 325 mg, and 30% in 425 mg groups).[28] Similar findings were observed in ERAFT (European Rythmol/Rytmonorm Atrial Fibrillation Trial).[29]

Flecainide may cause mild neurologic side effects, like headache and tremors. Propafenone can cause gastrointestinal symptoms, such as nausea, and should be avoided in chronic obstructive pulmonary disease.

Sotalol

Sotalol is a potassium channel blocker (I_{Kr}) with nonselective β-blocker properties. It is not used for cardioversion but can be used to prevent AF recurrence. In the Sotalol Amiodarone Atrial Fibrillation Efficacy Trial and Canadian Trial of Atrial Fibrillation studies, sotalol significantly reduced rates of AF compared with placebo with sinus rhythm maintenance at 1-year ranges between 30% and 50%.[21,29,30] Sotalol never showed benefit over amiodarone in preventing AF recurrence. Sotalol has near 100% renal excretion and should be used with caution in patients with chronic kidney disease or with unstable renal functions. Sotalol prolongs the QT interval and can cause torsades de pointes (TDP). It should not be used in patients who have significant left ventricular hypertrophy and HF. It is usually started

as an 80 mg twice a day regimen, unless creatinine clearance is between 30 and 60 mL/min, in which case it should be once a day.[31] The dose should be uptitrated, with careful attention paid to the corrected QT interval. The usual dose range is 160 mg to 480 mg a day, in divided doses. Most experts recommend starting sotalol in the inpatient setting with electrocardiographic (ECG) monitoring.

Dofetilide

Dofetilide is a class III AAD and a potassium channel blocker (I_{Kr}). It inhibits the delayed rectifier potassium current and increases the atrial and ventricular effective refractory period, without causing negative ionotropy. Its peak plasma concentration is achieved 2 to 3 hours after oral administration. Dofetilide is effective for sinus rhythm maintenance and for restoring sinus rhythm. The corrected QT interval lengthens in a dose-related linear pattern. Safety of dofetilide has been well studied in different settings. The DIAMOND (Danish Investigations of Arrhythmia and Mortality on Dofetalide) trial involved 2 large randomized control trials, DIAMOND-CHF and DIAMOND-AF.[28,32] DIAMOND-CHF enrolled 1518 patients, looking at mortality as a primary end point in patients with severe left ventricular systolic dysfunction receiving dofetilide or placebo. After a median follow-up of 18 months, there was no difference in survival between the 2 groups (41% vs 42%). DIAMOND-AF was a substudy of 506 patients with HF with baseline AF or atrial flutter and showed that 44% in the dofetilide group converted to sinus rhythm compared with 14% in the placebo group. After 1 year, 79% patients in the dofetilide group remained in sinus rhythm compared with 42% in the placebo. Incidence of TDP was 3.3% in DIAMOND-CHF, and 76% occurred within the first 3 days of initiating dofetalide; however, risk of TDP was reduced by dose adjusting dofetalide based on creatinine clearance.[32] Because of the increased risk of TDP with renal clearance, dofetilide requires mandatory inpatient ECG monitoring. Dofetilide by its QT prolonging effect and property of reverse use dependence promotes the development of the Ashman phenomenon in patients with AF.[33]

The SAFIRE-D (Symptomatic Atrial Fibrillation Investigative Research on Dofetilide) study[34] evaluated the safety and efficacy of dofetilide in 325 patients with persistent AF. The trial showed that 58% of patients maintained sinus rhythm at 1 year compared with 25% with placebo, with a lower incidence of TDP (0.8%) compared with the DIAMOND-AF study. In this trial, dofetilide dose was reduced for impaired renal functions and for corrected QT prolongation more than

15% from the baseline. It is approved in the United States, but not in Europe, for paroxysmal AF with a mandatory loading period of 3 days (or 5 doses) in hospital. Because of the complex dosing regimen and safety concerns of dofetilide, the US Food and Drug Administration (FDA) has restricted its prescription to registered physicians, nurses, and pharmacists who have completed specific training in the use of the drug. Dofetilide has shown reasonable safety in patients after myocardial infarction as well.[32]

Amiodarone

Amiodarone is the most effective AAD in preventing recurrence of paroxysmal as well as persistent AF.[22,30,35] Although it is not approved by the FDA for AF, it is still the most commonly prescribed AAD for AF, representing 45% of annual US drug prescriptions.[20] It is a complex iodinated compound, with action on multiple ion channels (I_{Na}, I_{Kur}, I_{to}, I_{CAL}, I_{KACh}, and I_f) and nonselective inhibition of α and β receptors.

In SAFE-T (Sotalol Amiodarone Atrial Fibrillation Efficacy Trial), 665 patients with persistent AF were randomized to receive amiodarone, sotalol, or placebo and were followed for 1 to 4.5 years. Recurrence rates at 1 year were 48%, 68%, and 87% in the amiodarone, sotalol, and placebo treated groups, respectively. There were higher bleeding rates in the amiodarone group, which is likely because of its interaction with warfarin.[29] Similar results were found in the Canadian Trial of Atrial Fibrillation, in which 403 patients were assigned to amiodarone, sotalol, or propafenone. After a mean follow-up of 16 months, the recurrence rate of AF in patients treated with amiodarone was 35%, compared with 63% in the sotalol or propafenone treated group. In a Veterans Affairs (VA) health system study,[36] amiodarone facilitated conversion to and maintenance of sinus rhythm in patients with left ventricular systolic dysfunction and decreased mortality in patients who remained in sinus rhythm, with no overall worsening of HF.

A study from Europe[37] compared the treatment of various AAD (amiodarone, sotalol, propafenone, dronedarone, and flecainide) for the treatment of AF or atrial flutter and found the largest reduction of AF recurrence in patients receiving amiodarone, but this benefit came at the expense of higher adverse effects and treatment withdrawals. In SCD HeFT (Sudden Cardiac Death in Heart Failure Trial),[38] amiodarone treatment was associated with more noncardiac deaths in patients with New York Heart Association (NYHA) class III HF.

Amiodarone is an iodine-rich lipid-soluble compound, with variable but generally poor bioavailability. Higher lipid solubility leads to extracardiac accumulation of amiodarone in fat, muscles, liver, skin, and lungs, causing multiple potential toxicities. Amiodarone should be avoided in younger patients, in whom other AAD can be useful (because of cumulative toxicity). Pulmonary toxicity of amiodarone is dose related and can be fatal. Amiodarone may be used as the initial AAD of choice in patients with left ventricular systolic dysfunction, left ventricular hypertrophy, and coronary artery disease (CAD) or previous myocardial infarction. Patients on chronic amiodarone therapy should be annually screened for the end organ damage (eg, liver, thyroid, lung, and eye). The most common cardiovascular effects is bradycardia, with the highest risk of pacemaker in women.[39] QT interval prolongation is common, but rarely associated with TDP ($\leq 0.5\%$).[40] Amiodarone is loaded in 600-mg to 1200-mg daily doses to a load of up to 10 g, before reducing the dose to a maintenance regimen of 200 mg or less a day. IV amiodarone does not have the same electrophysiologic effects as oral amiodarone. Use of oral amiodarone is associated with benefit of effective rate control, frequently eliminating the need for other drugs to control ventricular rates. Administration of the drug with food minimizes gastrointestinal side effects; however, grapefruit juice can inhibit amiodarone metabolism and can cause increased drug levels.[41] There is an increased risk of myositis when amiodarone is combined with a CYP3A4 substrate like simvastatin, which should be used at a dose of no more than 20 mg per day in patients treated with amiodarone. Amiodarone can also potentiate the anticoagulant effect of warfarin and inhibits P-glycoprotein transport, resulting in reduced digoxin clearance. Amiodarone is weakly effective for AF conversion into sinus rhythm.[24,42]

Dronedarone

Dronedarone is an amiodaronelike substance without the iodine moiety, which may be responsible for fewer extracardiac side effects than amiodarone.[43] Like amiodarone, dronedarone also carries complex antiarrhythmic properties, spanning all classes of Vaughan Williams classification. It inhibits sodium current I_{Na}, potassium current I_{Kr} and I_{KACh} and L-type calcium current, and carries α-receptor–blocking and β-receptor–blocking properties. Dronedarone prolongs the action potential in the atria and ventricles, with no major reverse use dependence.

The DAFNE (Dronedarone Atrial Fibrillation Study After Electrical Cardioversion) study[44] was formulated to study the most suitable dose of dronedarone for the prevention of AF after cardioversion. This trial showed that an 800-mg daily dose of dronedarone was the optimal dose. Extracardiac (thyroid, pulmonary, ocular, hepatic toxic) or proarrhythmic effects were not seen at any of the studied doses. EURIDIS (European Trial In Atrial Fibrillation or Flutter Patients Receiving Dronedarone for the Maintenance of Sinus Rhythm) and ADONIS (American-Australian Trial with Dronedarone in Atrial Fibrillation or Flutter Patients for the Maintenance of Sinus Rhythm) studied patients treated with dronedarone for AF and atrial flutter in maintaining sinus rhythm. These trials found that a dose of dronedarone of 400 mg twice a day was effective in preventing symptomatic and asymptomatic AF recurrences. The adverse events reported in both of these trials were similar in the dronedarone and placebo group, with more gastrointestinal toxicity associated with dronedarone.[44] Dronedarone was also tested in patients with symptomatic permanent AF for its effect on heart rate control. Dronedarone significantly reduced resting and maximal exercise heart rates compared with placebo.[45]

In the ATHENA trial,[46] patients with paroxysmal or persistent AF or atrial flutter with risk factors of thromboembolism, dronedarone reduced the combined end point of death and cardiovascular complications. This effect was largely seen by reducing hospitalization for AF. ANDROMEDA (Antiarrhythmic Trial with Dronedarone in Moderate to Severe Congestive Heart Failure Evaluating Morbidity Decrease)[47] evaluated tolerability of dronedarone in high-risk patients with HF and ventricular dysfunction in a double-blind, placebo-controlled fashion. The study was terminated prematurely because of excess risk of death in patients receiving dronedarone. The PALLAS trials[48] evaluated patients with persistent AF and found that dronedarone increases the combined end point of stroke, cardiovascular death, and hospitalization. As a result of these trials, dronedarone is contraindicated in patients with recent decompensated HF, depressed left ventricular function, or with NYHA class III or IV HF symptoms. It should be given for prevention of AF only to patients in whom sinus rhythm is already restored.

Dronedarone does not interact with warfarin. It increases serum creatinine levels through impaired tubular secretion, without an effect on renal function. Dronedarone, like amiodarone, interacts with P450 glycoprotein and CYP3A4 and therefore causes increase in digoxin levels and simvastatin induce myositis. There is generally a 10% risk of gastrointestinal side effects with the use of dronedarone. Like with warfarin, grapefruit juice increases dronedarone levels and should be avoided. The FDA has issued a warning to monitor liver function tests with the use of dronedarone, based on a few recent case reports of liver failure that occurred within 6 months of the start of dronedarone.[49]

After the start of dronedarone therapy, rhythm should be monitored at least every 3 to 6 months. Dronedarone may be considered as a rhythm control agent in patients without HF and when extracardiac side effects of amiodarone need to be avoided. Dronedarone should be avoided in patients with permanent AF.

Ibutilide

Ibutilide is an IV I_{Kr} blocker, which also enhances late inward sodium current.[50] It is metabolized by the cytochrome P450 isoenzyme of the liver other than CYP3A4 and CYP2D6, and its plasma concentration constitutes less than 10% of the administered ibutilide, with most of the drug (82% of a 0.01-mg/kg dose) quickly excreted in urine. After administration, it restores sinus rhythm in 50% of patients, with an average conversion time of less than 30 minutes. It converts atrial flutter, with a higher rate of success than AF,[51] and pretreatment with IV magnesium sulfate improves the efficacy of electrical cardioversion.[52] It prolongs the QT interval with a risk of TDP, and, therefore, ibutilide infusion must be carried out in the inpatient setting, with continuous monitoring of the ECG for greater than 4 hours after administration. Ibutilide should be avoided in patients with hypokalemia, baseline prolonged QT, and depressed left ventricular function (<30%), because of increased risk of proarrhythmia.[52] IV magnesium pretreatment may decrease the risk of proarrhythmia.[53]

Common Rules in AAD Selection

Selection of antiarrhythmic agents is based on the presence or absence of underlying cardiac disease (**Fig. 1**) and the cardiac or noncardiac toxicity profile of a chosen drug (**Table 1**) as well as contraindications and drug-drug interactions. Other factors that may play a role in AAD selection are risk of associated bradyarrhythmias, risk of QT prolongation and TDP, and renal or hepatic dysfunction. Class I antiarrhythmic agents are contraindicated in patients with marked left ventricular hypertrophy, CAD, or congestive HF, because of the risk of ventricular arrhythmia. In patients without underlying structural heart disease, almost all AAD can be selected; however, flecainide, propafenone, or sotalol are preferred first-line agents. Dronedarone can be used as a first-line maintenance therapy for AF in patients without structural heart disease, but because of the excess mortality in patients with HF and stroke in persistent AF, its market share is restricted. Among class III drugs, dofetilide and sotalol are

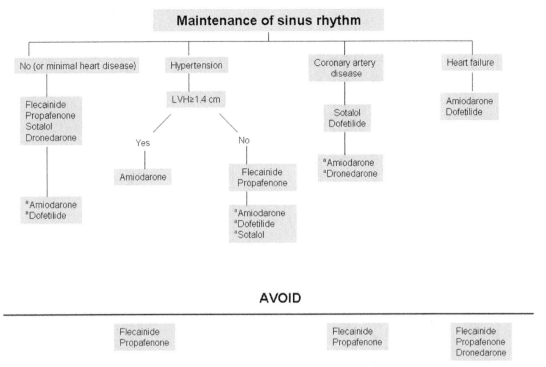

Fig. 1. Algorithm for AAD selection for maintenance of sinus rhythm. [a] Second-line drug therapy. LVH, left ventricular hypertrophy.

associated with QT prolongation and should be avoided in patients with marked left ventricular hypertrophy. Disopyramide, because of its negative ionotropic properties, is ideal for patients with HOCM, particularly if they already have a pacemaker or implantable cardioverter defibrillator.[25] In patients with congestive HF, only amiodarone and dofetilide are safe for use (see **Fig. 1**).

Our goal should be to use AAD in reducing AF symptoms. Occasional AF recurrences on AAD are expected and do not necessarily mean discontinuation of therapy. AAD for rhythm control should not be continued when AF becomes permanent. See **Table 1** for AAD dosage, side effects, and major drug-drug interactions.

OUTPATIENT VERSUS INPATIENT START OF ANTIARRHYTHMIC THERAPY

For paroxysmal AF, inpatient versus outpatient initiation of AAD therapy is an important consideration. Outpatient start of AAD is always desirable for patients, because it is less cumbersome and financially more feasible. Some controversy exists regarding the safety of outpatient start of AAD. This caution primarily relates to concerns of QT prolongation and risk of TDP, particular at the time of conversion from AF to sinus rhythm.[54] In patients with infrequent, and reasonably well-tolerated, symptomatic episodes of AF, the pill in

the pocket approach uses self-administration of a single dose of a drug shortly after the start of palpitations, therefore terminating an AF episode early and reducing the need for emergency room visits, hospitalization, and direct cardioversion. Flecainide and propafenone have been studied for this approach, and the expected effect is usually seen in 3 to 4 hours after administration.[55] However, this approach requires absence of any structural heart disease at baseline.[56]

Sotalol causes QT prolongation and may cause proarrhythmia. There is evidence of outpatient start of sotalol in patients with nearly no underlying structural heart disease with normal electrolytes and baseline QT interval of less than 450 milliseconds.[57] However, the package insert of sotalol has a black box warning against starting the medication in the outpatient setting. Patients treated with sotalol should be hospitalized with ECG monitoring if medication is to be initiated while the patient is in AF.[58] Data for outpatient AAD are strong for amiodarone and dronedarone. The decision to start AAD in an inpatient or outpatient setting should be carefully individualized.

UPSTREAM THERAPY FOR AF

The concept of upstream therapy is the use of drugs that can prevent atrial electric and mechanical remodeling, thereby reducing the likelihood of

Table 1
Currently available drugs for treatment of atrial fibrillation according to the Vaughan-Williams classification, their mechanism of action, and their main adverse effects

AAD	Dose/Metabolism	Drug Interactions/ Pharmacokinetics	Cardiovascular Toxicity	Noncardiovascular Toxicity
Vaughan Williams Class IA				
Quinidine	324–648 mg every 8 h; hepatic CYP3A4 (70%), renal (30%)	Inhibits P450: ↑ digoxin levels Inhibits CYP2D6: ↑ tricyclic antidepressant and metorpolol	QRS prolongation with toxic doses, TDP (non–dose- related)	Rash, thrombocytopenia, cinchonism, pruritus
Disopyramide	Immediate release: 100–200 mg once every 6 h Extended release: 200–400 mg once every 12 h; renal/hepatic CYP3A4; reduced dose for renal and hepatic dysfunction	Metabolized with CYP3A4: caution with inhibitors (verapamil, diltiazem, ketoconazole, macrolide antibiotics, protease inhibitors, grapefruit juice) and inducers (rifampin, phenobarbital, phenytoin)	TDP, congestive HF	Anticholinergic side effects: narrow angle glaucoma, dry mouth, constipation, urinary retention, blurry vision
Vaughan Williams Class IC				
Flecainide	50–200 mg every 12 h; renal/ hepatic CYP2D6	Metabolized by CYP2D6 (inhibitors include quinidine, fluoxetine, tricyclics; also genetically absent in 7%–10% of population) and renal excretion (dual impairment can increase plasma concentration)	Atrial flutter with 1:1 conduction, can unmask Brugada type ST elevation, contraindicated with CAD, ventricular tachycardia	Dizziness, headache, visual blurring
Propafenone	150–300 every 8 h or sustained release 225–425 twice a day; hepatic	Metabolized by CYP2D6 (inhibitors include quinidine, fluoxetine, tricyclics); genetically absent in 7%–10% of population—poor metabolizers have β blockade Inhibits P-glycoprotein: increases digoxin concentration Inhibits CYP2C9: increases warfarin concentration	Atrial flutter with 1:1 conduction, can unmask Brugada type ST elevation, contraindicated with CAD, ventricular tachycardia	Metallic taste, dizziness

Vaughan Williams Class III

Sotalol	40–160 mg once every 12 h; renal	None	TDP, bradycardia	Bronchospasm
Dofetilide	CrCl ≥60 (500 µg twice a day), CrCl 40–60 (250 µg twice a day), CrCl 20–39 (125 µg twice a day, CrCl<20 (not recommended); renal/hepatic CYP3A4	Metabolized by CYP3A: verapamil, hydrochlorothiazide, cimetidine, ketoconazole, trimethoprim, prochlorperazine, and megestrol are contraindicated; discontinue amiodarone at least 3 mo before initiation	TDP	None
Amiodarone	Half-life 50 days; oral: load 10 g over 7–10 d, 400–600 mg daily in divided doses for 2–4 wk; maintenance typically 100–200 mg every day IV: load 150–300 mg over 10 min; then 1 mg/min for 6 h; then 0.5 mg/min for 18 h or change to oral dosing; after 24 h, consider decreasing dose to 0.25 mg/min; hepatic	Inhibits most CYPs to cause drug interaction: increase concentrations of warfarin, statins, many other drugs Inhibits P-glycoprotein: increase digoxin concentration	Bradycardia	Pulmonary (acute hypersensitivity pneumonitis, chronic interstitial infiltrates); hepatitis; thyroid (hypothyroidism or hyperthyroidism); photosensitivity; skin discoloration with chronic high dose; nausea; ataxia; tremor; alopecia
Dronedarone	400 mg every 12 h; renal, hepatic	Metabolized by CYP3A: caution with inhibitors (verapamil, diltiazem, ketoconazole, macrolide antibiotics, protease inhibitors, grapefruit juice) and inducers (rifampin, phenobarbital, phenytoin) Inhibits CYP3A, CYP2D6, P-glycoprotein: increase concentrations of some statins, sirolimus, tacrolimus, β-blockers, digoxin	Bradycardia, avoid in congestive HF and permanent AF	Anorexia; nausea, liver failure
Ibutilide	IV 1 mg over 10 min; second dose 1 mg after 10 min if necessary; hepatic	No known drug interactions	TDP	Nausea

Abbreviation: CrCl: creatinine clearance.

AF. These drugs might arrest or delay the cellular process leading to AF either before (primary prevention) or after (secondary prevention) the development of AF. **Table 2** gives a summary of upstream therapy.

Angiotensin-Converting Enzyme Inhibitors and Angiotensin Receptor Blockers

Atrial tissue remodeling may contribute to the initiation and continuation of AF, especially in the population with HF. There are several studies, both in humans and animals, that have shown that inhibition of the renin angiotensin-aldosterone system (RAAS) may help prevent AF.[59,60] This finding could be because of the pleiotropic effects of RAAS blockade, which include prevention of left atrial dilatation and atrial fibrosis, slowing of atrial dilatation, and reduction of inflammation.[61,62]

Data for angiotensin-converting enzyme inhibitors (ACE-I) and angiotensin receptor blockers (ARB) for primary prevention (hypertensive heart disease without significant structural heart disease) are robust; however, secondary prevention has not been well shown.[60,63,64] A substudy of the Trandolapril Cardiac Evaluation trial[65] analyzed patients who had sinus rhythm at the time of randomization. After 2 to 4 years of follow-up, patients treated with trandolapril had significantly less AF compared with placebo. ACE-i have also been associated with reduced AF after myocardial infarction in patients with reduced LVEF.[66,67] Aldosterone inhibitors were compared with ACE-i in a randomized fashion, and they conferred the same reduction in AF recurrence rate in patients with paroxysmal AF.[68] A meta-analysis of AF studies[60] showed ACE-i and ARB use may be effective in reducing AF in patients with HF, and those with hypertension and left ventricular hypertrophy. However, the included retrospective studies were not designed to determine AF reduction as a primary outcome.

The ANTIPAF (Angiotensin II Antagonist in Paroxysmal Atrial Fibrillation) trial[69] is a prospective, randomized, placebo-controlled trial analyzing AF burden in patients with documented paroxysmal AF without baseline structural heart disease. In this trial, 430 patients received olmesartin 40 mg or placebo, and after 1 year of follow-up, ARB therapy failed to show any reduction in the primary outcome (ie, AF burden).

As per recent 2014 American College of Cardiology (ACC)/American Heart Association (AHA) Task Force on Practice Guidelines and the Heart Rhythm Society (HRS) AF guidelines,[10] upstream ACE-i and ARB are class IIa recommendations for primary prevention of new onset AF in patients with HF, and class IIb for primary prevention of new onset AF in the setting of hypertension.

3-Hydroxy-3-Methylglutaryl–Coenzyme A Reductase Inhibitors/Statins

Statins are known to have pleiotropic effects and may exert positive effects on AF by reducing inflammation by pathways other than 3-hydroxy-3-methylglutaryl–coenzyme A reductase inhibition.[70,71] Animal data show that simvastatin reduces electrical remodeling, atrial fibrosis by decreasing fibroblast proliferation, and reduces AF duration.[72,73] Most of the data evaluating statin effects on AF are retrospective and conflicting. Young-Xu and colleagues[74] studied 449 patients with chronic stable CAD, treated with any statin, followed for an average 5 years and showed a significant reduction in the risk of developing AF (odds ratio: 0.48; 95% confidence interval: 0.28–20.83). However, similar results were not seen in a VA study,[75] which looked at 5417 patients who received statin therapy (any brand) in a similar patient profile with CAD and failed to show any reduction in AF recurrence after 4.8 years of follow-up. Smaller randomized prospective studies have shown benefit of statins in reducing AF episodes; however, similar benefits are still to

---

Table 2
Upstream drug therapy for AF and its proposed mechanisms

Mechanism	Drugs/Agents	Effect on Atrial Fibrillation
RAAS inhibition	1. ACE-i/ARB	Inhibition of atrial fibrosis, remodeling, and antiinflammatory effect
	2. Aldosterone	Inhibition of atrial fibrosis, antiinflammatory effect
HMG-CoA reductase	Statins	Antiinflammatory effect, pleiotropic effects
Antiinflammatory drugs	1. Steroids	Antiinflammatory
	2. ω-3 PUFA	Unclear, may be direct antiarrhythmic effect

Abbreviations: ω-3 PUFA, ω-3 polyunsaturated fatty acids; ACE-i, angiotensin-converting enzyme inhibitors; ARB, angiotensin receptor blockers; HMG-CoA, 3-hydroxy-3-methylglutaryl–coenzyme A; RAAS, renin angiotensin-aldosterone system.

be determined in a larger prospective trial, PAFRIOSIES (Paroxysmal Atrial Fibrillation: Role of Inflammation, Oxidative Stress Injury and Effect of Statins) (ClinicalTrials.gov Identifier: NCT00321802), which is under way and awaiting results. Data are still unclear in regard to the effects of statins on clinical outcomes in AF. The clearest prospective data of statin in AF prevention are in the postoperative setting.[76] The ARMYDA-3 (Atorvastatin for Reduction of Myocardial Damage During Angioplasty 3) study[77] randomized 200 patients undergoing cardiothoracic surgery to receive either atorvastatin or placebo starting 7 days preoperatively. Atorvastatin showed a significant reduction in postoperative AF (POAF) versus placebo (P = .003) and significantly shorter length of hospital stay (P = .001).

Statin therapy may be reasonable for primary prevention of new onset AF in patients with CAD, but its routine use in preventing AF is not recommended.

Antiinflammatory Agents

Inflammation associated with or without postoperative setting has a clear association with AF.[78,79] The levels of inflammatory markers like C-reactive protein (CRP) are increased in patients with AF compared with sinus rhythm.[80] Inflammation seems to be involved in the early phase of electrical remodeling. However, it is not clear if inflammation is a precursor of AF and electrical remodeling or a marker of ongoing electrical remodeling.

- Corticosteroids: data for steroid use and reduction in AF burden and recurrence are sparse. Most of the steroid data evaluated steroids for POAF.[81] Studies evaluating beneficial effects of steroids in POAF are small or meta-analyses of smaller studies with heterogeneous patient pools.[82–85] The risk of long-term steroid use warrants their cautious prophylactic use. Judicious use of steroids for AF prevention and reduction of AF burden is not recommended.
- ω-3 polyunsaturated fatty acid (PUFA): Li and colleagues[86] reported that ω-3 PUFA inhibits transient outward (I_{to}), ultrarapid delayed rectifier potassium currents (I_{Kur}) and voltage gate sodium channel (I_{Na}) in human atrial myocyte, which may be responsible for decrease in AF with the use of ω-3 PUFA. Initial studies evaluated the use of ω-3 PUFA in sudden cardiac death and concluded with disappointing results. At the same time, a proof of concept open-label study showed a remarkable 65% reduction in AF occurrence after coronary

artery bypass graft,[87] and a search for antiarrhythmic effects of ω-3 PUFA in atrial tachyarrhythmias began. Despite positive results of ω-3 PUFA in various animal studies, similar results in large robust designed POAF trials and postelectrical cardioversion studies could not be replicated.[88,89] Kowey and colleagues[90] evaluated the safety and efficacy of ω-3 PUFA in a randomized, double-blind, placebo-controlled design in patients with paroxysmal or persistent AF without underlying structural heart disease. After 6 months of follow-up, there was no significant benefit of ω-3 PUFA in preventing recurrence of symptomatic AF in both AF strata.

Aldosterone Antagonists

Aldosterone is known to play an important role in angiotensin II–mediated inflammation and fibrosis. There is also a higher incidence of AF in patients with primary hyperaldosteronism. In an experimental model of HF, spironolactone and eplerenone decreased atrial fibrosis and vulnerability to AF. A substudy of the eplerenone in patients with mild systolic HF (EMPHASIS) trial showed that eplerenone treatment can prevent the first AF or atrial flutter episode. After 2 years of observation, 2.7% patients treated with eplerenone compared with 4.5% treated with placebo developed new AF.[91] The SPIR-AF trial evaluated the antiarrhythmic effect of spironolactone compared with ACE-i in 164 patients with an average 4-year recurrent AF history. It is a prospective, randomized 12-month trial, with 4 treatment arms: group A, spironolactone, enalapril, and a β-blocker; group B, spironolactone and a β-blocker; group C, enalapril plus a β-blocker; and group D, a β-blocker alone. There was a significant reduction in the incidences of symptomatic AF in both groups treated with spironolactone (group A and group B) ($P\leq.001$), at 3, 6, 9 and 12 months of treatment. However, no significant difference was seen in AF recurrences between group A and B.[68] Aldosterone antagonist treatment may be a simple and valuable additional option in the population with HF along with other approved antiarrhythmic agents for AF prevention. More robust data, especially in primary prevention, are required before recommending its upstream use (see **Table 2**).

FUTURE PHARMACOLOGIC THERAPY

Current AAD bring success with associated safety issues with their use, which has stimulated the development of AF pharmacologic agents in 2 directions: modification of existing compounds and designing drugs with new targets.

Vernakalant

Vernakalant is a complex class III electrophysiologic agent with the use-dependent or rate-dependent sodium inhibition and broad potassium channel inhibition (I_{to}, I_{KACh}, and I_{Kur}).[92,93] It has shown good safety both in animal studies as well as in initial phase 1 to 3 trials.[24,94,95] It is more effective in conversion of AF than atrial flutter, particularly if administered within 7 days of arrhythmia onset and AF of shorter duration. A phase 3 superiority study of Vernakalant Versus Amiodarone in Subjects With Recent Onset Atrial Fibrillation (AVRO), randomized 234 patients for AF conversion into an IV vernakalant and IV amiodarone strategy in a double-blind fashion. Conversion from AF to sinus rhythm within the first 90 minutes (primary end point) was achieved in 60 of 116 (51.7%) patients treated with vernakalant compared with 6 of 116 (5.2%) patients treated with amiodarone ($P<.0001$). Vernakalant showed efficacy superior to amiodarone for acute conversion of recent onset AF.[24] The IV formulation can cause hypotension and shock and is therefore not approved in the United States. An IV form is available in Europe, and an oral formulation is in development.

Ranolazine

Ranolazine is a new drug approved for refractory chronic angina. Preclinical data showed that as well as being anti-ischemic, ranolazine also reduced supraventricular arrhythmia, including AF. It blocks several ion channels, including peak and late I_{Na}, I_{CAL}, and I_{Kr}. Inhibition of I_{Na} with ranolazine or vernakalant may reduce the risk of TDP associated with I_{Kr} inhibition. It is still to be determined if combination of ranolazine or vernakalant with I_{Kr} blockers (sotalol or dofetilide) decreases the risk of TDP.

Nonclinical studies showed that dronedarone in combination with ranolazine works synergistically, which is likely caused by a multichannel ion effect, resulting in inhibition of peak and late I_{Na}, I_{KACh}, and I_{Kr} in atrial myocyte. A synergistic effect of low-dose dronedarone with ranolazine was studied in a recently presented phase 2 study (HARMONY trial, ClinicalTrials.gov Identifier: NCT01522651), evaluating AF reduction with the combination drug. After a 12-week treatment, in patients treated with ranolazine/dronedarone 750 mg/150 mg twice a day and 750 mg/225 mg twice a day, there was a 45% and 59% AF reduction, respectively ($P = .072$ and $P = .008$), versus placebo.[96] These results are consistent with preclinical findings of a synergistic effect when these therapies are used in combination.

Miscellaneous

Atrial tissue has a predominance of I_{Kur} and I_{KACh}, and therefore, inhibiting these ion channels selectively prolongs action potential duration in the atria. AVE0118 selectively blocks the I_{Kur} and showed some efficacy in the early phase of development.[97] Tertiapin-Q is a nonselective inhibitor of I_{KACh} and is derived from honeybee. Tertiapin-Q terminated AF in a vagally induced AF model, as well as reducing AF inducibility.[98,99] NTC-801 is the only available selective I_{KACh} inhibitor.[100] There are still limited human data of specific potassium channel blockers, but there is promise for future growth in AAD development for AF. Oral vanoxerine was initially in clinical development for Parkinson disease, but recent preclinical data showed its prominent antiarrhythmic effects.

SUMMARY

AF is a complex disease, requiring better understanding and a multifaceted approach. Research is needed to develop, subclassify, and identify new therapeutic targets, with promise that precise therapies aimed at preventing or reversing AF will be developed. Antiarrhythmic therapeutic strategies for AF should be focused on controlling pathophysiologic remodeling, with better prevention and disease-modifying strategies. Large randomized controlled trials are required in order to develop improved clinically relevant guidelines for AF.[101]

REFERENCES

1. Jaïs P, Hocini M, Macle L, et al. Distinctive electrophysiological properties of pulmonary veins in patients with atrial fibrillation. Circulation 2002;106: 2479–85.
2. Takahashi Y, Iesaka Y, Takahashi A, et al. Reentrant tachycardia in pulmonary veins of patients with paroxysmal atrial fibrillation. J Cardiovasc Electrophysiol 2003;14:927–32.
3. Mandapati R, Skanes A, Chen J, et al. Stable microreentrant sources as a mechanism of atrial fibrillation in the isolated sheep heart. Circulation 2000; 101:194–9.
4. Saeed W, Kusick JW, Sardar MR, et al. Stroke prevention in atrial fibrillation: pharmacologic update. Am Med J 2013;4(2):143–9. http://dx.doi.org/10.3844/amjsp.2013.143.149.
5. Naccarelli GV, Varker H, Lin J, et al. Increasing prevalence of atrial fibrillation and flutter in the

United States. Am J Cardiol 2009;104:1534–9. http://dx.doi.org/10.1016/j.amjcard.2009.07.022.

6. Skanes AC, Mandapati R, Berenfeld O, et al. Spatiotemporal periodicity during atrial fibrillation in the isolated sheep heart. Circulation 1998;98: 1236–48.

7. Atienza F, Almendral J, Moreno J, et al. Activation of inward rectifier potassium channels accelerates atrial fibrillation in humans: evidence for a reentrant mechanism. Circulation 2006;114:2434–42. http://dx.doi.org/10.1161/CIRCULATIONAHA.106.633735.

8. Toma M, Ezekowitz JA, Bakal JA, et al. The relationship between left ventricular ejection fraction and mortality in patients with acute heart failure: insights from the ASCEND-HF Trial. Eur J Heart Fail 2014;16:334–41. http://dx.doi.org/10.1002/ejhf.19.

9. Tsai CF, Tai CT, Hsieh MH, et al. Initiation of atrial fibrillation by ectopic beats originating from the superior vena cava: electrophysiological characteristics and results of radiofrequency ablation. Circulation 2000;102:67–74.

10. January CT, Wann LS, Alpert JS, et al. 2014 AHA/ACC/HRS guideline for the management of patients with atrial fibrillation: a report of the American College of Cardiology/American Heart Association Task Force on Practice Guidelines and the Heart Rhythm Society. J Am Coll Cardiol 2014. http://dx.doi.org/10.1016/j.jacc.2014.03.022.

11. Van Gelder IC, Hagens VE, Bosker HA, et al. A comparison of rate control and rhythm control in patients with recurrent persistent atrial fibrillation. N Engl J Med 2002;347:1834–40. http://dx.doi.org/10.1056/NEJMoa021375.

12. Wyse DG, Waldo AL, DiMarco JP, et al. A comparison of rate control and rhythm control in patients with atrial fibrillation. N Engl J Med 2002;347:1825–33. http://dx.doi.org/10.1056/NEJMoa021328.

13. Hohnloser SH, Kuck KH, Lilienthal J. Rhythm or rate control in atrial fibrillation–Pharmacological Intervention in Atrial Fibrillation (PIAF): a randomised trial. Lancet 2000;356:1789–94.

14. Carlsson J, Miketic S, Windeler J, et al. Randomized trial of rate-control versus rhythm-control in persistent atrial fibrillation: the Strategies of Treatment of Atrial Fibrillation (STAF) study. J Am Coll Cardiol 2003;41:1690–6.

15. Corley SD, Epstein AE, DiMarco JP, et al. Relationships between sinus rhythm, treatment, and survival in the Atrial Fibrillation Follow-Up Investigation of Rhythm Management (AFFIRM) Study. Circulation 2004;109:1509–13. http://dx.doi.org/10.1161/01.CIR.0000121736.16643.11.

16. Chung MK, Shemanski L, Sherman DG, et al. Functional status in rate- versus rhythm-control strategies for atrial fibrillation: results of the Atrial Fibrillation Follow-Up Investigation of Rhythm Management (AFFIRM) Functional Status Substudy.

J Am Coll Cardiol 2005;46:1891–9. http://dx.doi.org/10.1016/j.jacc.2005.07.040.

17. Roy D, Talajic M, Nattel S, et al. Rhythm control versus rate control for atrial fibrillation and heart failure. N Engl J Med 2008;358:2667–77. http://dx.doi.org/10.1056/NEJMoa0708789.

18. Opolski G, Torbicki A, Kosior DA, et al. Rate control vs rhythm control in patients with nonvalvular persistent atrial fibrillation: the results of the Polish How to Treat Chronic Atrial Fibrillation (HOT CAFE) Study. Chest 2004;126:476–86. http://dx.doi.org/10.1378/chest.126.2.476.

19. Martin-Doyle W, Essebag V, Zimetbaum P, et al. Trends in US hospitalization rates and rhythm control therapies following publication of the AFFIRM and RACE trials. J Cardiovasc Electrophysiol 2011;22:548–53. http://dx.doi.org/10.1111/j.1540-8167.2010.01950.x.

20. Zimetbaum P. Antiarrhythmic drug therapy for atrial fibrillation. Circulation 2012;125:381–9. http://dx.doi.org/10.1161/CIRCULATIONAHA.111.019927.

21. Naccarelli GV, Wolbrette DL, Bhatta L, et al. A review of clinical trials assessing the efficacy and safety of newer antiarrhythmic drugs in atrial fibrillation. J Interv Card Electrophysiol 2003;9: 215–22.

22. Nattel S, Opie LH. Controversies in atrial fibrillation. Lancet 2006;367:262–72. http://dx.doi.org/10.1016/S0140-6736(06)68037-9.

23. Belhassen B, Glick A, Viskin S. Efficacy of quinidine in high-risk patients with Brugada syndrome. Circulation 2004;110:1731–7. http://dx.doi.org/10.1161/01.CIR.0000143159.30585.90.

24. Camm AJ, Capucci A, Hohnloser SH, et al. A randomized active-controlled study comparing the efficacy and safety of vernakalant to amiodarone in recent-onset atrial fibrillation. J Am Coll Cardiol 2011;57:313–21. http://dx.doi.org/10.1016/j.jacc.2010.07.046.

25. Sherrid MV, Barac I, McKenna WJ, et al. Multicenter study of the efficacy and safety of disopyramide in obstructive hypertrophic cardiomyopathy. J Am Coll Cardiol 2005;45:1251–8. http://dx.doi.org/10.1016/j.jacc.2005.01.012.

26. Sardar MR, Saeed W, Wong K. Class I antiarrhythmic medications. In: Daoud E, Kalbfleisch S, editors. Color atlas and synopsis of electrophysiology (SET). 1st edition. McGraw-Hill Ryerson; 2015.

27. Echt DS, Liebson PR, Mitchell LB, et al. Mortality and morbidity in patients receiving encainide, flecainide, or placebo. The Cardiac Arrhythmia Suppression Trial. N Engl J Med 1991;324:781–8. http://dx.doi.org/10.1056/NEJM199103213241201.

28. Pritchett EL, Page RL, Carlson M, et al. Efficacy and safety of sustained-release propafenone (propafenone SR) for patients with atrial fibrillation. Am J Cardiol 2003;92:941–6.

29. Singh BN, Singh SN, Reda DJ, et al. Amiodarone versus sotalol for atrial fibrillation. N Engl J Med 2005;352:1861–72. http://dx.doi.org/10.1056/NEJMoa041705.

30. Lafuente-Lafuente C, Mouly S, Longás-Tejero MA, et al. Antiarrhythmic drugs for maintaining sinus rhythm after cardioversion of atrial fibrillation: a systematic review of randomized controlled trials. Arch Intern Med 2006;166:719–28. http://dx.doi.org/10.1001/archinte.166.7.719.

31. Nabar A, Rodriguez LM, Timmermans C, et al. Class IC antiarrhythmic drug induced atrial flutter: electrocardiographic and electrophysiological findings and their importance for long term outcome after right atrial isthmus ablation. Heart 2001;85:424–9.

32. Torp-Pedersen C, Møller M, Bloch-Thomsen PE, et al. Dofetilide in patients with congestive heart failure and left ventricular dysfunction. Danish Investigations of Arrhythmia and Mortality on Dofetilide Study Group. N Engl J Med 1999;341:857–65. http://dx.doi.org/10.1056/NEJM199909163411201.

33. Sardar MR, Khaji A, Robert J, et al. The Ashman phenomenon in patients with atrial fibrillation treated with an IKr blocker, dofetilide. Circulation 2013;128:A10380.

34. Singh S, Zoble RG, Yellen L, et al. Efficacy and safety of oral dofetilide in converting to and maintaining sinus rhythm in patients with chronic atrial fibrillation or atrial flutter: the Symptomatic Atrial Fibrillation Investigative Research on Dofetilide (SAFIRE-D) study. Circulation 2000;102:2385–90.

35. Roy D, Talajic M, Dorian P, et al. Amiodarone to prevent recurrence of atrial fibrillation. Canadian Trial of Atrial Fibrillation Investigators. N Engl J Med 2000;342:913–20. http://dx.doi.org/10.1056/NEJM200003303421302.

36. Deedwania PC, Singh BN, Ellenbogen K, et al. Spontaneous conversion and maintenance of sinus rhythm by amiodarone in patients with heart failure and atrial fibrillation: observations from the Veterans Affairs Congestive Heart Failure Survival Trial of Antiarrhythmic Therapy (CHF-STAT). The Department of Veterans Affairs CHF-STAT Investigators. Circulation 1998;98:2574–9.

37. Freemantle N, Lafuente-Lafuente C, Mitchell S, et al. Mixed treatment comparison of dronedarone, amiodarone, sotalol, flecainide, and propafenone, for the management of atrial fibrillation. Europace 2011;13:329–45. http://dx.doi.org/10.1093/europace/euq450.

38. Bardy GH, Lee KL, Mark DB, et al. Amiodarone or an implantable cardioverter-defibrillator for congestive heart failure. N Engl J Med 2005;352:225–37. http://dx.doi.org/10.1056/NEJMoa043399.

39. Kaufman ES, Zimmermann PA, Wang T, et al. Risk of proarrhythmic events in the Atrial Fibrillation Follow-up Investigation of Rhythm Management (AFFIRM) study: a multivariate analysis. J Am Coll Cardiol 2004;44:1276–82. http://dx.doi.org/10.1016/j.jacc.2004.06.052.

40. Meng X, Mojaverian P, Doedée M, et al. Bioavailability of amiodarone tablets administered with and without food in healthy subjects. Am J Cardiol 2001;87:432–5.

41. Libersa CC, Brique SA, Motte KB, et al. Dramatic inhibition of amiodarone metabolism induced by grapefruit juice. Br J Clin Pharmacol 2000;49:373–8.

42. Galve E, Rius T, Ballester R, et al. Intravenous amiodarone in treatment of recent-onset atrial fibrillation: results of a randomized, controlled study. J Am Coll Cardiol 1996;27:1079–82. http://dx.doi.org/10.1016/0735-1097(95)00595-1.

43. Piccini JP, Hasselblad V, Peterson ED, et al. Comparative efficacy of dronedarone and amiodarone for the maintenance of sinus rhythm in patients with atrial fibrillation. J Am Coll Cardiol 2009;54:1089–95. http://dx.doi.org/10.1016/j.jacc.2009.04.085.

44. Touboul P, Brugada J, Capucci A, et al. Dronedarone for prevention of atrial fibrillation: a dose-ranging study. Eur Heart J 2003;24:1481–7.

45. Singh BN, Connolly SJ, Crijns HJ, et al. Dronedarone for maintenance of sinus rhythm in atrial fibrillation or flutter. N Engl J Med 2007;357:987–99. http://dx.doi.org/10.1056/NEJMoa054686.

46. Hohnloser SH, Crijns HJ, van Eickels M, et al. Effect of dronedarone on cardiovascular events in atrial fibrillation. N Engl J Med 2009;360:668–78. http://dx.doi.org/10.1056/NEJMoa0803778.

47. Køber L, Torp-Pedersen C, McMurray JJ, et al. Increased mortality after dronedarone therapy for severe heart failure. N Engl J Med 2008;358:2678–87. http://dx.doi.org/10.1056/NEJMoa0800456.

48. Connolly SJ, Camm AJ, Halperin JL, et al. Dronedarone in high-risk permanent atrial fibrillation. N Engl J Med 2011;365:2268–76. http://dx.doi.org/10.1056/NEJMoa1109867.

49. Center for Drug Evaluation and Research and Drug Safety and Availability. FDA Drug Safety Communication. Severe liver injury associated with the use of dronedarone (marketed as Multaq). Available at: http://www.fda.gov/Drugs/DrugSafety/ucm240011.htm. Accessed June 15, 2014.

50. Stambler BS, Wood MA, Ellenbogen KA, et al. Efficacy and safety of repeated intravenous doses of ibutilide for rapid conversion of atrial flutter or fibrillation. Ibutilide Repeat Dose Study Investigators. Circulation 1996;94:1613–21.

51. Murray KT. Ibutilide. Circulation 1998;97:493–7.

52. Oral H, Souza JJ, Michaud GF, et al. Facilitating transthoracic cardioversion of atrial fibrillation with ibutilide pretreatment. N Engl J Med 1999;340:1849–54. http://dx.doi.org/10.1056/NEJM199906173402401.

53. Patsilinakos S, Christou A, Kafkas N, et al. Effect of high doses of magnesium on converting ibutilide to

a safe and more effective agent. Am J Cardiol 2010; 106:673–6. http://dx.doi.org/10.1016/j.amjcard.2010. 04.020.

54. Kozhevnikov DO, Yamamoto K, Robotis D, et al. Electrophysiological mechanism of enhanced susceptibility of hypertrophied heart to acquired torsade de pointes arrhythmias: tridimensional mapping of activation and recovery patterns. Circulation 2002;105:1128–34.

55. Boriani G, Diemberger I, Biffi M, et al. Pharmacological cardioversion of atrial fibrillation: current management and treatment options. Drugs 2004; 64:2741–62.

56. Alboni P, Botto GL, Baldi N, et al. Outpatient treatment of recent-onset atrial fibrillation with the "pill-in-the-pocket" approach. N Engl J Med 2004;351:2384–91. http://dx.doi.org/10.1056/NEJMoa041233.

57. European Heart Rhythm Association, Heart Rhythm Society, Fuster V, et al. ACC/AHA/ESC 2006 guidelines for the management of patients with atrial fibrillation–executive summary: a report of the American College of Cardiology/American Heart Association Task Force on Practice Guidelines and the European Society of Cardiology Committee for Practice Guidelines (Writing Committee to Revise the 2001 Guidelines for the Management of Patients with Atrial Fibrillation). J Am Coll Cardiol 2006;48:854–906. http://dx.doi.org/10.1016/j.jacc. 2006.07.009.

58. De Vos CB, Pisters R, Nieuwlaat R, et al. Progression from paroxysmal to persistent atrial fibrillation clinical correlates and prognosis. J Am Coll Cardiol 2010;55:725–31. http://dx.doi.org/10.1016/j.jacc. 2009.11.040.

59. Shi Y, Li D, Tardif JC, et al. Enalapril effects on atrial remodeling and atrial fibrillation in experimental congestive heart failure. Cardiovasc Res 2002;54: 456–61.

60. Schneider MP, Hua TA, Böhm M, et al. Prevention of atrial fibrillation by renin-angiotensin system inhibition a meta-analysis. J Am Coll Cardiol 2010;55:2299–307. http://dx.doi.org/10. 1016/j.jacc.2010.01.043.

61. Xiao HD, Fuchs S, Campbell DJ, et al. Mice with cardiac-restricted angiotensin-converting enzyme (ACE) have atrial enlargement, cardiac arrhythmia, and sudden death. Am J Pathol 2004;165:1019–32. http://dx.doi.org/10.1016/S0002-9440(10)63363-9.

62. Boos CJ, Lip GY. Targeting the renin-angiotensin-aldosterone system in atrial fibrillation: from pathophysiology to clinical trials. J Hum Hypertens 2005;19:855–9. http://dx.doi.org/10.1038/sj.jhh. 1001933.

63. GISSI-AF Investigators, Disertori M, Latini R, et al. Valsartan for prevention of recurrent atrial fibrillation. N Engl J Med 2009;360:1606–17. http://dx. doi.org/10.1056/NEJMoa0805710.

64. Wachtell K, Lehto M, Gerdts E, et al. Angiotensin II receptor blockade reduces new-onset atrial fibrillation and subsequent stroke compared to atenolol: the Losartan Intervention for End Point Reduction in Hypertension (LIFE) study. J Am Coll Cardiol 2005;45: 712–9. http://dx.doi.org/10.1016/j.jacc.2004.10.068.

65. Pedersen OD, Bagger H, Kober L, et al. Trandolapril reduces the incidence of atrial fibrillation after acute myocardial infarction in patients with left ventricular dysfunction. Circulation 1999;100:376–80.

66. Murray KT, Rottman JN, Arbogast PG, et al. Inhibition of angiotensin II signaling and recurrence of atrial fibrillation in AFFIRM. Heart Rhythm 2004;1:669–75. http://dx.doi.org/10.1016/j.hrthm.2004.08.008.

67. Pedersen OD, Bagger H, Køber L, et al. The occurrence and prognostic significance of atrial fibrillation/-flutter following acute myocardial infarction. TRACE Study group. TRAndolapril Cardiac Evaluation. Eur Heart J 1999;20:748–54.

68. Dabrowski R, Borowiec A, Smolis-Bak E, et al. Effect of combined spironolactone-β-blocker ± enalapril treatment on occurrence of symptomatic atrial fibrillation episodes in patients with a history of paroxysmal atrial fibrillation (SPIR-AF study). Am J Cardiol 2010;106:1609–14. http://dx.doi.org/ 10.1016/j.amjcard.2010.07.037.

69. Goette A, Schön N, Kirchhof P, et al. Angiotensin II-antagonist in paroxysmal atrial fibrillation (ANTIPAF) trial. Circ Arrhythm Electrophysiol 2012;5:43–51. http://dx.doi.org/10.1161/CIRCEP.111.965178.

70. Lahoti A, Saeed W, Badri M, et al. Impact of statins on long term mortality in heart failure with preserved ejection fraction (HFPEF). J Am Coll Cardiol 2012;59:E1010. http://dx.doi.org/10.1016/S0735-1097(12)61011-0.

71. Salamon JN, Mazurek J, Sardar MR, et al. Mortality benefit of statins in patients with atrial fibrillation. J Card Fail 2011;17:S55.

72. Shiroshita-Takeshita A, Brundel BJ, Burstein B, et al. Effects of simvastatin on the development of the atrial fibrillation substrate in dogs with congestive heart failure. Cardiovasc Res 2007;74:75–84. http://dx.doi.org/10.1016/j.cardiores.2007.01.002.

73. Shiroshita-Takeshita A, Schram G, Lavoie J, et al. Effect of simvastatin and antioxidant vitamins on atrial fibrillation promotion by atrial-tachycardia remodeling in dogs. Circulation 2004;110:2313–9. http:// dx.doi.org/10.1161/01.CIR.0000145163.56529.D1.

74. Young-Xu Y, Jabbour S, Goldberg R, et al. Usefulness of statin drugs in protecting against atrial fibrillation in patients with coronary artery disease. Am J Cardiol 2003;92:1379–83.

75. Adabag AS, Nelson DB, Bloomfield HE. Effects of statin therapy on preventing atrial fibrillation in coronary disease and heart failure. Am Heart J 2007; 154:1140–5. http://dx.doi.org/10.1016/j.ahj.2007. 07.018.

76. Fauchier L, Clementy N, Babuty D. Statin therapy and atrial fibrillation: systematic review and updated meta-analysis of published randomized controlled trials. Curr Opin Cardiol 2013;28:7–18. http://dx.doi.org/10.1097/HCO.0b013e32835b0956.

77. Patti G, Chello M, Candura D, et al. Randomized trial of atorvastatin for reduction of postoperative atrial fibrillation in patients undergoing cardiac surgery: results of the ARMYDA-3 (Atorvastatin for Reduction of Myocardial Dysrhythmia after cardiac surgery) study. Circulation 2006;114:1455–61. http://dx.doi.org/10.1161/CIRCULATIONAHA.106.621763.

78. Aviles RJ, Martin DO, Apperson-Hansen C, et al. Inflammation as a risk factor for atrial fibrillation. Circulation 2003;108:3006–10. http://dx.doi.org/10.1161/01.CIR.0000103131.70301.4F.

79. Sardar MR, Saeed W, Wertan M, et al. Incidence of postoperative atrial fibrillation (POAF) after robotic CABG versus traditional CABG and its associated mortality and morbidity. J Am Coll Cardiol 2014. http://dx.doi.org/10.1016/S0735-1097(14)60431-9.

80. Chung MK, Martin DO, Sprecher D, et al. C-reactive protein elevation in patients with atrial arrhythmias: inflammatory mechanisms and persistence of atrial fibrillation. Circulation 2001; 104:2886–91.

81. Dernellis J, Panaretou M. Relationship between C-reactive protein concentrations during glucocorticoid therapy and recurrent atrial fibrillation. Eur Heart J 2004;25:1100–7. http://dx.doi.org/10.1016/j.ehj.2004.04.025.

82. Halonen J, Halonen P, Järvinen O, et al. Corticosteroids for the prevention of atrial fibrillation after cardiac surgery: a randomized controlled trial. JAMA 2007;297:1562–7. http://dx.doi.org/10.1001/jama.297.14.1562.

83. Halvorsen P, Raeder J, White PF, et al. The effect of dexamethasone on side effects after coronary revascularization procedures. Anesth Analg 2003; 96:1578–83 [table of contents].

84. Marik PE, Fromm R. The efficacy and dosage effect of corticosteroids for the prevention of atrial fibrillation after cardiac surgery: a systematic review. J Crit Care 2009;24:458–63. http://dx.doi.org/10.1016/j.jcrc.2008.10.016.

85. Prasongsukarn K, Abel JG, Jamieson WR, et al. The effects of steroids on the occurrence of postoperative atrial fibrillation after coronary artery bypass grafting surgery: a prospective randomized trial. J Thorac Cardiovasc Surg 2005;130:93–8. http://dx.doi.org/10.1016/j.jtcvs.2004.09.014.

86. Li GR, Sun HY, Zhang XH, et al. Omega-3 polyunsaturated fatty acids inhibit transient outward and ultra-rapid delayed rectifier K+ currents and Na+ current in human atrial myocytes. Cardiovasc Res 2009;81:286–93. http://dx.doi.org/10.1093/cvr/cvn322.

87. Calò L, Bianconi L, Colivicchi F, et al. N-3 Fatty acids for the prevention of atrial fibrillation after coronary artery bypass surgery: a randomized, controlled trial. J Am Coll Cardiol 2005;45:1723–8. http://dx.doi.org/10.1016/j.jacc.2005.02.079.

88. Savelieva I, Kakouros N, Kourliouros A, et al. Upstream therapies for management of atrial fibrillation: review of clinical evidence and implications for European Society of Cardiology guidelines. Part I: primary prevention. Europace 2011;13:308–28. http://dx.doi.org/10.1093/europace/eur002.

89. Bianconi L, Calò L, Mennuni M, et al. n-3 polyunsaturated fatty acids for the prevention of arrhythmia recurrence after electrical cardioversion of chronic persistent atrial fibrillation: a randomized, double-blind, multicentre study. Europace 2011;13:174–81. http://dx.doi.org/10.1093/europace/euq386.

90. Kowey PR, Reiffel JA, Ellenbogen KA, et al. Efficacy and safety of prescription omega-3 fatty acids for the prevention of recurrent symptomatic atrial fibrillation: a randomized controlled trial. JAMA 2010;304:2363–72. http://dx.doi.org/10.1001/jama.2010.1735.

91. Zannad F, McMurray JJ, Krum H, et al. Eplerenone in patients with systolic heart failure and mild symptoms. N Engl J Med 2011;364:11–21. http://dx.doi.org/10.1056/NEJMoa1009492.

92. Burashnikov A, Barajas-Martinez H, Hu D, et al. Atrial-selective prolongation of refractory period with AVE0118 is due principally to inhibition of sodium channel activity. J Cardiovasc Pharmacol 2012;59:539–46. http://dx.doi.org/10.1097/FJC.0b013e31824e1b93.

93. Kozlowski D, Budrejko S, Lip GY, et al. Vernakalant hydrochloride for the treatment of atrial fibrillation. Expert Opin Investig Drugs 2009;18:1929–37. http://dx.doi.org/10.1517/13543780903386246.

94. Kowey PR, Dorian P, Mitchell LB, et al. Vernakalant hydrochloride for the rapid conversion of atrial fibrillation after cardiac surgery: a randomized, double-blind, placebo-controlled trial. Circ Arrhythm Electrophysiol 2009;2:652–9. http://dx.doi.org/10.1161/CIRCEP.109.870204.

95. Roy D, Pratt CM, Torp-Pedersen C, et al. Vernakalant hydrochloride for rapid conversion of atrial fibrillation: a phase 3, randomized, placebo-controlled trial. Circulation 2008;117:1518–25. http://dx.doi.org/10.1161/CIRCULATIONAHA.107.723866.

96. Kowey PR, Reiffel JA, Camm J. The effect of the combination of ranolazine and low dose dronedarone on atrial fibrillation burden in patients with paroxysmal atrial fibrillation (HARMONY trial). Presented paper at 35th Annual Scientific Sessions for the Late Breaking Clinical Trials III. San Francisco, May 10, 2014.

97. De Haan S, Greiser M, Harks E, et al. AVE0118, blocker of the transient outward current (I(to)) and

ultrarapid delayed rectifier current (I(Kur)), fully restores atrial contractility after cardioversion of atrial fibrillation in the goat. Circulation 2006;114: 1234–42. http://dx.doi.org/10.1161/CIRCULATION AHA.106.630905.

98. Hashimoto N, Yamashita T, Tsuruzoe N. Tertiapin, a selective IKACh blocker, terminates atrial fibrillation with selective atrial effective refractory period prolongation. Pharmacol Res 2006;54:136–41. http://dx.doi.org/10.1016/j.phrs.2006.03.021.

99. Ravens U, Poulet C, Wettwer E, et al. Atrial selectivity of antiarrhythmic drugs. J Physiol 2013;591: 4087–97. http://dx.doi.org/10.1113/jphysiol.2013. 256115.

100. Machida T, Hashimoto N, Kuwahara I, et al. Effects of a highly selective acetylcholine-activated K+ channel blocker on experimental atrial fibrillation. Circ Arrhythm Electrophysiol 2011;4:94–102. http://dx.doi.org/10.1161/CIRCEP.110.951608.

101. Sardar MR, Badri M, Prince C, et al. How representative of the general population are the cohorts included in the clinical trials that drive our guidelines? Circulation 2013;128(suppl): A14780.

Catheter Ablation of Atrial Fibrillation

Rakesh Latchamsetty, MD*, Fred Morady, MD

KEYWORDS

- Atrial fibrillation • Catheter ablation • Outcomes

KEY POINTS

- When performed by experienced operators, catheter ablation is a safe and effective option for the management of atrial fibrillation (AF).
- Further understanding of the pathophysiologic mechanisms of AF would facilitate development of novel strategies and technologies to improve ablation outcomes.
- Postprocedure clinical follow-up and management are critical to achieve the full benefits of ablation.

INTRODUCTION

Catheter ablation was introduced as a therapeutic option for the management of atrial fibrillation (AF) in the late 1990s and is now readily available in many middle-volume to large-volume cardiovascular centers worldwide. Its growth has been accompanied by changes in procedural strategy, advances in mapping and ablation technologies, refinement in periprocedural management, and a better understanding of the mechanisms driving and perpetuating AF. Rates of sinus rhythm maintenance have remained stable over the past 15 years despite inclusion of a broader selection of patients with persistent and long-standing persistent AF as well as multiple cardiac and other comorbidities including cardiomyopathy, valvular disease, and renal failure. Long-term benefits of sinus rhythm maintenance in addition to symptomatic relief are also under investigation.

PREOPERATIVE PLANNING
Patient Selection

Current American Heart Association (AHA)/American College of Cardiology (ACC)/Heart Rhythm Society (HRS) guidelines endorse catheter ablation as a class I recommendation for patients with symptomatic paroxysmal AF refractory or intolerant to at least 1 class I or III antiarrhythmic drugs (AADs), or a class IIa recommendation when offered before initiation of an AAD.[1] In patients with symptomatic persistent AF refractory or intolerant to at least 1 class I or III AAD, catheter ablation is considered a class IIa recommendation.[1] Although not considered contraindications to ablation, other patient characteristics to consider include significant left atrial dilatation, prolonged duration of AF, and patient age and comorbidities. Ablation should not be considered in patients who cannot receive anticoagulation during the periprocedural period.

The primary goal of ablation remains symptomatic improvement, although some studies suggest other benefits such as improved left ventricular function or reduced stroke risk. Ablation should not be performed with the goal of eliminating the need for long-term anticoagulation.

Preprocedure Testing

Before scheduled AF ablation, patients should have documentation of their arrhythmia. Long-term

This article originally appeared in Cardiology Clinics, Volume 32, Issue 4, November 2014.
Disclosure: The authors have no relevant financial relationships to disclose.
Department of Electrophysiology, University of Michigan Hospital, 1500 East Medical Center Drive, Ann Arbor, MI 48109-5853, USA
* Corresponding author. CVC, SPC 5853, Department of Electrophysiology, 1500 East Medical Center Drive, Ann Arbor, MI 48109-5853.
E-mail address: rakeshl@umich.edu

monitoring may reveal an inciting supraventricular tachycardia or single-focus ectopy that degenerates into or triggers AF. Such patients may simply require a more targeted ablation for their primary arrhythmia.

Patients should be anticoagulated before ablation. In patients with persistent AF, transesophageal echocardiography should be performed to rule out left atrial or left atrial appendage clot or the patient should be verified to be therapeutically anticoagulated for at least 3 consecutive weeks before ablation. Cardiac computed tomography or magnetic resonance imaging to delineate left atrial and pulmonary vein (PV) anatomy can be helpful.

Anticoagulation

Perioperative anticoagulation with warfarin or target-specific oral anticoagulants (TSOACs; ie, dabigatran, rivaroxaban, or apixaban) is usually maintained for at least 1 month before and at least 3 months following catheter ablation. In the recent COMPARE (Role of Coumadin in Preventing Thromboembolism in Atrial Fibrillation Patients Undergoing Catheter Ablation)[2] trial, patients randomized to uninterrupted warfarin had fewer periprocedural stroke and minor bleeding episodes compared with those who discontinued warfarin before the procedure. Bleeding complications can also be managed effectively despite therapeutic anticoagulation. In patients who have tamponade during ablation, early recognition and management results in favorable outcomes even among those with uninterrupted warfarin.[3] With the available safety data and potential to avoid the inconvenience and cost of bridging with heparin-based products, maintaining warfarin throughout the perioperative period may be the optimal strategy. Without reliable reversal agents for the TSOAC, most patients discontinue these medications before their ablation. However, early data suggest that uninterrupted TSOAC use may also be safe without increased bleeding or thromboembolic complications in the perioperative period.[4] These data need to be verified in larger scale, prospective studies.

ABLATION STRATEGY
AF Mechanisms

Reliable elimination of AF by ablation requires an understanding of the mechanisms by which AF is induced and perpetuated. Although considerable progress in this endeavor has been achieved over the past century, significant questions remain. Multiple mechanisms have been shown in vivo as well as in simulated models and varying mechanisms are likely to be predominant in different patients (**Fig. 1**).[5–7]

Early hypotheses for the mechanisms of AF include rapidly firing foci (1907),[8] so-called circus movement or reentry (1913),[9] and the multiple wavelets theory (1960s).[10] Recognition of rapid depolarizations from the PVs initiating and perpetuating AF was instrumental in providing an effective target for catheter-based therapy, and PV isolation (PVI) has remained a key component of most ablation strategies.[11] Other areas recognized to possess arrhythmogenic properties that may contribute to AF include the superior vena cava, inferior vena cava, coronary sinus, and ligament of Marshall. These seem to be less commonly arrhythmogenic than PVs, but may serve as adjunctive targets in select patients.[12–14]

In addition to focal triggers, high-frequency sources described as rotors have been identified in both animal and human models, supporting their role in maintaining AF.[5] These organized areas of electrical activity may or may not remain stationary and have been shown to produce wavebreak and fibrillatory conduction at their periphery, leading to disorganized activity throughout the remainder of the atria.[15,16] Identifying these elusive targets has been the focus of some recent ablation strategies to map more specific electrogram-guided and not purely anatomic targets. In addition, the role of the autonomic system through both sympathetic and parasympathetic influences has been widely described.[17] In particular, stimulation of atrial ganglionated plexi (GPs) has been shown to trigger PV arrhythmias and increase AF inducibility.[18]

PVI

The emergence of catheter ablation as a viable strategy to treat AF began with showing the efficacy of targeting focal PV triggers by electrically isolating the PVs.[11] With recognition of antral tissue harboring critical atrial substrate[19] as well as to avoid PV stenosis, PVI has evolved from an ostial to an antral approach (**Fig. 2**).[20] Despite high acute rates in achieving PVI (>95%),[21] reconnection of some veins can be shown in most patients regardless of clinical arrhythmia recurrence.[22] Adenosine infusion following isolation has been suggested as a means to unmask dormant PV connection and prompt further ablation; however, whether this translates into long-term clinical improvement is unclear. Newer technologies such as real-time monitoring of catheter contact force or real-time lesion visualization need to be evaluated in terms of their ability to produce more durable lesions. At present, antral PVI remains the most widely used strategy in ablation of both paroxysmal and

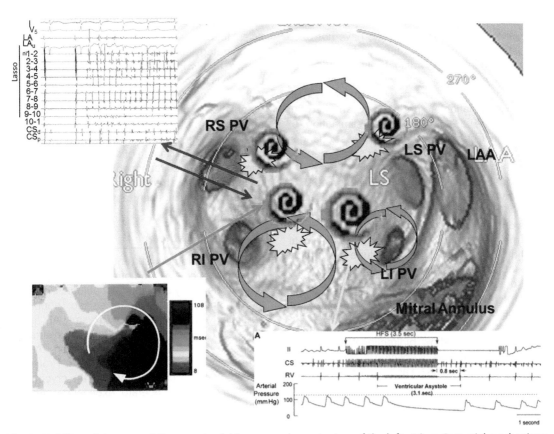

Fig. 1. Multifactorial nature of the genesis of AF on an endoscopic view of the left atrium. Potential mechanisms of AF include PV tachycardias that initiate and perpetuate AF (*left upper insert*), rotors (*magnified phase map in the left lower insert*), multiple reentrant circuits (*green circles*), and autonomic modulation through ganglion-ated plexi (*yellow patches* and *right lower inset*). There is a dynamic interplay between the PVs and other drivers of AF such that they continually activate and perpetuate each other. LAA, left atrial appendage; LI, left inferior; LS, left superior; RI, right inferior; RS, right superior. (*Reproduced from* Zipes D, Jalife J. Cardiac electrophysiology, from cell to bedside. Philadelphia: Saunders Elsevier; 2013, p. 740, with permission; *Adapted from* Jalife J. Rotors and spiral waves in atrial fibrillation. J Cardiovasc Electrophysiol 2003;14:777, with permission; and Po SS, Nakagawa H, Jackman WM. Localization of left atrial ganglionated plexi in patients with atrial fibrillation. J Cardiovasc Electrophysiol 2009;20:1187, with permission.)

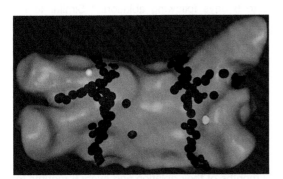

Fig. 2. Electroanatomic image of a posterior view of the left atrium and PVs following antral PVI. *Red dots* indicate ablation sites. Occasional more ostial lesions depicted in yellow were delivered to facilitate elimination of specific pulmonary vein fascicles. Lesions directly over the esophagus (*blue dots*) were avoided.

nonparoxysmal AF. PVI alone has been associated with freedom from recurrent atrial arrhythmias in greater than 80% of patients with paroxysmal AF at 1-year follow-up.[23,24]

Additional Strategies

Common adjunctive strategies to PVI include linear ablation, elimination of complex fractionated atrial electrograms (CFAEs), ablation of sites harboring GPs, ablation of specific focal triggers, and more specific strategies designed to identify and eliminate sites of AF rotors.

CFAE ablation involves targeting areas of rapid, fractionated, or continuous atrial electrograms. An early study describing ablation of CFAEs as a potential stand-alone strategy in patients with persistent AF reported a high incidence of AF termination during ablation (67% without ibutilide and 95% with ibutilide) as well as 91% AF-free survival at 1 year.[25] These results have not been consistently replicated and targeting of CFAEs is most commonly used adjunctively to PVI. Sites of CFAEs are usually selected subjectively and can be nonspecific. The mechanisms of benefit from CFAE ablation are not firmly established but likely include a combination of elimination or containment of high-frequency sources, changes in autonomic input into the atria, or simple debulking of the atrial substrate.[16,26,27]

Linear ablation can facilitate termination of AF to sinus rhythm incrementally to PVI and CFAE ablation.[28] The most common sites of linear ablation are along the left atrial roof and mitral isthmus. The mechanisms of AF termination with linear ablation are unknown but may include interruption of reentrant circuits, compartmentalization of the atria, or ablation of nearby structures (eg, the ligament of Marshall along the mitral isthmus).[29,30] A concern with linear ablation is the potential for recurrent macroreentrant circuits and it is therefore important to show bidirectional conduction block across the lines of ablation.[31]

Targeting of GPs can be accomplished by either ablating at typical anatomic locations near the PV ostia and septum or by identifying locations with vagal responses to rapid stimuli. Although GP ablation alone is unlikely to be sufficient, some studies have reported improvement in sinus rhythm maintenance when used in addition to PVI.[32]

In addition, more recent strategies sought to identify sites harboring AF rotors based on real-time atrial electrogram analysis. Previous work showed that sites where ablation terminated AF tended to have higher dominant frequencies and elimination of frequency gradients within or between the atria can be predictive of procedural success.[33–35] A recent technique described as the focal impulse and rotor modulation (FIRM) method uses a proprietary algorithm to identify electrical activation patterns during AF and localize optimal ablation targets (**Fig. 3**).[36] Results from this method are promising and have shown acute termination of AF with a median of 2.5 minutes of ablation time (interquartile range, 1.0–3.1 minutes) and improved long-term freedom from atrial arrhythmias for paroxysmal and persistent AF at 890 days' follow-up using the FIRM method versus standard ablation techniques (70.4% vs 36.9%; $P = .003$).[37]

In paroxysmal AF, antral PVI alone is a reasonable ablation strategy with favorable clinical outcomes. After PVI, any further triggers that either spontaneously manifest or are revealed through pacing or intravenous drug infusion should be targeted. For persistent AF, PVI alone seems insufficient for optimal long-term results and an adjunctive strategy is recommended. Studies have shown that conversion to sinus rhythm during ablation is associated with improved long-term results[38]; however, whether a prospective strategy of ablation until conversion to sinus rhythm is beneficial is not known. Following ablation of intended targets, and depending on the patient's clinical status and length of the procedure, cardioversion may be reasonable to restore sinus rhythm. Further attempts at induction may also be performed to identify any coexisting arrhythmias or AF triggers.

Cryoballoon Catheter

The most common current ablation technique uses irrigated-tip radiofrequency catheters. Among the newly available technologies, cryoballoon therapy has recently gained popularity, particularly in patients with paroxysmal AF. Immediate and 1-year outcomes for paroxysmal AF seem to be similar with cryoballoon therapy compared with radiofrequency.[39,40] Procedure times and complication rates with the cryoballoon catheter depend on operator experience, although a higher incidence of phrenic nerve injury is seen with cryoballoon ablation. Acute phrenic nerve injury was reported to be as high as 11% in the STOP AF (Sustained Treatment of Paroxysmal Atrial Fibrillation) trial[41] and 6.38% in a prior meta-analysis of 1349 procedures.[42] Most of these injuries resolve clinically, with about 0.4% persisting at 1 year. Atrioesophageal fistula has also been reported with the use of cryoballoon ablation[43] and a recent study with the second-generation 28-mm cryoballoon showed a 12% incidence of healing esophageal thermal lesions 2 to 6 days following ablation.[44] Similar to the use of radiofrequency, visualization of the esophagus may help in limiting esophageal injury. The question of durability of cryoballoon lesions needs to be answered in studies evaluating longer-term follow-up. When more targeted ablation beyond PVI is considered, additional radiofrequency ablation is also needed.

POSTPROCEDURE CARE AND FOLLOW-UP

Patients should be seen in follow-up within 3 months of their ablation and every 6 months for the first 2 years with electrocardiograms (ECGs) obtained at each visit.[45] Longer-term monitoring is decided on an individual basis but may be performed routinely when patients are evaluated as part of a research protocol. Patients with symptomatic complaints warrant longer-term

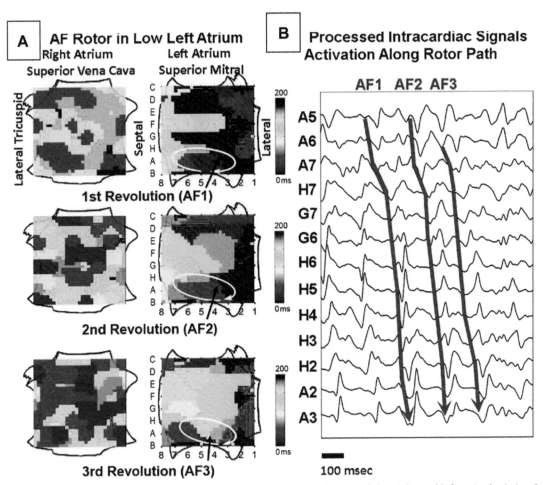

Fig. 3. Mapping of an electrical rotor during AF. (*A*) Computational maps of the right and left atria depicting 3 cycles of a left atrial rotor during AF with clockwise revolution (activation time scale coded from red to blue). (*B*) Processed and filtered intracardiac signals showing sequential activation over the rotor path for the 3 cycles. (*From* Narayan SM, Krummen DE, Shivkumar K, et al. Treatment of atrial fibrillation by the ablation of localized sources: confirm (conventional ablation for atrial fibrillation with or without focal impulse and rotor modulation) trial. J Am Coll Cardiol 2012;60(7):631; with permission.)

monitoring to document the frequency and type of arrhythmia recurrence. Asymptomatic patients may also benefit from long-term monitoring if long-term management decisions are affected by the presence of atrial arrhythmias. Early recurrences within the first 3 months are common and are often transient, and long-term monitoring is usually performed after this period. Anticoagulation should be continued for at least the first 3 months following ablation and long-term use should be based on clinical stroke risk factors. Assessment of a patient's rhythm status should also be performed to address the need for continuation of AAD therapy. Following an ablation, without documented recurrence, efforts should be made to discontinue long-term AAD use when possible.

ABLATION OUTCOMES
Procedural Success

Catheter ablation has been shown to be superior to AAD for the maintenance of sinus rhythm.[20] Measures of ablation success are variable and depend heavily on patient populations being studied, type and duration of AF, and length of ECG monitoring following ablation. Overall, successful maintenance of sinus rhythm without use of AAD at 1 year following ablation generally ranges from 75% to 93% for paroxysmal AF[23,24,46–48] and 63% to 74% for nonparoxysmal AF.[20,25,48,49] Repeat ablations are frequently required for long-term success and a mean of 1.3 procedures per patient were reported in one multicenter study,[48] and the rate can be higher for persistent AF. At 3 to 5 years, long-term success off AAD following ablation of paroxysmal AF decreases to about 57% to 65%, but with the use of AAD it is about 80%. Success rates are lower following ablation of persistent AF, for which, at 5 years, maintenance of sinus rhythm is slightly less than 50% inclusive of AAD use.[50]

However, these reported success rates are based on complete elimination of AF and may underestimate the potential clinical benefit of ablation for several reasons. First, categorizing an ablation that significantly reduces a patient's symptoms or even eliminates them for 1 or more years as unsuccessful likely undervalues its benefit. Furthermore, several studies have reported symptomatic improvement in a subset of patients who experienced AF recurrence, even in cases of persistent AF.[20,51,52] In addition, other benefits not directly measured by AF symptoms or arrhythmia recurrence, such as a decrease in stroke risk, may also be present.

Stroke Benefit

The association with AF and stroke risk is well documented,[53] but it is not clear whether AF directly causes this increased risk or whether it is a secondary marker of an alternative mechanism. Data evaluating the benefit of successful catheter ablation in mitigating this risk are also conflicting. A recent single-center retrospective analysis of 3058 patients following ablation showed that reduced AF burden following catheter ablation failed to predict improvement in stroke risk over a total follow-up period of 11,347 patient years.[54] However, the patients in this study may have

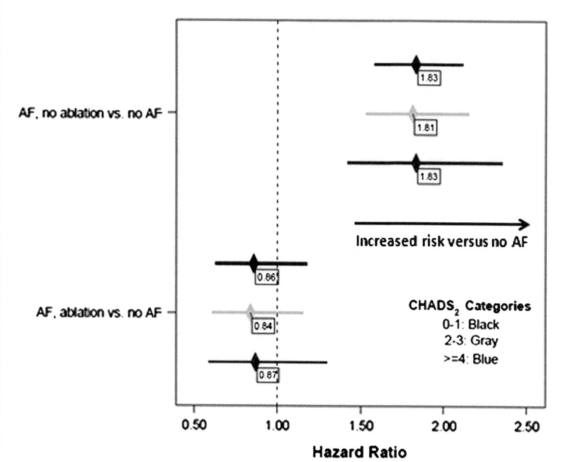

Fig. 4. Multivariate hazard ratios (HRs) for patients with AF who did not undergo ablation (top 3) and patients with AF who underwent ablation (bottom 3) versus patients with no known history of AF. An HR greater than 1.0 indicates an increased risk of stroke in patients with AF not treated with ablation. HRs are displayed by CHADS₂ risk scores. Across all categories and subcategories, HRs greater than 1.0 are noted in patients with AF ablation who did not undergo ablation versus patients with no AF. Across all categories and subcategories, HR crossed 1.0 in patients who had AF ablation versus patients with no AF. (*From* Bunch TJ, May HT, Bair TL, et al. Atrial fibrillation ablation patients have long-term stroke rates similar to patients without atrial fibrillation regardless of chads2 score. Heart Rhythm 2013;10:1276; with permission.)

represented a lower-risk cohort with nearly 75% of patients having a CHADS$_2$ (congestive heart failure, hypertension, age $\geq$ 75 years, diabetes mellitus, stroke or transient ischemic attack)[55] score of 0 or 1. This finding led to an insufficiently low stroke rate (2.3%) to show differences among the groups. Also, the groups in this study were not directly compared with patients who did not receive ablation.

Another recent study showed that 4212 patients who underwent AF ablation and were followed for at least 3 years had a significantly decreased stroke risk compared with matched controls with AF who did not undergo ablation, and were similar

to matched controls without AF.[56] This was true for patients across all CHADS$_2$ score levels in this study (**Fig. 4**). Another prior retrospective study of 2692 patients who discontinued oral anticoagulation following successful AF ablation in patients without PV stenosis or severe left atrial dysfunction showed that only 2 patients had ischemic strokes over a 2-year follow-up compared with 3 patients who remained on anticoagulation (0.07% vs 0.45%; $P = .06$).[57] No patients off anticoagulation and a CHADS$_2$ score greater than or equal to 2 had an ischemic stroke in this study. Although not compared directly with patients without ablation, this study did reveal the potential for reduced

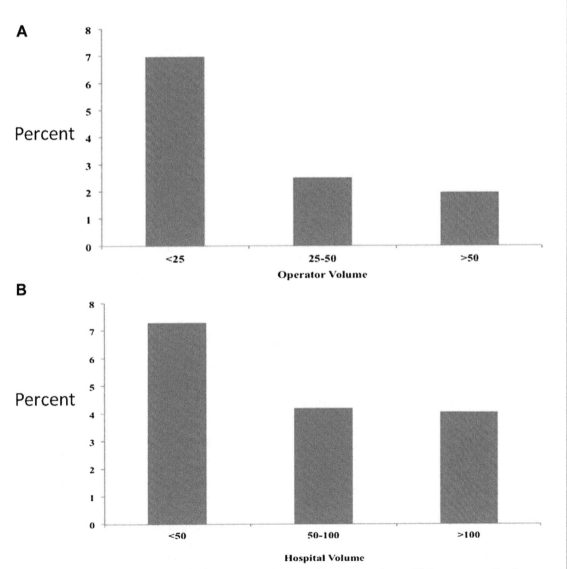

Fig. 5. (*A*) Percent complication rate for AF ablations by annual operator volume. (*B*) Percent complication rate for AF ablations by annual hospital volume. (*Adapted from* Deshmukh A, Patel NJ, Pant S, et al. In-hospital complications associated with catheter ablation of atrial fibrillation in the United States between 2000 and 2010: analysis of 93 801 procedures. Circulation 2013;128:2109, 2110; with permission.)

stroke risk following successful ablation even off anticoagulation.

Long-term, large-scale prospective studies are needed to accurately assess the degree of reduction in stroke risk following ablation. However, existing evidence suggests the potential for reduced long-term stroke risk in certain patients following ablation, and this benefit may or may not depend on complete elimination of AF. Populations that warrant specific attention include those at higher risk for stroke as well as very young patients whose cumulative duration of benefit could span several decades. Current ACC/AHA/HRS guidelines on AF management do not advocate altering anticoagulation management decisions based on outcomes of catheter ablation.[1] Choice of long-term anticoagulation should be based on stroke risk stratification scores (ie, CHA_2DS_2-VASc [congestive heart failure, hypertension, age $\geq$ 75 years, diabetes mellitus, stroke or transient ischemic attack or thromboembolism, vascular disease, age 65-64 years, sex category][58]) with closer monitoring of patients at higher risk of bleeding, identified through available bleeding risk scores (ie, HAS-BLED [hypertension [uncontrolled], abnormal renal/liver function, stroke, bleeding history or predisposition [anemia], labile international normalized ratio, elderly, drugs/alcohol concomitantly]).[59]

Mortality Benefit

A history of AF is a known risk factor for mortality (OR, 1.5; 95% confidence interval [CI], 1.2–1.8 in men; OR, 1.9; 95% CI, 1.5–2.2 in women).[60] This risk has not been shown to be decreased with the use of AAD therapy, and whether catheter ablation can decrease AF-related mortality remains to be seen. A recent retrospective single-center study showed an associated improvement in cardiovascular mortality (hazard ratio [HR], 0.41; 95% CI, 0.20–0.84)[54] following successful maintenance of sinus rhythm but no significant decrease in all-cause mortality. Prospective large-scale and long-term clinical trials such as CABANA (the Catheter Ablation versus Antiarrhythmic Drug Therapy for Atrial Fibrillation) and EAST (Early Treatment of Atrial Fibrillation for Stroke Prevention Trial) are designed to provide more definitive answers to this important question, particularly in young patients undergoing ablation.

Complications

Procedural complication rates are subject to the experience and volume of the centers and operators performing the ablations. A study published in 2010 compiled self-reported complications for 20,825 procedures performed at 521 centers from 2003 to 2006 and reported a major complication rate of 4.5%.[48] Despite the inclusion of more patients with persistent and long-standing persistent AF, larger atria, and other cardiac comorbidities, this was similar to a rate of 4.2% in a previous version of this survey published in 2005 for procedures performed between 1995 and 2002.[61] Pericardial tamponade and cerebrovascular event rates were similar over this time period at 1.22% to 1.31% and 0.94%, respectively. Important differences include the decrease in PV stenosis requiring intervention, from 0.74% to 0.29% (likely attributable to a shift from ostial to antral ablation), and the recognition of atrioesophageal fistulas in the 2010 survey (0.04% incidence, with 71% of cases leading to mortality).

A recent analysis using data from a national inpatient sample registry reported in-hospital complications among 93,801 AF ablations performed between 2000 and 2010. This registry captured events at low-volume and large-volume centers and showed a higher overall in-hospital complication rate of 6.29%. Most disturbing among these findings is an in-hospital mortality of 0.46%,[62] which is exclusive of atrioesophageal fistulas, which typically present following discharge. Complication rates were significantly affected by operator experience and annual hospital volume (**Fig. 5**), with 81% of total procedures performed by operators performing fewer than 25 AF ablations annually and in hospitals with annual volumes of fewer than 50 procedures. This finding highlights the importance of the experience necessary to safely perform this procedure.

SUMMARY

Catheter ablation continues to offer an important therapeutic option in the management of paroxysmal and persistent AF. Current management and procedural techniques are described in this article but these continue to evolve. With the continued growth in the frequency of catheter ablation for AF as well as adaptation of new technologies, a constant reevaluation of procedural outcomes and safety profiles is necessary. Although success rates have remained stable despite an increased range of patients being offered ablation, the lack of steady improvement in overall outcomes should compel clinicians to seek a more complete understanding of the pathophysiologic mechanisms of AF and continue to drive innovations to improve ablation.

However, attempts to seek technological advancements should be accompanied adherence to known standards of follow-up care. A recent European registry evaluated practice patterns in 72 centers conducting 1410 AF ablations between 2010 and 2011 without any imposed management guidelines.[63] The report identified that anticoagulation was continued at 1 year in 48% of patients with a CHA_2DS_2-VASc of 0 and discontinued in 24% of patients with a CHA_2DS_2-VASc greater than or equal to 2. AAD use was also continued in most patients despite lack of documented arrhythmia recurrence. Clinical follow-up also did not conform to recommendations, with only 78% of patients having a cardiology clinic follow-up during the 12 months following ablation. This registry highlights the importance of clinical follow-up and medical decision making beyond the time of ablation. Only with strict adherence to established standards of clinical care can the clinical benefits of catheter ablation be accurately determined in the management of AF.

REFERENCES

1. January CT, Wann LS, Alpert JS, et al. 2014 AHA/ACC/HRS guideline for the management of patients with atrial fibrillation: executive summary: a report of the American College of Cardiology/American Heart Association Task Force on Practice Guidelines and the Heart Rhythm Society. Circulation 2014. [Epub ahead of print].
2. Di Biase L, Burkhardt D, Santangeli P, et al. Periprocedural stroke and bleeding complications in patients undergoing catheter ablation of atrial fibrillation with different anticoagulation management: results from the "COMPARE" randomized trial. Circulation 2014;129(25):2638–44.
3. Latchamsetty R, Gautam S, Bhakta D, et al. Management and outcomes of cardiac tamponade during atrial fibrillation ablation in the presence of therapeutic anticoagulation with warfarin. Heart Rhythm 2011;8:805–8.
4. Lakkireddy D, Reddy YM, Di Biase L, et al. Feasibility and safety of uninterrupted rivaroxaban for periprocedural anticoagulation in patients undergoing radiofrequency ablation for atrial fibrillation: results from a multicenter prospective registry. J Am Coll Cardiol 2014;63:982–8.
5. Jalife J. Rotors and spiral waves in atrial fibrillation. J Cardiovasc Electrophysiol 2003;14:776–80.
6. Po SS, Nakagawa H, Jackman WM. Localization of left atrial ganglionated plexi in patients with atrial fibrillation. J Cardiovasc Electrophysiol 2009;20:1186–9.
7. Zipes D, Jalife J. Cardiac electrophysiology, from cell to bedside. Philadelphia: Saunders Elsevier; 2013.
8. H W. Studien über herzflimmern. I. Über die wirkung des n. Vagus und accelerans auf das flimmern des herzens. Bonn: M. Hager; 1907. p. 223–56.
9. Mines GR. On dynamic equilibrium in the heart. J Physiol 1913;46:349–83.
10. Moe GK. A conceptual model of atrial fibrillation. J Electrocardiol 1968;1:145–6.
11. Haïssaguerre M, Jaïs P, Shah DC, et al. Spontaneous initiation of atrial fibrillation by ectopic beats originating in the pulmonary veins. N Engl J Med 1998;339:659–66.
12. Oral H, Ozaydin M, Chugh A, et al. Role of the coronary sinus in maintenance of atrial fibrillation. J Cardiovasc Electrophysiol 2003;14:1329–36.
13. Kim DT, Lai AC, Hwang C, et al. The ligament of Marshall: a structural analysis in human hearts with implications for atrial arrhythmias. J Am Coll Cardiol 2000;36:1324–7.
14. Lin WS, Tai CT, Hsieh MH, et al. Catheter ablation of paroxysmal atrial fibrillation initiated by non-pulmonary vein ectopy. Circulation 2003;107:3176–83.
15. Jalife J, Berenfeld O, Mansour M. Mother rotors and fibrillatory conduction: a mechanism of atrial fibrillation. Cardiovasc Res 2002;54:204–16.
16. Kalifa J, Tanaka K, Zaitsev AV, et al. Mechanisms of wave fractionation at boundaries of high-frequency excitation in the posterior left atrium of the isolated sheep heart during atrial fibrillation. Circulation 2006;113:626–33.
17. Bettoni M, Zimmermann M. Autonomic tone variations before the onset of paroxysmal atrial fibrillation. Circulation 2002;105:2753–9.
18. Po SS, Scherlag BJ, Yamanashi WS, et al. Experimental model for paroxysmal atrial fibrillation arising at the pulmonary vein-atrial junctions. Heart Rhythm 2006;3:201–8.
19. Douglas YL, Jongbloed MR, Gittenberger-de Groot AC, et al. Histology of vascular myocardial wall of left atrial body after pulmonary venous incorporation. Am J Cardiol 2006;97:662–70.
20. Oral H, Pappone C, Chugh A, et al. Circumferential pulmonary-vein ablation for chronic atrial fibrillation. N Engl J Med 2006;354:934–41.
21. Oral H, Chugh A, Yoshida K, et al. A randomized assessment of the incremental role of ablation of complex fractionated atrial electrograms after antral pulmonary vein isolation for long-lasting persistent atrial fibrillation. J Am Coll Cardiol 2009;53:782–9.
22. Jiang RH, Po SS, Tung R, et al. Incidence of pulmonary vein conduction recovery in patients without clinical recurrence after ablation of paroxysmal atrial fibrillation: mechanistic implications. Heart Rhythm 2014;11:969–76.
23. Pappone C, Augello G, Sala S, et al. A randomized trial of circumferential pulmonary vein ablation

versus antiarrhythmic drug therapy in paroxysmal atrial fibrillation: the APAF study. J Am Coll Cardiol 2006;48:2340–7.

24. Wazni OM, Marrouche NF, Martin DO, et al. Radiofrequency ablation vs antiarrhythmic drugs as first-line treatment of symptomatic atrial fibrillation: a randomized trial. JAMA 2005;293: 2634–40.

25. Nademanee K, McKenzie J, Kosar E, et al. A new approach for catheter ablation of atrial fibrillation: mapping of the electrophysiologic substrate. J Am Coll Cardiol 2004;43:2044–53.

26. Lin J, Scherlag BJ, Zhou J, et al. Autonomic mechanism to explain complex fractionated atrial electrograms (CFAE). J Cardiovasc Electrophysiol 2007;18:1197–205.

27. Segerson NM, Daccarett M, Badger TJ, et al. Magnetic resonance imaging-confirmed ablative debulking of the left atrial posterior wall and septum for treatment of persistent atrial fibrillation: rationale and initial experience. J Cardiovasc Electrophysiol 2010;21:126–32.

28. Knecht S, Hocini M, Wright M, et al. Left atrial linear lesions are required for successful treatment of persistent atrial fibrillation. Eur Heart J 2008;29:2359–66.

29. Nishida K, Sarrazin JF, Fujiki A, et al. Roles of the left atrial roof and pulmonary veins in the anatomic substrate for persistent atrial fibrillation and ablation in a canine model. J Am Coll Cardiol 2010; 56:1728–36.

30. Hwang C, Chen PS. Ligament of Marshall: why it is important for atrial fibrillation ablation. Heart Rhythm 2009;6:S35–40.

31. Matsuo S, Wright M, Knecht S, et al. Peri-mitral atrial flutter in patients with atrial fibrillation ablation. Heart Rhythm 2010;7:2–8.

32. Zhou Q, Hou Y, Yang S. A meta-analysis of the comparative efficacy of ablation for atrial fibrillation with and without ablation of the ganglionated plexi. Pacing Clin Electrophysiol 2011;34:1687–94.

33. Atienza F, Almendral J, Jalife J, et al. Real-time dominant frequency mapping and ablation of dominant frequency sites in atrial fibrillation with left-to-right frequency gradients predicts long-term maintenance of sinus rhythm. Heart Rhythm 2009;6:33–40.

34. Lin YJ, Tsao HM, Chang SL, et al. Role of high dominant frequency sites in nonparoxysmal atrial fibrillation patients: insights from high-density frequency and fractionation mapping. Heart Rhythm 2010;7:1255–62.

35. Sanders P, Berenfeld O, Hocini M, et al. Spectral analysis identifies sites of high-frequency activity maintaining atrial fibrillation in humans. Circulation 2005;112:789–97.

36. Narayan SM, Krummen DE, Shivkumar K, et al. Treatment of atrial fibrillation by the ablation of localized sources: CONFIRM (Conventional Ablation for Atrial Fibrillation With or Without Focal Impulse and Rotor Modulation) trial. J Am Coll Cardiol 2012;60(7):628–36.

37. Narayan SM, Baykaner T, Clopton P, et al. Ablation of rotor and focal sources reduces late recurrence of atrial fibrillation compared with trigger ablation alone: extended follow-up of the CONFIRM trial (Conventional Ablation for Atrial Fibrillation With or Without Focal Impulse and Rotor Modulation). J Am Coll Cardiol 2014;63:1761–8.

38. Faustino M, Pizzi C, Capuzzi D, et al. The impact of atrial fibrillation termination mode during catheter ablation procedure on maintenance of sinus rhythm. Heart Rhythm 2014. [Epub ahead of print].

39. Schmidt M, Dorwarth U, Andresen D; et al. Cryoballoon versus RF ablation in paroxysmal atrial fibrillation: results from the German ablation registry. J Cardiovasc Electrophysiol 2014;25:1–7.

40. Kojodjojo P, O'Neill MD, Lim PB, et al. Pulmonary venous isolation by antral ablation with a large cryoballoon for treatment of paroxysmal and persistent atrial fibrillation: medium-term outcomes and non-randomised comparison with pulmonary venous isolation by radiofrequency ablation. Heart 2010; 96:1379–84.

41. Packer DL, Kowal RC, Wheelan KR, et al. Cryoballoon ablation of pulmonary veins for paroxysmal atrial fibrillation: first results of the North American Arctic Front (STOP AF) pivotal trial. J Am Coll Cardiol 2013;61:1713–23.

42. Andrade JG, Khairy P, Guerra PG, et al. Efficacy and safety of cryoballoon ablation for atrial fibrillation: a systematic review of published studies. Heart Rhythm 2011;8:1444–51.

43. Stöckigt F, Schrickel JW, Andrié R, et al. Atrioesophageal fistula after cryoballoon pulmonary vein isolation. J Cardiovasc Electrophysiol 2012;23: 1254–7.

44. Metzner A, Burchard A, Wohlmuth P, et al. Increased incidence of esophageal thermal lesions using the second-generation 28-mm cryoballoon. Circ Arrhythm Electrophysiol 2013;6:769–75.

45. Calkins H, Kuck KH, Cappato R, et al. 2012 HRS/EHRA/ECAS expert consensus statement on catheter and surgical ablation of atrial fibrillation: recommendations for patient selection, procedural techniques, patient management and follow-up, definitions, endpoints, and research trial design: a report of the Heart Rhythm Society (HRS) Task Force on Catheter and Surgical Ablation of Atrial Fibrillation. Developed in partnership with the European Heart Rhythm Association (EHRA), a registered branch of the European Society of Cardiology (ESC) and the European Cardiac Arrhythmia Society (ECAS); and in collaboration with the American College of Cardiology (ACC),

American Heart Association (AHA), the Asia Pacific Heart Rhythm Society (APHRS), and the Society of Thoracic Surgeons (STS). Endorsed by the governing bodies of the American College of Cardiology Foundation, the American Heart Association, the European Cardiac Arrhythmia Society, the European Heart Rhythm Association, the Society of Thoracic Surgeons, the Asia Pacific Heart Rhythm Society, and the Heart Rhythm Society. Heart Rhythm 2012;9:632–96.e21.

46. Jaïs P, Cauchemez B, Macle L, et al. Catheter ablation versus antiarrhythmic drugs for atrial fibrillation: the A4 study. Circulation 2008;118:2498–505.

47. Oral H, Chugh A, Good E, et al. A tailored approach to catheter ablation of paroxysmal atrial fibrillation. Circulation 2006;113:1824–31.

48. Cappato R, Calkins H, Chen SA, et al. Updated worldwide survey on the methods, efficacy, and safety of catheter ablation for human atrial fibrillation. Circ Arrhythm Electrophysiol 2010;3:32–8.

49. Brooks AG, Stiles MK, Laborderie J, et al. Outcomes of long-standing persistent atrial fibrillation ablation: a systematic review. Heart Rhythm 2010; 7:835–46.

50. Latchamsetty R, Morady F. Long-term benefits following catheter ablation of atrial fibrillation. Circ J 2013;77:1091–6.

51. Ouyang F, Tilz R, Chun J, et al. Long-term results of catheter ablation in paroxysmal atrial fibrillation: lessons from a 5-year follow-up. Circulation 2010; 122:2368–77.

52. Medi C, Sparks PB, Morton JB, et al. Pulmonary vein antral isolation for paroxysmal atrial fibrillation: results from long-term follow-up. J Cardiovasc Electrophysiol 2011;22:137–41.

53. Benjamin EJ, Wolf PA, D'Agostino RB, et al. Impact of atrial fibrillation on the risk of death: the Framingham Heart Study. Circulation 1998;98:946–52.

54. Ghanbari H, Baser K, Jongnarangsin K, et al. Mortality and cerebrovascular events after radiofrequency catheter ablation of atrial fibrillation. Heart Rhythm 2014. [Epub ahead of print].

55. Gage BF, Waterman AD, Shannon W, et al. Validation of clinical classification schemes for predicting stroke: results from the National Registry of Atrial Fibrillation. JAMA 2001;285:2864–70.

56. Bunch TJ, May HT, Bair TL, et al. Atrial fibrillation ablation patients have long-term stroke rates similar to patients without atrial fibrillation regardless of CHADS2 score. Heart Rhythm 2013;10: 1272–7.

57. Themistoclakis S, Corrado A, Marchlinski FE, et al. The risk of thromboembolism and need for oral anticoagulation after successful atrial fibrillation ablation. J Am Coll Cardiol 2010;55:735–43.

58. Lip GY, Nieuwlaat R, Pisters R, et al. Refining clinical risk stratification for predicting stroke and thromboembolism in atrial fibrillation using a novel risk factor-based approach: the Euro Heart Survey on Atrial Fibrillation. Chest 2010;137:263–72.

59. Pisters R, Lane DA, Nieuwlaat R, et al. A novel user-friendly score (HAS-BLED) to assess 1-year risk of major bleeding in patients with atrial fibrillation: the Euro Heart Survey. Chest 2010;138:1093–100.

60. Roger VL, Go AS, Lloyd-Jones DM, et al. Heart disease and stroke statistics–2012 update: a report from the American Heart Association. Circulation 2012;125:e2–220.

61. Cappato R, Calkins H, Chen SA, et al. Worldwide survey on the methods, efficacy, and safety of catheter ablation for human atrial fibrillation. Circulation 2005;111:1100–5.

62. Deshmukh A, Patel NJ, Pant S, et al. In-hospital complications associated with catheter ablation of atrial fibrillation in the united states between 2000 and 2010: analysis of 93 801 procedures. Circulation 2013;128:2104–12.

63. Arbelo E, Brugada J, Hindricks G, et al, Atrial Fibrillation Ablation Pilot Study Investigators. The Atrial Fibrillation Ablation Pilot Study: a European survey on methodology and results of catheter ablation for atrial fibrillation conducted by the European Heart Rhythm Association. Eur Heart J 2014;35(22): 1466–78.

Surgery for Atrial Fibrillation

Christopher P. Lawrance, MD, Matthew C. Henn, MD, Ralph J. Damiano Jr, MD*

KEYWORDS

- Cox-Maze • Atrial fibrillation • Surgical ablation • Minimally invasive

KEY POINTS

- The Cox-Maze procedure is the current gold standard in the surgical ablation of atrial fibrillation.
- Failure to isolate the entire posterior left atrium and the pulmonary veins greatly increases atrial fibrillation recurrence.
- Advances in minimally invasive techniques and technologies have allowed for a less-invasive Cox-Maze procedure to be performed through a right mini thoracotomy.

INTRODUCTION

Atrial fibrillation (AF) remains the most common arrhythmia, affecting more than 5 million people in the United States alone. With the aging population, the prevalence of AF has increased over the last decade and is expected to double by the year 2030.[1] Despite advances in treatment, AF still carries significant morbidity and mortality that stem from 2 major mechanisms: (1) asynchronous atrioventricular contractions, which result in varying degrees of hemodynamic compromise, and (2) stasis of blood in the atria that predisposes patients to clotting and subsequent thromboemboli.[2] The risk of stroke in patients with AF is increased by as much as 5-fold.[3] Most AF patients require anticoagulation, and despite the introduction of direct factor Xa inhibitors, anticoagulation predisposes to other major morbidities including gastrointestinal bleeding and hemorrhagic stroke.[4]

The treatment of AF represents a significant economic burden, with an estimated $26 billion spent annually in the United States.[5] Antiarrhythmic medications have been the mainstay of treatment for nearly 100 years, but their use has been limited by systemic toxicity, low efficacy, and arrhythmogenicity.[6] Pharmacotherapy is routinely directed at either controlling the patient's rhythm or ventricular rate. The Atrial Fibrillation Follow-up Investigation of Rhythm Management (AFFIRM) study found that management with rhythm control had no survival benefit over rate control in anticoagulated patients[7]; however, there was a clear survival benefit for patients that were able to achieve normal sinus rhythm.[8] The pharmacologic inadequacies of treating atrial fibrillation have justified a role for interventional management of atrial fibrillation.

Starting in the 1980s, several procedures were developed in an effort to treat atrial fibrillation, including left atrial isolation,[9] corridor operation,[10] and atrial transection.[11] However, these procedures were abandoned because of their inability to reliably prevent or cure atrial fibrillation in humans. It was not until 1987 that a team led by Dr James Cox devised the Maze procedure, now known as the Cox-Maze Procedure, which reliably and successfully treated AF.[11] This review discusses the indications for surgical ablation of AF

This article originally appeared in Cardiology Clinics, Volume 32, Issue 4, November 2014.

Disclosure of Funding: Support in part by National Institutes of Health grants R01 HL032257 and T32 HL007776. R.J. Damiano is a consultant for AtriCure and receives grant support from Edwards. All other authors have no disclosures.

Division of Cardiothoracic Surgery, Barnes-Jewish Hospital, Washington University School of Medicine, 660 South Euclid Avenue, Campus Box 8234, St Louis, MO 63110, USA

* Corresponding author.

E-mail address: damianor@wustl.edu

1551-7136/16/$ – see front matter © 2016 Elsevier Inc. All rights reserved.

and the technique and results of the Cox-Maze IV (CMIV) procedure.

INDICATIONS FOR SURGICAL ABLATION OF ATRIAL FIBRILLATION

In 2007, a task force that included the Society of Thoracic Surgeons, American College of Cardiology, Heart Rhythm Society, European Heart Rhythm Association, and European Cardiac Arrhythmia Society was established to create a consensus statement on AF surgical and catheter-based treatment.[12] Over the last several years, a large volume of literature has evaluated the efficacy and safety of not only catheter-based ablation but also surgical ablation. Also, the advent of ablation technology has allowed for greater flexibility of the surgical approach and has expanded the indications, particularly for concomitant AF procedures, in patients undergoing other cardiac surgery.

The task force reconvened in 2012 and released the consensus indications for surgical ablation divided into 2 separate categories: those patients undergoing concomitant cardiac surgery and those having stand-alone surgical treatment of their AF.[13] For those undergoing other cardiac surgical procedures, all patients with symptomatic atrial fibrillation should be considered for surgical ablation, regardless of whether antiarrhythmic medications have been started. Ablation should also be considered in selected asymptomatic patients in whom adding an ablation procedure would not add to operative morbidity or mortality. However, stand-alone surgical ablation is generally indicated in patients with symptomatic AF who do not respond to medical therapy and have had one or more failed catheter ablations or prefer surgical therapy.[13]

SURGICAL TECHNIQUE: COX-MAZE IV PROCEDURE
Preoperative Planning

To simplify the CMIII, our group at Washington University replaced most of the cut-and-sew lesions that comprised the CMIII with a combination of bipolar radiofrequency ablation and cryoablation and have termed the revision the *CMIV*. All patients receive a transthoracic echocardiogram to determine left atrial (LA) LA size and the presence of valvular disease. LA size in particular is important because LA diameter is a strong predictor of procedural success, with a diameter of ≥8 cm associated with a failure rate of greater than 50%.[14] Although transthoracic echocardiogram also can be used to evaluate for the presence of LA clot, this finding needs to be confirmed intraoperatively with transesophageal echocardiography. In patients do not respond to catheter ablation, a contrast chest computed tomography scan is obtained to evaluate the pulmonary veins.

This procedure can be performed through either a sternotomy or a less-invasive right mini thoracotomy (RMT). Our group prefers an RMT approach in the absence of contraindications, which include previous right thoracotomy, severe atherosclerotic disease of the aorta, iliac or femoral vessels, and severely decreased left ventricular ejection fraction (≤20%). All patients scheduled to have an RMT receive a computed tomography angiogram of the thoracic and abdominal aorta as well as the femoral arteries if they are older than 40 years, have risk factors for the development of peripheral vascular disease, or have demonstrate evidence of peripheral vascular disease on physical examination. An RMT approach can be used in patients receiving a concomitant mitral or tricuspid valve procedure. Other concomitant procedures, such as aortic valve replacement, are performed through a sternotomy approach.

Positioning

Positioning is dependent on the approach being used. In a sternotomy approach, patients are placed supine with both arms tucked. In an RMT procedure, the patient is intubated using a bronchial blocker placed in the right main stem bronchus allowing for right lung deflation. The patient is then placed supine with the hips flat but the right chest elevated 30° to 45°. The right arm is placed over the head in anatomic position with the aid of an arm board, and the left arm is tucked. Both groins are prepped with antiseptic solution in the RMT approach in preparation for femoral cannulation (**Fig. 1**).

Operative Technique

There are several important differences between the sternotomy and RMT approaches. An outline of each approach and its lesions sets are listed below followed by a description of the key operative steps. Each RF ablation line is created by performing 2 to 3 firings of the bipolar RF clamp. This is done to assure a transmural lesion.[15]

Sternotomy approach

- Median sternotomy, central cannulation of superior vena cava (SVC), inferior vena cava (IVC), and aorta and initiation of cardiopulmonary bypass (CPB)
- Right and left pulmonary vein isolation (PVI)
- Right atrial (RA) lesion set (**Figs. 2**A and **3**)

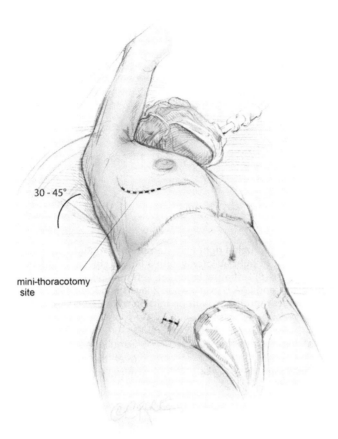

Fig. 1. Positioning for right mini thoracotomy approach. (Images reproduced with permission from Bioperspective.)

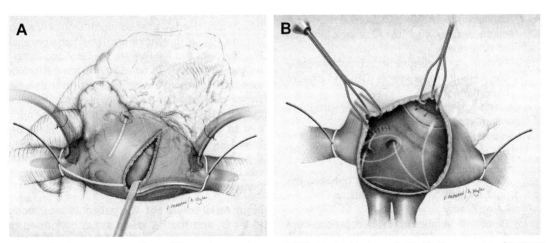

Fig. 2. CMIV lesion set as performed through a sternotomy. (*A*) Right atrial lesion set. RF ablations consist of SVC/IVC ablation and RA free wall ablation. Cryoablations include linear cryoablations through a purse-string suture to the 10'oclock position of the tricuspid valve annulus and through the superior aspect of the atriotomy to the 2'oclock position of tricuspid valve annulus. (*B*) Left atrial lesion set. Bipolar RF ablation lines consist of bilateral pulmonary vein isolations, ablations between the left superior pulmonary vein and amputated atrial appendage, pulmonary vein roof and floor connecting ablations, and ablation between the inferior aspect of the atriotomy to mitral valve annulus. Cryoablations include linear epicardial cryoablation over the coronary sinus and at the mitral valve annulus.

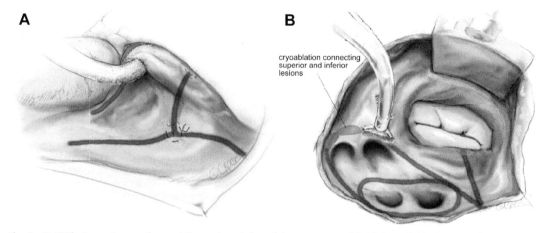

A

B

cryoablation connecting
superior and inferior
lesions

Fig. 3. CMIV lesion set as performed through a right mini sternotomy. (*A*) Right atrial lesion set. Three separate purse-string sutures and replacement of right atriotomy with a line of bipolar RF ablation. All other lesions are identical to the sternotomy approach. (*B*) Left atrial lesion set. Left pulmonary vein isolation is achieved through sequential endocardial cryoablation, and LAA is oversewn in 2 layers endocardially. All other lesion are identical to the sternotomy approach. (Images reproduced with permission from Bioperspective.)

- ○ Purse-string suture at the base of the RA appendage
- ○ Bipolar RF ablation line through this purse-string suture toward SVC on the aortic side of the appendage
- ○ Right vertical atriotomy
- ○ Bipolar RF ablation lines from the inferior aspect of the atriotomy up to the SVC and down to the IVC
- ○ Linear endocardial cryoablation from superior aspect of atriotomy to 2'oclock position of the tricuspid valve (TV) annulus
- ○ Linear endocardial cryoablation from RA purse-string suture to 10'oclock position of TV annulus
- ○ Placement of retrograde cardioplegia catheter in the coronary sinus (CS) and closure of right atriotomy
- • Cardioplegic arrest with antegrade/retrograde cardioplegia
- • Left atrial (LA) lesion set (see **Fig. 2**B)
  - ○ LA appendage amputation and bipolar RF ablation to left superior PV
  - ○ Mark CS with methylene blue between the right and left coronary circulations
  - ○ LA atriotomy
  - ○ Bipolar RF ablation connecting lesions from the inferior aspect of the atriotomy into the left inferior PV and from the superior aspect of the atriotomy into the superior PV
  - ○ Bipolar RF ablation from inferior aspect of atriotomy toward mitral valve (MV) annulus and across the CS
  - ○ Endocardial cryoablation to connect the end of this bipolar RF ablation to the MV annulus
  - ○ Simultaneous epicardial linear cryoablation over the coronary sinus to complete the mitral isthmus ablation

Pulmonary Vein Isolation Intraoperatively, the absence of LA clot is confirmed with transesophageal echo in all patients. A median sternotomy is performed and cardiopulmonary bypass is initiated. Both the right and left PVs are bluntly dissected after the initiation of normothermic CPB. If a patient happens to be in AF at the time of the surgery and there is no LA clot, they are electrically cardioverted after administration of IV amiodarone. Pacing thresholds are measured from each PV. The right and left PVs are then isolated using a bipolar RF clamp. Three ablations are performed for each lesion, and the clamp is moved slightly between each ablation to ensure electrical isolation between the PVs and the rest of the LA. It is important to clamp a generous cuff of atrial tissue between the jaws of bipolar RF clamp to complete the PVI. Isolation is confirmed by documenting exit block demonstrated by a failure to epicardially pace from each of the pulmonary veins.

Right Atrial Lesion Set The patient is then cooled to 34°C, and the RA lesion set is performed on the beating heart (see **Fig. 2**A). A small purse-string suture is placed at the base of the RA appendage, wide enough to accommodate one jaw of the bipolar RF ablation clamp. An ablation lesion is created with the bipolar clamp across the free wall of the RA down toward the SVC on the aortic side of the right atrial appendage. A vertical atriotomy then is made from the intra-atrial septum up toward the AV groove near the free margin of the heart. This incision should be at least 2 cm from the first free wall ablation to avoid an area of slow conduction. A linear cryoprobe is used to create an endocardial cryoablation from the superior aspect of this incision down to the tricuspid annulus at the 2'oclock position. All cryoablations are performed for 3 minutes at a temperature less than 40°C. Cryoablation is ideal to complete lesions over annular tissues because it preserves the fibrous skeleton of the heart, therefore, maintaining valve competency. The linear cryoprobe is then inserted through the previously placed purse-string suture, and an endocardial cryoablation is created down to the tricuspid valve annulus at the 10'oclock position. The RF ablation clamp is used to create ablation lines running from the inferior aspect of the right atriotomy up along the lateral aspect of the SVC and down to the IVC.

Left Atrial Lesion Set At this point, the LA lesion set is performed (see **Fig. 2**B). The aorta is cross-clamped, and the heart is arrested using cold blood cardioplegia. The heart is retracted, and the LA appendage (LAA) is amputated. Through the amputated LAA, the bipolar RF clamp is used to create an ablation line to either of the left PVs. The LAA is oversewn in 2 layers with a 4-0 Prolene suture. The CS is marked with methylene blue at a position between the posterior descending artery and the terminal branch of the circumflex artery. A standard left atriotomy is performed connecting to the previous right pulmonary vein isolation. The entire posterior left atrium is then isolated by using the bipolar RF ablation clamp. The first ablation line is placed from the inferior aspect of the atriotomy across the floor of the LA into the left inferior PV. A second ablation line is created from the superior aspect of the atriotomy across the roof of the LA into the left superior PV. A final bipolar RF ablation is placed from the inferior aspect of the atriotomy, across the atrial floor of the LA, toward the mitral valve annulus. This ablation is aimed toward the P2 scallop of the posterior mitral leaflet in most patients who have a right dominant circulation and should cross the coronary sinus at the area previously marked with methylene blue. An endocardial cryoablation is then performed to connect this ablation line to the mitral valve annulus at the end of the mitral isthmus lesion. To complete the LA isthmus ablation, a simultaneous epicardial cryoablation is performed over the coronary sinus in line with the endocardial lesion.

Right mini-thoracotomy approach

Right Mini-Thoracotomy Approach Outline
- Subinguinal incision and femoral cannulation
- A 5- to 6-mm RMT at fourth intercostal space
- Initiation of CPB
  - Right lung deflation
  - Insertion of 5-mm port in posterior-axillary line at the sixth intercostal space for 30° endoscope
- Right PVI
  - Right PVI using bipolar RF clamp. Three ablations are recommended.
  - Pacing is used to document exit block from each of the right PVs
- RA lesion set
  - RA purse-string #1 between SVC/IVC; bipolar RF ablation lines are made up to SVC and down to IVC
  - The bipolar RF clamp is placed through purse-string #1 to create an ablation line up the RA free wall toward the AV groove, approximately at the free margin of the heart.
  - RA purse-string #2 is placed at the superior aspect of this free wall bipolar RF ablation
  - A linear endocardial cryoablation through purse-string #2 down to the 2 o'clock position of TV annulus
  - RA purse-string #3 at base of RA appendage, bipolar RF ablation of RA free wall toward SVC along the aortic side of the RA appendage
  - A second linear endocardial cryoablation through purse-string #3 down to the 10 o'clock position of TV annulus
- Aortic cross-clamp placed through right lateral chest wall
  - Antegrade cardioplegia needle in the proximal ascending aorta
  - Cold anterograde cardioplegic arrest
- LA lesion set
  - Right anterior chest wall stab incision for placement of left atrial lift system through fourth intercostal space
  - Left atriotomy and placement of left atrial lift system
  - Endocardial LA appendage closure
  - Bipolar RF ablation connecting lesions from the inferior aspect of the atriotomy into the left inferior PV and from the superior aspect of the atriotomy into the superior PV
  - Endocardial cryoablation to connect these to ablation lines going behind the left PVs, isolating the entire posterior LA.
  - Bipolar RF ablation from inferior aspect of atriotomy toward MV annulus and across the CS
  - Endocardial cryoablation to connect the end of this bipolar RF ablation to the MV annulus
  - Simultaneous epicardial linear cryoablation over the coronary sinus to complete the mitral isthmus ablation

A video and illustrated description of our RMT approach was published previously.[16,17] Although there are several obvious differences between the sternotomy and RMT approaches, the lesion set in the RMT approach remains the same. Initial differences between these approaches are establishment of femoral cannulation for CPB under transesophageal echo guidance and the need to deflate the right lung to facilitate a minimally invasive exposure. The RA lesion set has been modified with replacement of the atriotomy with a line of bipolar RF ablation while the other RA lesions are performed through 3 separate purse-string sutures. The LA lesion set is identical with 2 exceptions. Left pulmonary vein isolation is achieved by sequential endocardial cryoablation connecting the superior and inferior connecting box lesions behind the left pulmonary veins usually along the lateral ridge, because epicardial isolation of the left pulmonary veins is difficult through a right mini thoracotomy. Lastly, exclusion of the LAA in the RMT approach is achieved by oversewing endocardially in 2 layers as opposed to epicardial amputation, which is performed in the sternotomy approach.

PERIOPERATIVE AND POSTOPERATIVE MANAGEMENT

Perioperative management is similar for both approaches. Considerations unique to the CMIV procedure include postoperative arrhythmias, including junctional and atrial tachyarrhythmias (ATAs). Epicardial pacing wires that are left on the RA and right ventricle at the end of the procedure are used to pace the atria at 80 to 100 beats per minute. The atrial wires are helpful in diagnosing atrial arrhythmias, because the p wave can be small and difficult to see after a CM procedure. If heart block develops, AV sequential pacing (DDD mode) is used. Junctional rhythms, which are present in most patients postoperatively, usually resolve without intervention after several days. Antiarrhythmic medications should not be started until the patients develop sinus rhythm, particularly in patients with bradyarrhythmias. Approximately 5% of patients will fail to recover sinus rhythm and require a permanent pacemaker after a CMIV procedure and the incidence of pacemaker implantation increases with patient age.[18] Approximately half of patients will have ATAs postoperatively, which usually resolve after the first postoperative month. Patients with stable ATAs are usually rate controlled pharmacologically and are DC cardioverted if ATAs persist. It is best to wait 1 to 3 weeks after surgery before cardioversion, if possible, to allow the inflammation to subside.

The final consideration is the initiation of anticoagulation. Warfarin is started postoperatively in all patients receiving a CMIV procedure and is continued for at least 3 months postoperatively in the absence of contraindications. If, after a 3-month blanking period the patient has no ATAs off antiarrhythmic medications on prolonged monitoring (at least a 24-hour Holter) and shows no atrial stasis on echocardiography, we recommend the discontinuation of warfarin.[19] Using this approach, we have had a low stroke risk after the CM procedure even in patients with high CHADS$_2$ scores.

SURGICAL RESULTS: CMPIV

The CMP has long been considered the gold standard in surgical ablation and continues to be the interventional procedure with the single highest success rate of terminating ATA. There are several studies documenting the long-term efficacy of the CMPIII. One study from our own institution looked at the results of 187 patients who received the CMPIII. This study showed a 97% freedom from symptomatic AF at 5.4 years. This same study showed no difference in recurrence when comparing patients who received a stand-alone CMPIII versus patients who received a concomitant procedure.[20]

The excellent long-term efficacy of the CMPIV has also been reported. Our group prospectively followed 100 patients who received a lone CMPIV procedure. Follow-up was scheduled at 3-, 6-, and 12-month intervals and annually thereafter. Most patients were evaluated with 24-hour Holter monitoring and, when not available, an electrocardiogram. Patients were considered to have late recurrence if there was any episode of AF, atrial flutter, or atrial tachycardia lasting longer than 30 seconds. The mean follow-up time was 17 ± 10 months. Thirty-one percent of patients had paroxysmal AF, 6% had persistent AF, and 63% had longstanding persistent AF. This study found that at both 12 and 24 months, 90% of patients were free from ATAs, whereas 82% were free from ATAs and off antiarrhythmic medications.[21] In a separate study, this same group was then retrospectively compared with 112 patients who had a lone CMPIII procedure from 1992 to 2002. In the CMPIII group, late recurrence was determined by measuring only symptomatic AF at follow-up, which likely overestimated the procedure's success. This comparison showed no difference in freedom from AF off antiarrhythmic medications between the CMPIII group and CMPIV group (83% vs 82%).[22]

The CMIV procedure was also found to be advantageous in the perioperative setting when compared with the CMPIII. Mean aortic cross-clamp times were significantly decreased with a lone CMPIV compared with a lone CMPIII (39 minutes vs 90 minutes). Mean concomitant cross-clamp times are also found to be shorter when comparing the CMPIV with the CMPIII (99 ± 30 minutes vs 122 ± 37 minutes).[20,23] In addition, the CMPIV does have a significantly lower major complication rate compared with the CMPIII. In our previous series comparing the CMPIII with the CMPIV, major complication was defined as reoperation for bleeding, early stroke, renal failure, mediastinitis, and need for intra-aortic balloon pump (10% vs 1%).[22] There were no differences in 3-month pacemaker implantation rate or 30-day mortality rate when comparing both versions of the procedure, which were 7% to 8% and 1% to 2%, respectively.[22]

Originally, the CMPIV lacked a posterior left atrial box lesion set, which was used in 2005. Before this, only a single connecting lesion was used between the left and right inferior pulmonary veins. This was because there was initially concern that complete electrical exclusion of the entire posterior LA might have a detrimental effect on LA function. This thought has since been disproven with aid of cardiac magnetic resonance imaging showing LA function is maintained with the addition of a box lesion.[24] However, studies from our group comparing 78 patients who had a true box lesion set with 22 patients without, showed an increase in freedom from AF off antiarrhythmic medications (85% vs 47%) at greater than 1 year follow-up.[21] Because of this, all CMPIV at our institution now use the full box lesion.

Atrial fibrillation is frequently coincident with other cardiac disease processes including coronary artery disease and valvular disease. The development of new ablation technologies associated with the CMIV took a technically difficult and time-consuming operation and made it easy for all cardiac surgeons to perform. Whereas few patients (<1%) with AF undergoing cardiac surgery before 2000 underwent a concomitant CMP, a study has shown that more than 40% of patients with AF undergoing cardiac surgery had a concomitant ablation procedure in 2006.[25] More recent studies have found similar CMIV outcomes in patients with lone AF compared with receiving concomitant mitral procedures.[26] Specifically, freedom from AF and antiarrhythmic drugs at 12 and 24 months were nearly identical between the 2 groups (73% vs 76% at 12 months; 77% vs 78% at 24 months).[27]

Although there are reports of less-invasive surgical ablation approaches, few groups have evaluated the long-term outcomes using these approaches. Our group has developed a minimally invasive approach to the CMIV using a right mini thoracotomy (RMT) approach. Early results using this approach have been promising when compared with the CMIV performed through a sternotomy.[28] More recent unpublished data have shown freedom from AF off antiarrhythmic drugs was not significantly different between the 2 groups 1 and 2 years postoperatively. Furthermore, patients who underwent RMT had fewer complications, and both decreased intensive care unit and hospital lengths of stay when compared with those patients who underwent a CMIV through a sternotomy. These results show that the CMIV performed through an RMT approach is as effective as sternotomy in the treatment of atrial fibrillation.

Risk factors for recurrence after performing a CMIV procedure at 1 year include (1) failure to perform a box lesion, (2) increasing left atrial size, and (3) early ATAs.[14] As discussed earlier, our group found previously that a full left atrial isolation via a box lesion significantly reduced the recurrence of AF. This finding is in agreement with data from the electrophysiology laboratory, which showed that a wide area circumferential ablation involving a large portion of the posterior left atrium is more effective than pulmonary vein isolation alone.[13,29,30] Increased left atrial size was found by multiple groups to be a significant risk factor for recurrence, with a probability of recurrence exceeding 50% once the left atrium approaches 8 cm.[14,31–33] Finally, early ATAs was found previously by our group to be a risk factor for recurrence.[14] It is likely that early ATAs are likely a marker of more advanced pathology within the atrial substrate itself; therefore, it would make sense that these patients would be more likely to have a late AF recurrence.

SUMMARY

The surgical treatment of atrial fibrillation has undergone many evolutions. The CMPIV helped solve some of the limitations of the CMPIII. With the use of ablation technology to replace the surgical incisions, similar cure rates have been achieved despite more stringent follow-up criteria. Because of advances in minimally invasive technologies, the CMIV operation can now be performed through a less-invasive RMT approach in properly selected patients, resulting in a shorter hospital stay with equivalent 2-year outcomes. As the mechanisms for AF are better understood and technology continues to improve, surgical treatments will likely become less invasive with improved cure rates as procedures are tailored to patient-specific pathology.

REFERENCES

1. Colilla S, Crow A, Petkun W, et al. Estimates of current and future incidence and prevalence of atrial

fibrillation in the U.S. Adult population. Am J Cardiol 2013;112(8):1142–7.

2. Badheka AO, Rathod A, Kizilbash MA, et al. Comparison of mortality and morbidity in patients with atrial fibrillation and heart failure with preserved versus decreased left ventricular ejection fraction. Am J Cardiol 2011;108:1283–8.

3. Wolf PA, Abbott RD, Kannel WB. Atrial fibrillation as an independent risk factor for stroke: the framingham study. Stroke 1991;22:983–8.

4. Mitchell SA, Simon TA, Raza S, et al. The efficacy and safety of oral anticoagulants in warfarin-suitable patients with nonvalvular atrial fibrillation: systematic review and meta-analysis. Clin Appl Thromb Hemost 2013;19(6):619–31.

5. Kim MH, Johnston SS, Chu BC, et al. Estimation of total incremental health care costs in patients with atrial fibrillation in the united states. Circulation 2011;4:313–20.

6. Zimetbaum P. Antiarrhythmic drug therapy for atrial fibrillation. Circulation 2012;125:381–9.

7. Wyse DG, Waldo AL, DiMarco JP, et al, Atrial Fibrillation Follow-up Investigation of Rhythm Management (AFFIRM) Investigators. A comparison of rate control and rhythm control in patients with atrial fibrillation. N Engl J Med 2002;347:1825–33.

8. Corley SD, Epstein AE, DiMarco JP, et al, AFFIRM Investigators. Relationships between sinus rhythm, treatment, and survival in the atrial fibrillation follow-up investigation of rhythm management (affirm) study. Circulation 2004;109:1509–13.

9. Williams JM, Ungerleider RM, Lofland GK, et al. Left atrial isolation: new technique for the treatment of supraventricular arrhythmias. J Thorac Cardiovasc Surg 1980;80:373–80.

10. Defauw JJ, Guiraudon GM, van Hemel NM, et al. Surgical therapy of paroxysmal atrial fibrillation with the "corridor" operation. Ann Thorac Surg 1992;53:564–70 [discussion: 571].

11. Cox JL. The surgical treatment of atrial fibrillation. IV. Surgical technique. J Thorac Cardiovasc Surg 1991; 101:584–92.

12. European Heart Rhythm Association (EHRA), European Cardiac Arrhythmia Society (ECAS), American College of Cardiology (ACC), et al. HRS/EHRA/ECAS expert consensus statement on catheter and surgical ablation of atrial fibrillation: recommendations for personnel, policy, procedures and follow-up. A report of the heart rhythm society (HRS) task force on catheter and surgical ablation of atrial fibrillation. Heart Rhythm 2007;4:816–61.

13. Calkins H, Kuck KH, Cappato R, et al, Heart Rhythm Society Task Force on Catheter and Surgical Ablation of Atrial Fibrillation. 2012 HRS/EHRA/ECAS expert consensus statement on catheter and surgical ablation of atrial fibrillation: recommendations for patient selection, procedural techniques, patient management and follow-up, definitions, endpoints, and research trial design: a report of the Heart Rhythm Society (HRS) task force on catheter and surgical ablation of atrial fibrillation. Developed in partnership with the European Heart Rhythm Association (EHRA), a registered branch of the European Society of Cardiology (ESC) and the European Cardiac Arrhythmia Society (ECAS); and in collaboration with the american College of Cardiology (ACC), American Heart Association (AHA), the Asia Pacific Heart Rhythm Society (APHRS), and the Society of Thoracic Surgeons (STS). Endorsed by the governing bodies of the American College of Cardiology foundation, the American Heart Association, the European Cardiac Arrhythmia Society, the European Heart Rhythm Association, the Society of Thoracic Surgeons, the Asia Pacific Heart Rhythm Society, and the Heart Rhythm Society. Heart Rhythm 2012;9:632–96.e21.

14. Damiano RJ Jr, Schwartz FH, Bailey MS, et al. The cox maze iv procedure: predictors of late recurrence. J Thorac Cardiovasc Surg 2011;141:113–21.

15. Voeller RK, Zierer A, Schuessler RB, et al. Performance of a novel dual-electrode bipolar radiofrequency ablation device: a chronic porcine study. Innovations (Phila) 2011;6:17–22.

16. Saint LL, Lawrance CP, Leidenfrost JE, et al. How I do it: minimally invasive Cox-Maze IV procedure. Ann Cardiothorac Surg 2014;3:117–9.

17. Robertson JO, Saint LL, Leidenfrost JE, et al. Illustrated techniques for performing the cox-maze iv procedure through a right mini-thoracotomy. Ann Cardiothorac Surg 2014;3:105–16.

18. Robertson JO, Cuculich PS, Saint LL, et al. Predictors and risk of pacemaker implantation after the cox-maze iv procedure. Ann Thorac Surg 2013;95: 2015–20 [disussion: 2020–1].

19. Pet M, Robertson JO, Bailey M, et al. The impact of chads2 score on late stroke after the cox maze procedure. J Thorac Cardiovasc Surg 2013;146:85–9.

20. Prasad SM, Maniar HS, Camillo CJ, et al. The cox maze III procedure for atrial fibrillation: long-term efficacy in patients undergoing lone versus concomitant procedures. J Thorac Cardiovasc Surg 2003; 126:1822–8.

21. Weimar T, Bailey MS, Watanabe Y, et al. The cox-maze iv procedure for lone atrial fibrillation: a single center experience in 100 consecutive patients. J Interv Card Electrophysiol 2011;31:47–54.

22. Weimar T, Schena S, Bailey MS, et al. The cox-maze procedure for lone atrial fibrillation: a single-center experience over 2 decades. Circ Arrhythm Electrophysiol 2012;5:8–14.

23. Rosenberg MA, Samuel M, Thosani A, et al. Use of a noninvasive continuous monitoring device in the management of atrial fibrillation: a pilot study. Pacing Clin Electrophysiol 2013;36:328–33.

24. Voeller RK, Zierer A, Lall SC, et al. The effects of the cox maze procedure on atrial function. J Thorac Cardiovasc Surg 2008;136:1257–64, 1264.e1–3.

25. Gammie JS, Haddad M, Milford-Beland S, et al. Atrial fibrillation correction surgery: lessons from the society of thoracic surgeons national cardiac database. Ann Thorac Surg 2008;85:909–14.

26. Saint LL, Bailey MS, Prasad S, et al. Cox-Maze IV results for patients with lone atrial fibrillation versus concomitant mitral disease. Ann Thorac Surg 2012; 93:789–94 [discussion: 794–5].

27. Lawrance CP, Henn MC, Miller JR, et al. Comparison of the stand-alone cox-maze iv procedure to the concomitant cox-maze iv and mitral valve procedure for atrial fibrillation. Ann Cardiothorac Surg 2014;3:55–61.

28. Lee AM, Clark K, Bailey MS, et al. A minimally invasive cox-maze procedure: operative technique and results. Innovations (Phila) 2010;5:281–6.

29. Oral H, Scharf C, Chugh A, et al. Catheter ablation for paroxysmal atrial fibrillation: segmental pulmonary vein ostial ablation versus left atrial ablation. Circulation 2003;108:2355–60.

30. Pappone C, Oreto G, Rosanio S, et al. Atrial electroanatomic remodeling after circumferential radiofrequency pulmonary vein ablation: efficacy of an anatomic approach in a large cohort of patients with atrial fibrillation. Circulation 2001;104: 2539–44.

31. Kamata J, Kawazoe K, Izumoto H, et al. Predictors of sinus rhythm restoration after cox maze procedure concomitant with other cardiac operations. Ann Thorac Surg 1997;64:394–8.

32. Kobayashi J, Kosakai Y, Nakano K, et al. Improved success rate of the maze procedure in mitral valve disease by new criteria for patients' selection. Eur J Cardiothorac Surg 1998;13:247–52.

33. Gillinov AM, Sirak J, Blackstone EH, et al. The cox maze procedure in mitral valve disease: predictors of recurrent atrial fibrillation. J Thorac Cardiovasc Surg 2005;130:1653–60.

Atrioventricular Junction Ablation for Atrial Fibrillation

Dilesh Patel, MD[a], Emile G. Daoud, MD, FHRS[a,b,*]

KEYWORDS

- Atrioventricular junction • Atrioventricular node • Ablation • Ablate and pace • Rate control
- Atrial fibrillation

KEY POINTS

- Atrioventricular junction (AVJ) ablation and pacing therapy is a safe and effective method to control heart rate in patients with atrial fibrillation and rapid ventricular rates who have failed other therapies.
- AVJ ablation and pacing strategy is associated with improvement in symptoms, quality of life, and exercise capacity.
- After AVJ ablation and pacing, improvement in ejection fraction can be seen in patients with tachycardia-associated cardiomyopathy.
- Biventricular pacing systems should be implanted in patients undergoing AVJ ablation who have reduced cardiac function.
- Mortality benefit is associated with AVJ ablation in patients with heart failure and atrial fibrillation who are undergoing implantation of cardiac resynchronization therapy devices.

INTRODUCTION

Atrial fibrillation (AF) is the most common arrhythmia in clinical practice. Among Medicare beneficiaries, AF is in the top 15 chronic medical conditions, leading to almost half a million hospitalizations with AF as the primary diagnosis.[1–3]

Management of medically refractory AF has included atrioventricular junction (AVJ) ablation since the first human AVJ ablation performed on April 9, 1981, using high-energy direct current in a retired male oil worker with frequent episodes of AF with rapid ventricular rate and associated pulmonary edema.[4] Since that successful procedure, ablation therapy for AF has significantly evolved, and pulmonary vein isolation has become the cornerstone therapy for eliminating medically refractory AF. However, with the onset of left atrial flutters and the recurrence of AF following pulmonary vein isolation, particularly in patients with persistent and long-standing persistent AF, patients still require AVJ ablation. The goal of this procedure is to create complete atrioventricular (AV) conduction block and, in this manner, the patient finds freedom from the symptoms associated with AF caused by a rapid ventricular rate and an irregular ventricular rhythm.

This article reviews the indications for, and advances in, AVJ ablation as well as the implications for device therapy when using this technique.

This article originally appeared in Cardiology Clinics, Volume 32, Issue 4, November 2014.

Disclosures: The authors have no pertinent conflicts of interest related to this work.

[a] Electrophysiology Section, Division of Cardiology, Ross Heart Hospital, Wexner Medical Center at The Ohio State University, Columbus, OH 43210, USA; [b] Internal Medicine, Wexner Medical Center at The Ohio State University, 473 West 12th Avenue, DHLRI, Suite 200, Columbus, OH 43210, USA

* Corresponding author. Internal Medicine, 473 West 12th Avenue, DHLRI, Suite 200, Columbus, OH 43210.

E-mail address: emile.daoud@osumc.edu

heartfailure.theclinics.com

INDICATIONS FOR AVJ ABLATION

In general, 2 groups of patients are referred for AVJ ablation.

Refractory AF/Atrial Flutter and Rapid Ventricular Rates

The first group is the most common and consists of patients with AF and/or left atrial flutter associated with rapid ventricular rates.[2] In these patients, AVJ ablation is often the last resort; it often implies that both rhythm control and medical rate control strategies have been unsuccessful. Most patients have usually tried β-blockers, calcium channel blockers, multiple antiarrhythmic medications, and multiple cardioversions, and may have failed pulmonary vein isolation to maintain sinus rhythm. The rapid ventricular rate, even with paroxysmal AF, is the source of symptoms and, if long lasting, may result in a tachycardia-induced cardiomyopathy.[5,6] Because it is permanent and mandates lifelong pacing, AVJ ablation is only considered once these therapies have failed or have resulted in side effects.

It is worthwhile to highlight a subset of patients who undergo AVJ ablation for management of new-onset left atrial flutter following left atrial ablation for management of AF.[7] Following left atrial ablation for AF, there is a potential for a proarrhythmic effect from the ablation therapy. After ablation, patients may experience their first episode of sustained left atrial flutter. Because of the more organized atrial activity, the ventricular rate with this flutter can be greater and more challenging to control compared with when the patient was experiencing AF.[8,9] Although a repeat left atrial ablation to eliminate the left atrial flutter should be pursued and is often successful, in some patients repeat ablation is unsuccessful and these patients require AVJ ablation to control symptoms. Therefore, some patients who present with paroxysmal AF can develop a proarrhythmic effect from left atrial ablation and transition to a subsequent need for AVJ ablation. This potential outcome should be considered when planning a strategy for ablation of AF.

Patients whose sole arrhythmia is isthmus-dependent right atrial flutter rarely require AVJ ablation because this tachyarrhythmia has a high success rate for curative ablation. Curative ablation of this flutter should be pursued, even if multiple procedures are required, rather than AVJ ablation.

AF and Cardiac Resynchronization Therapy

The second group of patients referred for AVJ ablation consists of those who require biventricular pacing for management of systolic heart failure and who also have a high burden of AF despite a rhythm control approach. Even though the ventricular rate may be well controlled with medical therapy, AVJ ablation has been recommended for these patients to ensure a high degree of biventricular pacing without fusion from AF impulses conducted through the AV node. Dong and colleagues,[10] showed that, in patients who require cardiac resynchronization therapy (CRT), the rate of heart failure hospitalization and the need for heart transplantation are significantly less when biventricular pacing is greater than 96% and there is no fusion with native conduction through the AVJ. Based on this report and others,[11] many electrophysiologists and heart failure experts recommend AVJ ablation for patients who require CRT and who have a high burden of AF despite attempts to maintain sinus rhythm, even if the ventricular rate during AF is controlled (see Long-term Outcomes After AVJ Ablation section).

AVJ ABLATION PROCEDURE

The anatomy and physiology of the AV node region is complex (**Fig. 1**) and has evolved significantly since the original description by Tawara in 1906.[12,13] The compact AV node is located at the

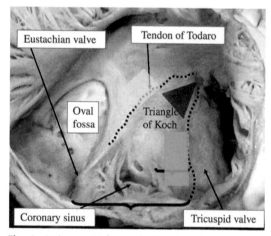

Fig. 1. Atrioventricular node (AVN) and surrounding anatomy. The compact AVN (*blue area*) is found at the apex of the triangle of Koch. The tendon of Todaro and the tricuspid valve annulus form the sides and the ostium of the coronary sinus forms the base of the triangle. The approximate location of the slow pathway (*green*) and fast pathway (*yellow*) inputs into the AVN are shown. The red circle is the location of the central fibrous body, which is where the His electrogram is usually recorded. The large bracket identifies the cavotricuspid isthmus and the small bracket identifies the septal isthmus. (*Adapted from* Anderson RH, Cook AC. The structure and components of the atrial chambers. Europace 2007;9(Suppl 6):vi3; with permission.)

apex of the triangle of Koch, defined by the anterior portion of the tricuspid valve annulus, the tendon of Todaro, and the ostium of the coronary sinus. Slow pathway input is located adjacent to the coronary sinus and the tricuspid annulus and the fast pathway is adjacent to the superior aspect of the tendon of Todaro, near the compact AV node.

AVJ radiofrequency ablation is accomplished via right femoral vein access and ablation lesions are directed by intracardiac electrograms. The preferred site of ablation is at the compact AV node (not the His bundle) penetrating the most proximal portion of the His bundle. The goal is to preserve automaticity distal to the site of ablation so to achieve a stable junctional escape rhythm and prevent pacemaker dependence. An ideal location for ablation is identified by recording a large atrial electrogram with a ventricular electrogram and a His potential. A common pitfall to ablating the AVJ is applying radiofrequency lesion at sites with a right bundle potential. A right bundle potential appears similar to a His potential, but there is a large ventricular signal, no atrial electrogram, and the interval between the right bundle potential and the surface QRS is too short to be consistent with a His potential recording (**Fig. 2**). The ideal outcome for a successful AVJ ablation is a stable junctional rhythm with complete AV block. A permanent pacing device is then required for adequate heart rate response.

Complete AV block is successfully achieved by a right-sided ablation approach in 95% to 97% of patients.[4,14] In less than 5% of patients with structural heart disease, prior attempted ablations, or aortic root dilation, right-sided ablation is not successful because of atypical AV node location or catheter instability[14] when using a 4-mm tip ablation catheter. For these patients, a retrograde aortic approach via femoral arterial access is used; however, with the development of catheters able to generate larger/deeper lesions (8 mm and irrigated tip catheters), left-side AVJ ablation is becoming uncommon.[15] With a left-sided approach, specific ablation of the AVJ is rarely feasible. Ablation in the left ventricle (LV) most often ablates the His bundle, resulting in complete heart block without an escape rhythm. In the presence of mechanical aortic valve or significant aortic atherosclerotic debris, a transseptal approach is also feasible. Overall, the recurrence of AV conduction after AVJ ablation is approximately 4%.[13,16]

COMPLICATIONS

Because AVJ ablation and pacemaker implantation are invasive procedures, various procedure-related complications have been reported, but the complication rate is low. Reported complications include access site vascular injury leading to bleeding or thrombosis, infection, pneumothorax, cardiac injury or perforation, tricuspid regurgitation caused by right ventricular (RV) lead placement, mitral valve regurgitation exacerbated by single-site RV apical pacing,[17,18] arrhythmias including polymorphic ventricular tachycardia,

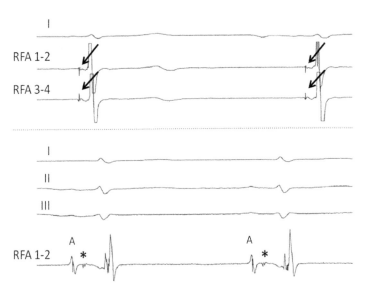

Fig. 2. Right bundle potential versus His potential. Top panel shows the tracings of surface lead I and intracardiac ablation (radiofrequency ablation [RFA]) catheter (distal 1–2 and proximal 3–4) electrodes at the time of AVJ ablation. The RFA intracardiac tracings show a right bundle potential (*arrows*), which is not a His potential as confirmed by the short interval between the potential and the onset of the surface QRS, and the absence of an atrial electrogram recorded on the RFA catheter. Ablating at this location would lead to right bundle branch block and would not result in AVJ conduction block. Bottom panel shows tracings of surface leads I, II, and III and intracardiac tracing of distal RFA (electrodes 1–2) catheter at the time of AVJ ablation. The RFA intracardiac tracing shows local atrial electrogram (A) and a His potential (*asterisk*), confirmed by an appropriate HV interval. Ablation at this site resulted in complete heart block with a stable narrow QRS escape rhythm of 38 beats per minute. (Tracings obtained at 200 mm/s sweep speed.)

and (rarely) death. In the North American Society of Pacing and Electrophysiology prospective voluntary registry, severe complications occurred in 5 (0.8%) out of 646 patients.[16] In the Multicenter European Radiofrequency Survey (MERFS), the serious complication rate was 1.8% and total complication rate was 3.2% in 900 patients who underwent ablation of the AVJ.[19]

The most feared complication after AVJ ablation is sudden death. Since the early days of the technique, there has been a small but well-characterized risk of sudden cardiac death in the immediate postablation period.[20–23] The rate of sudden death has been reported to be as high as 6%, although this occurred during the early experience with AVJ ablation. In the setting of relative bradycardia, along with altered activation of the ventricle (activation from the RV apex, rather than via the His-Purkinje system), altered global repolarization pattern, and changes in local dispersion of repolarization, there is a transient increased risk of polymorphic ventricular tachycardia. This complication has been almost eliminated by programming a higher postablation pacing rate (typically 80 pulses per minute [ppm]) for about 8 to 12 weeks[21,23]; thereafter, the lower pacing rate can be programmed to the desired rate because the risk of ventricular tachyarrhythmia is significantly lessened.

HEMODYNAMICS OF AVJ ABLATION

In addition to rate control, AVJ ablation and subsequent ventricular pacing results in regularization of the rhythm and has a positive impact on hemodynamics. In a study by Daoud and colleagues,[24] irregular ventricular pacing resulted in an approximately 12% decrease in invasively measured cardiac output after just 2 minutes of pacing compared with regular interval pacing at the same mean cycle length. Several underlying mechanisms help explain the reduced cardiac output. In patients with AF, there is no effective atrial contraction and ventricular filling is compromised at baseline. With irregular ventricular rhythm, the periods with short RR intervals have reduced ventricular filling and forward flow. The increased filling during longer RR intervals may not necessarily compensate for the reduced filling attributed to short RR intervals, considering alterations in contractility based on the Frank-Starling mechanism.[25] In addition, ventricular mechanics are inefficient with an irregular rhythm.[24,26]

The effects of AVJ ablation and pacing on cognitive function and brain perfusion were recently assessed in patients with medically refractory AF.[27] Brain perfusion was quantified before and after AVJ ablation via single-photon emission computed tomography. After AVJ ablation and pacemaker therapy, there was significant improvement in perfusion of the right inferior frontal, left superior frontal, and the left temporal cortex compared with pre-AVJ ablation and native conduction. This enhanced perfusion resulted in improvement in cognition in verbal memory, visual memory, attention, and psychomotor speed and learning.

In addition to measurable increases in cardiac and brain function, the benefits of AVJ ablation and pacing have translated to overall improvement in clinical symptoms. In the Ablate and Pace trial, symptomatic patients with AF refractory to medical management reported an improvement in quality of life after AVJ ablation and pacing.[22]

TACHYCARDIA-INDUCED CARDIOMYOPATHY

A common problem associated with rapid ventricular rates caused by atrial arrhythmias is the development of a tachycardia-induced cardiomyopathy. The mechanism of the cardiomyopathy is related to excessive ventricular rate with subsequent intracellular calcium overload, alteration of mitochondrial function, and subsequent reduced contractility.[28] However, once the cause of the calcium overload is managed (ie, elimination of the rapid ventricular rates), after a period of 3 to 4 months the LV ejection fraction (LVEF) should improve significantly.[28] Prospective evaluation of this effect was assessed in the Ablate and Pace trial.[22] In this study of 156 patients, those with a reduced LV function had the greatest and most sustained improvement in LV function at 12 months (baseline mean ejection fraction [EF] of 31% increased to mean EF of 41% at 12 months after the procedure). This finding correlates with other studies that have shown improvement in systolic function after rate control in patients with AF-related tachycardia-induced cardiomyopathy. A meta-analysis of almost 1181 patients across 21 studies reported a mean absolute improvement in LVEF of 4.4% across all patients, including those with mild or no myocardial dysfunction.[29] In addition, this meta-analysis showed favorable outcomes in 17 other clinical parameters, including improvement in symptoms (measured by well-being scale, activity scale, and general quality-of-life scale), number of admissions and outpatient visits, duration of exercise on treadmill or bicycle, New York Heart Association (NYHA) classification, and heart rate (**Fig. 3**).[29]

Overall, in those patients with AF and rapid ventricular rates with reduced cardiac function, tachycardia-induced cardiomyopathy may play a role, and rate control with AVJ ablation results in

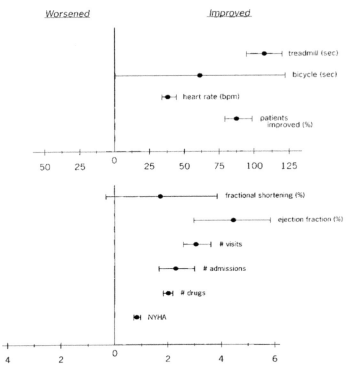

Fig. 3. Benefits of AVJ ablation. Forrest plots showing the effect size (*dark circles*) and 95% confidence intervals (*error bars*). In the top plot, 80% of the patients reported improvement in symptoms; plus improvements were noted in exercise duration with treadmill or bicycle. The bottom plot shows the improvements in EF, number of health care visits, admissions, number of drugs in the medication regimen, and NYHA classification associated with AVJ ablation. (*Adapted from* Wood MA, Brown-Mahoney C, Kay GN, et al. Clinical outcomes after ablation and pacing therapy for atrial fibrillation: a meta-analysis. Circulation 2000;101(10):1141; with permission.)

improvement in cardiac function. However, this approach to managing patients with atrial arrhythmias and rapid ventricular rates should be used when other therapies for rhythm control and medical rate control have failed.

DEVICE SELECTION AFTER AVJ ABLATION

Patients undergoing AVJ ablation require a permanent pacing device and can either have a conventional single-chamber or biventricular (right and left ventricular pacing for CRT) device implanted before or at the time of the ablation procedure. In those patients who still have periods of sinus rhythm, an atrial electrode may also be indicated.

In the early experience with AVJ ablation, single-site RV pacing was the standard treatment. However, long-term RV pacing is not free from complications. In some models, it leads to negative inotropic effects, abnormal histologic changes with thinning of the myocardial wall, and fibrosis.[30,31] In humans, clinical studies have suggested that long-term RV pacing can also be detrimental because of regional wall motion abnormalities and adverse LV

hemodynamics related to pacing-induced dyssynchrony, from pacing-related left bundle branch block activation of the ventricles. In a study by Tse and colleagues,[32] long-term RV apical pacing resulted in myocardial perfusion defects on thallium nuclear studies, and these findings were associated with impaired LVEF in patients free from significant coronary artery disease or other structural heart disease. In the Dual Chamber and VVI Implantable Defibrillator (DAVID) trial, there was an increase in mortality with dual-chamber pacing at a rate of 70 ppm compared with ventricular pacing at a backup rate of 40 ppm, presumably because pacing at 70 ppm resulted in a high degree of RV pacing and subsequent LV dyssynchrony.[33] These findings led to the growing concern regarding adverse effects of long-term RV pacing. Similar findings of worsening mortality associated with high percentage of RV pacing were found in patients in the Multicenter Automatic Defibrillator Implantation Trial II (MADIT II) trial.[34] However, these studies were not in patients who had undergone AVJ ablation and most patients in these studies had underlying ischemic disease.

Selection of the appropriate pacing system for patients after AVJ ablation is influenced by the favorable results of the use of biventricular pacing systems among patients with heart failure. Numerous studies have shown the adverse effects of native left bundle branch block conduction and the improvement in mortality, hospitalization, LV function, exercise tolerance, and quality of life with the use of biventricular pacing in patients with heart failure with broad QRS native conduction (**Figs. 4** and **5**).[35–41] Although these studies did not include patients who had undergone AVJ ablation, these data suggest that biventricular pacing may be preferred in patients after AVJ ablation to avoid LV dyssynchrony from chronic RV apical pacing.

In a study by Chen and colleagues,[42] long-term effects of RV pacing in patients who had AVJ ablation were evaluated in 286 patients. Overall, there was no change in mean LVEF in the group followed for a mean of 36 months (EF of 49% before vs 48% after). Only 1% of patients with an EF less than 40% developed any significant reduction in cardiac function. There was no significant change in heart failure hospitalization pattern in patients after initiation of RV pacing.

The impact of biventricular pacing after AVJ ablation was first studied by Doshi and colleagues[43] in the Post AV Nodal ablation Evaluation (PAVE) study. In this study, 184 patients with medically refractory AF and who underwent AVJ ablation were randomized to either biventricular

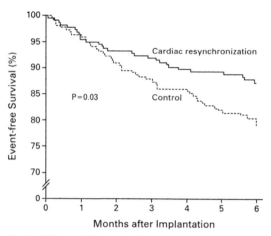

Fig. 5. Effect of biventricular pacing/CRT on time to death or first hospitalization with worsening heart failure. The risk of an event was 40% lower in the CRT group. (*From* Abraham WT, Fisher WG, Smith AL, et al. Cardiac resynchronization in chronic heart failure. N Engl J Med 2002;346(24):1851; with permission.)

pacing or RV pacing. At 6 months after ablation, there was an overall improvement in the primary end point of 6-minute walk test in both study groups. In subgroup analysis, when outcomes were stratified by EF, the overall improvement in 6-minute walk test was more prominent in those with an EF less than 45% who were randomized to CRT than in those randomized to RV pacing. There was no difference in improvement in the 6-minute walk test between the CRT group and

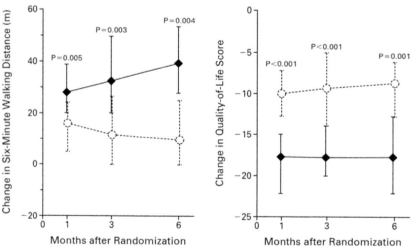

Fig. 4. Changes in 6-minute walking distance and Minnesota Living With Heart Failure Score (MLWHFS) after implantation of biventricular pacing systems in patients with heart failure. Open circles represent the control group and solid diamonds represent patients with biventricular pacing. The 6-minute walking distance was greater at 1 month after randomization and continued to increase throughout the follow-up period in the group with the biventricular devices (*left*). The quality-of-life benefits of biventricular pacing were present at 1 month and were sustained throughout follow-up. A lower score on the MLWHFS represents a higher quality of life (*right*). (*From* Abraham WT, Fisher WG, Smith AL, et al. Cardiac resynchronization in chronic heart failure. N Engl J Med 2002;346(24):1849; with permission.)

the RV group in those with an EF greater than 45%. The mean LVEF at the end of 6 months remained stable in the CRT group and was reduced in the RV pacing group (EF of 46% vs 41%; $P = .03$). A recent meta-analysis by Chatterjee and colleagues[44] included 4 randomized controlled trials assessing outcomes of biventricular versus RV pacing after AVJ ablation in 534 patients. This analysis also reported a better LVEF and improved symptoms with CRT among patients with a depressed EF (mean of 41%).

Considering these studies, the recommendation is to proceed with CRT after AVJ ablation in patients with left ventricular dysfunction (EF<45%). An RV pacing system is recommended in those patients with preserved left ventricular function. After a procedure, if the EF declines, patients with an RV pacing system may require revision to a CRT system.[45]

LONG-TERM OUTCOMES AFTER AVJ ABLATION

Overall, AVJ ablation has proved to be effective in improving symptoms and may improve LVEF in those patients with depressed cardiac function. Long-term survival after AVJ ablation and RV pacing was studied by Ozcan and colleagues[46] in 350 patients with a mean follow-up of 36 months. There was no difference in survival in patients with AF managed with drug therapy compared with patients managed with AVJ ablation (Fig. 6). However, patients with AF, compared with sex-matched and age-matched control subjects without AF, had worse survival. This survival

difference was attributed to the presence of other comorbid conditions (see Fig. 6). When assessing total mortality among patients with lone AF (no structural heart disease), there was no difference in survival compared with sex-matched and age-matched control subjects free from AF (Fig. 7).

Long-term survival in patients with heart failure and biventricular pacing system/CRT is improved with greater duration of biventricular pacing. In a large registry of more than 36,000 patients (not inclusive of patients who had undergone AVJ ablation), the duration of biventricular pacing over time predicted mortality (Fig. 8).[11] These data emphasize the need to ensure a high degree of biventricular pacing. Therefore, in patients with heart failure, a wide QRS, and AF, and who undergo implantation of a biventricular pacing system, AVJ ablation with subsequent complete AV conduction block leads to maximal biventricular pacing. This benefit of AVJ block in patients with heart failure, AF, and CRT was shown in a systematic review by Ganesan and colleagues.[47] In this analysis of 6 studies involving 768 patients with heart failure with CRT and AF, AVJ ablation was associated with significant reduction in all-cause mortality (Fig. 9) and cardiovascular mortality, and improvement in NYHA functional class (Fig. 10). Therefore, it is common to proceed with AVJ ablation at the time of CRT implantation for patients with heart failure and AF.

ALTERNATIVES

An alternative to AVJ ablation is AVJ modification. The goal of the modification procedure is

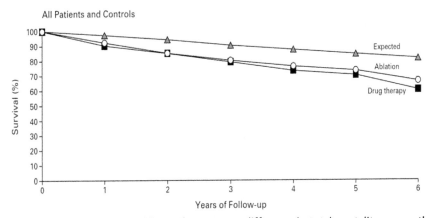

Fig. 6. Long-term outcome in patients with AF. There was no difference in total mortality among those patients with AF managed with AVJ ablation (*open circles*) versus drug therapy (*solid squares*) at 6 years. However, patients with AF, compared with the sex-matched and age-matched control subjects without AF (*solid triangles*), had a worse survival. This reduced survival difference was attributable to the presence of other comorbid conditions. (*From* Ozcan C, Jahangir A, Friedman PA, et al. Long-term survival after ablation of the atrioventricular node and implantation of a permanent pacemaker in patients with atrial fibrillation. N Engl J Med 2001;344(14):1046; with permission.)

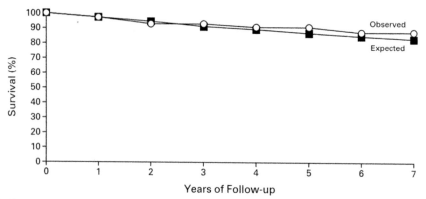

Fig. 7. Survival with lone AF. No difference in survival between those with lone AF (*open circles*) and sex-matched and age-matched control subjects without AF (*solid squares*) in the absence of congestive heart failure or coronary artery disease. (*From* Ozcan C, Jahangir A, Friedman PA, et al. Long-term survival after ablation of the atrioventricular node and implantation of a permanent pacemaker in patients with atrial fibrillation. N Engl J Med 2001;344(14):1049; with permission.)

to ablate in the slow pathway region to prolong the AV nodal refractory period, to achieve a net decrease in ventricular rate during AF and to avoid the need for a permanent pacing system. The procedure success rate was approximately 70% in the short-term and long-term follow-up.[48,49] However, this approach was limited by poor rate control and sometimes unintended complete AV block. As a result, AVJ modification is now rarely performed.

NEW TECHNOLOGY

With a conventional 8-mm tip ablation catheter, radiofrequency energy is delivered 8 mm distal to the recording of the His potential, thus increasing the likelihood of ablating the His bundle rather than the AVJ. However, with a recently available 8-mm tip ablation catheter that provides imbedded electrodes at the distal tip, these microelectrodes can record a His potential at the distal aspect of the ablation electrode surface area. Ablation

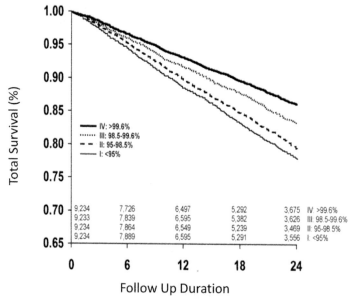

Fig. 8. Survival and percentage of biventricular pacing. Subjects in the highest quartile of biventricular pacing (with >99.6% of biventricular pacing) had a 24% relative reduction in mortality compared with other quartile groups. (*From* Hayes DL, Boehmer JP, Day JD, et al. Cardiac resynchronization therapy and the relationship of percent biventricular pacing to symptoms and survival. Heart Rhythm 2011;8(9):1472; with permission.)

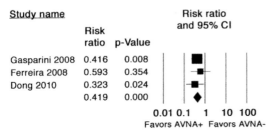

Study name	Risk ratio	p-Value	Risk ratio and 95% CI
Gasparini 2008	0.416	0.008	
Ferreira 2008	0.593	0.354	
Dong 2010	0.323	0.024	
	0.419	0.000	

0.01 0.1 1 10 100
Favors AVNA+ Favors AVNA-

Fig. 9. All-cause mortality in patients with heart failure, AF, and CRT devices. Survival is favored in those who underwent AV node ablation (AVNA+) compared with those who did not (AVNA−). CI, confidence interval. (*From* Ganesan AN, Brooks AG, Roberts-Thomson KC, et al. Role of AV nodal ablation in cardiac resynchronization in patients with coexistent atrial fibrillation and heart failure a systematic review. J Am Coll Cardiol 2012;59(8):723; with permission.)

mapped to this location with the embedded electrodes means that radiofrequency energy is delivered proximal to the His recording and thus is more likely to result in AVJ ablation.

Another important advance in technology is the advent of the leadless pacing system. In the LEADLESS trial, a self-contained leadless cardiac pacemaker device (**Fig. 11**) was implanted in 33 patients and followed for 90 days.[50] The device was designed to address poor clinical outcomes associated with complications, including fractures and erosions associated with conventional leads used in current pacemakers. The overall complication-free rate in this nonrandomized prospective trial was 94%. At 90 months, adequate sensing and pacing thresholds were met in all patients. A leadless pacing system may become part of the ablate and pace strategy for patients with AF.

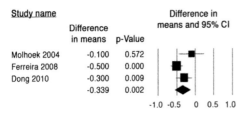

Study name	Difference in means	p-Value	Difference in means and 95% CI
Molhoek 2004	-0.100	0.572	
Ferreira 2008	-0.500	0.000	
Dong 2010	-0.300	0.009	
	-0.339	0.002	

-1.0 -0.5 0 0.5 1.0

Favors AVNA+   Favors AVNA-

Fig. 10. Changes in NYHA classification in patients with heart failure, AF, and CRT devices. Patients who underwent ablation (AVNA+) experienced an improvement in their NYHA classification (represented by a reduction in value) compared with those without ablation (AVNA−). (*From* Ganesan AN, Brooks AG, Roberts-Thomson KC, et al. Role of AV nodal ablation in cardiac resynchronization in patients with coexistent atrial fibrillation and heart failure a systematic review. J Am Coll Cardiol 2012;59(8):723; with permission.)

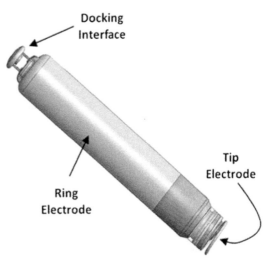

Fig. 11. Leadless cardiac pacing device. Length is 42 mm and maximum diameter is 5.99 mm. This device contains the entire programmable pacing system, inclusive of battery source. (*From* Reddy VY, Knops RE, Sperzel J, et al. Permanent leadless cardiac pacing: results of the leadless trial. Circulation 2014;129(14):1467; with permission.)

SUMMARY

AVJ ablation and pacing strategy is indicated for patients who have failed rhythm control and medical rate control strategies for AF. It is a safe and effective way to reduce symptoms, and is associated with an increase in EF in patients with tachycardia-induced cardiomyopathy. A survival benefit has been reported in patients with heart failure who undergo AVJ and have a CRT device implanted.

REFERENCES

1. Go AS, Mozaffarian D, Roger VL, et al. Heart disease and stroke statistics–2014 update: a report from the American Heart Association. Circulation 2014;129:e28–292.
2. January CT, Wann LS, Alpert JS, et al. 2014 AHA/ACC/HRS Guideline for the management of patients with atrial fibrillation: executive summary. A report of the American College of Cardiology/American Heart Association Task Force on Practice Guidelines and the Heart Rhythm Society. J Am Coll Cardiol 2014. Available at: http://doi.dx.org/10.1016/j.jacc.2014.03.022.
3. Centers for Medicare and Medicaid Services. Chronic conditions among Medicare beneficiaries, Chartbook, 2012 Edition. Baltimore (MD); 2012.
4. Hoffmayer KS, Scheinman M. Current role of atrioventricular junction (AVJ) ablation. Pacing Clin Electrophysiol 2013;36(2):257–65.

5. Grogan M, Smith HC, Gersh BJ, et al. Left ventricular dysfunction due to atrial fibrillation in patients initially believed to have idiopathic dilated cardiomyopathy. Am J Cardiol 1992;69(19):1570–3.

6. Shinbane JS, Wood MA, Jensen DN, et al. Tachycardia-induced cardiomyopathy: a review of animal models and clinical studies. J Am Coll Cardiol 1997;29(4):709–15.

7. Ejima K, Arai K, Suzuki T, et al. Long-term outcome and preprocedural predictors of atrial tachyarrhythmia recurrence following pulmonary vein antrum isolation-based catheter ablation in patients with non-paroxysmal atrial fibrillation. J Cardiol 2013;64(1):57–63.

8. Daoud EG, Weiss R, Augostini R, et al. Proarrhythmia of circumferential left atrial lesions for management of atrial fibrillation. J Cardiovasc Electrophysiol 2006;17(2):157–65.

9. Chugh A. Atrial tachycardia after ablation of persistent atrial fibrillation: is it us or them? Circ Arrhythm Electrophysiol 2013;6(6):1047–9.

10. Dong K, Shen WK, Powell BD, et al. Atrioventricular nodal ablation predicts survival benefit in patients with atrial fibrillation receiving cardiac resynchronization therapy. Heart Rhythm 2010;7(9):1240–5.

11. Hayes DL, Boehmer JP, Day JD, et al. Cardiac resynchronization therapy and the relationship of percent biventricular pacing to symptoms and survival. Heart Rhythm 2011;8(9):1469–75.

12. Tawara S, Aschoff L. The conduction system of the mammalian heart. London, UK: Imperial College Press; 2000.

13. Wit AL. Atrioventricular nodal electrophysiology: still exciting after all these years. Circ Res 2003; 93(11):1018–9.

14. Feld GK. Atrioventricular node modification and ablation for ventricular rate control in atrial fibrillation. Heart Rhythm 2007;4(Suppl 3):S80–3.

15. Sousa J, el-Atassi R, Rosenheck S, et al. Radiofrequency catheter ablation of the atrioventricular junction from the left ventricle. Circulation 1991;84(2): 567–71.

16. Scheinman MM, Huang S. The 1998 NASPE prospective catheter ablation registry. Pacing Clin Electrophysiol 2000;23(6):1020–8.

17. Twidale N, Manda V, Holliday R, et al. Mitral regurgitation after atrioventricular node catheter ablation for atrial fibrillation and heart failure: acute hemodynamic features. Am Heart J 1999;138(6 Pt 1): 1166–75.

18. Vanderheyden M, Goethals M, Anguera I, et al. Hemodynamic deterioration following radiofrequency ablation of the atrioventricular conduction system. Pacing Clin Electrophysiol 1997;20(10 Pt 1):2422–8.

19. Hindricks G. The Multicentre European Radiofrequency Survey (MERFS): complications of radiofrequency catheter ablation of arrhythmias. The Multicentre European Radiofrequency Survey (MERFS) investigators of the Working Group on Arrhythmias of the European Society of C. Eur Heart J 1993;14(12):1644–53.

20. Ozcan C, Jahangir A, Friedman PA, et al. Sudden death after radiofrequency ablation of the atrioventricular node in patients with atrial fibrillation. J Am Coll Cardiol 2002;40(1):105–10.

21. Geelen P, Brugada J, Andries E, et al. Ventricular fibrillation and sudden death after radiofrequency catheter ablation of the atrioventricular junction. Pacing Clin Electrophysiol 1997;20(2 Pt 1):343–8.

22. Kay GN, Ellenbogen KA, Giudici M, et al. The Ablate and Pace Trial: a prospective study of catheter ablation of the AV conduction system and permanent pacemaker implantation for treatment of atrial fibrillation. APT Investigators. J Interv Card Electrophysiol 1998;2(2):121–35.

23. Wang RX, Lee HC, Hodge DO, et al. Effect of pacing method on risk of sudden death after atrioventricular node ablation and pacemaker implantation in patients with atrial fibrillation. Heart Rhythm 2013;10(5):696–701.

24. Daoud EG, Weiss R, Bahu M, et al. Effect of an irregular ventricular rhythm on cardiac output. Am J Cardiol 1996;78(12):1433–6. Available at: http://www.ncbi.nlm.nih.gov/pubmed/8970422. Accessed April 21, 2014.

25. Gosselink AT, Blanksma PK, Crijns HJ, et al. Left ventricular beat-to-beat performance in atrial fibrillation: contribution of Frank-Starling mechanism after short rather than long RR intervals. J Am Coll Cardiol 1995;26(6):1516–21.

26. Herbert WH. Cardiac output and the varying R-R interval of atrial fibrillation. J Electrocardiol 1973; 6(2):131–5.

27. Efimova I, Efimova N, Chernov V, et al. Ablation and pacing: improving brain perfusion and cognitive function in patients with atrial fibrillation and uncontrolled ventricular rates. Pacing Clin Electrophysiol 2012;35(3):320–6.

28. Gupta S, Figueredo VM. Tachycardia mediated cardiomyopathy: pathophysiology, mechanisms, clinical features and management. Int J Cardiol 2014;172(1):40–6.

29. Wood MA, Brown-Mahoney C, Kay GN, et al. Clinical outcomes after ablation and pacing therapy for atrial fibrillation: a meta-analysis. Circulation 2000; 101(10):1138–44.

30. Bedotto JB, Grayburn PA, Black WH, et al. Alterations in left ventricular relaxation during atrioventricular pacing in humans. J Am Coll Cardiol 1990;15(3):658–64.

31. Karpawich PP, Rabah R, Haas JE. Altered cardiac histology following apical right ventricular pacing in patients with congenital atrioventricular block. Pacing Clin Electrophysiol 1999;22(9):1372–7.

32. Tse HF, Lau CP. Long-term effect of right ventricular pacing on myocardial perfusion and function. J Am Coll Cardiol 1997;29(4):744–9.

33. Wilkoff BL, Cook JR, Epstein AE, et al. Dual-chamber pacing or ventricular backup pacing in patients with an implantable defibrillator: the Dual Chamber and VVI Implantable Defibrillator (DAVID) Trial. JAMA 2002;288(24):3115–23.

34. Brenyo A, Goldenberg I, Barsheshet A. The downside of right ventricular apical pacing. Indian Pacing Electrophysiol J 2012;12(3):102–13.

35. Abraham WT, Fisher WG, Smith AL, et al. Cardiac resynchronization in chronic heart failure. N Engl J Med 2002;346(24):1845–53.

36. Bristow MR, Saxon LA, Boehmer J, et al. Cardiac-resynchronization therapy with or without an implantable defibrillator in advanced chronic heart failure. N Engl J Med 2004;350(21):2140–50.

37. Cazeau S, Leclercq C, Lavergne T, et al. Effects of multisite biventricular pacing in patients with heart failure and intraventricular conduction delay. N Engl J Med 2001;344(12):873–80.

38. Gras D, Leclercq C, Tang AS, et al. Cardiac resynchronization therapy in advanced heart failure the multicenter InSync clinical study. Eur J Heart Fail 2002;4(3):311–20.

39. Higgins SL, Hummel JD, Niazi IK, et al. Cardiac resynchronization therapy for the treatment of heart failure in patients with intraventricular conduction delay and malignant ventricular tachyarrhythmias. J Am Coll Cardiol 2003;42(8):1454–9.

40. Linde C, Leclercq C, Rex S, et al. Long-term benefits of biventricular pacing in congestive heart failure: results from the MUltisite STimulation in cardiomyopathy (MUSTIC) study. J Am Coll Cardiol 2002;40(1):111–8.

41. Young JB, Abraham WT, Smith AL, et al. Combined cardiac resynchronization and implantable cardioversion defibrillation in advanced chronic heart failure: the MIRACLE ICD Trial. JAMA 2003;289(20):2685–94.

42. Chen L, Hodge D, Jahangir A, et al. Preserved left ventricular ejection fraction following atrioventricular junction ablation and pacing for atrial fibrillation. J Cardiovasc Electrophysiol 2008;19(1):19–27.

43. Doshi RN, Daoud EG, Fellows C, et al. Left ventricular-based cardiac stimulation post AV nodal ablation evaluation (the PAVE study). J Cardiovasc Electrophysiol 2005;16(11):1160–5.

44. Chatterjee NA, Upadhyay GA, Ellenbogen KA, et al. Atrioventricular nodal ablation in atrial fibrillation: a meta-analysis of biventricular vs. right ventricular pacing mode. Eur J Heart Fail 2012;14(6):661–7.

45. Leon AR, Greenberg JM, Kanuru N, et al. Cardiac resynchronization in patients with congestive heart failure and chronic atrial fibrillation: effect of upgrading to biventricular pacing after chronic right ventricular pacing. J Am Coll Cardiol 2002;39(8):1258–63.

46. Ozcan C, Jahangir A, Friedman PA, et al. Long-term survival after ablation of the atrioventricular node and implantation of a permanent pacemaker in patients with atrial fibrillation. N Engl J Med 2001;344(14):1043–51.

47. Ganesan AN, Brooks AG, Roberts-Thomson KC, et al. Role of AV nodal ablation in cardiac resynchronization in patients with coexistent atrial fibrillation and heart failure a systematic review. J Am Coll Cardiol 2012;59(8):719–26.

48. Williamson BD, Man KC, Daoud E, et al. Radiofrequency catheter modification of atrioventricular conduction to control the ventricular rate during atrial fibrillation. N Engl J Med 1994;331(14):910–7.

49. Morady F, Hasse C, Strickberger SA, et al. Long-term follow-up after radiofrequency modification of the atrioventricular node in patients with atrial fibrillation. J Am Coll Cardiol 1997;29(1):113–21.

50. Reddy VY, Knops RE, Sperzel J, et al. Permanent leadless cardiac pacing: results of the leadless trial. Circulation 2014;129(14):1466–71.

Antithrombotic and Anticoagulant Therapy for Atrial Fibrillation

Mikhail S. Dzeshka, MD[a,b], Gregory Y.H. Lip, MD[a,*]

KEYWORDS

- Atrial fibrillation • Stroke risk • Bleeding risk • Antithrombotic prophylaxis • Oral anticoagulants
- Antiplatelet drugs

KEY POINTS

- Prophylaxis of stroke and other thromboembolic events is central to the management of patients with atrial fibrillation (AF).
- All patients with AF, but with low risk of stroke (nonvalvular AF and CHA_2DS_2-VASc score = 0 in males or 1 in females), require treatment with oral anticoagulants (OACs) unless they are contraindicated.
- Vitamin K antagonists (VKAs) and non-VKA OACs (eg, dabigatran, rivaroxaban, apixaban) can be administered depending on the clinical situation.
- Antiplatelet drugs, either alone or in combination, are inferior to OACs for antithrombotic prophylaxis but have to be used in combination with OACs in AF patients undergoing percutaneous intervention with stent implantation.
- In high-risk patients with contraindications for anticoagulation, left atrial appendage exclusion is an alternative option.

INTRODUCTION

Atrial fibrillation (AF) is the most common sustained cardiac arrhythmia associated with high morbidity and mortality. The upward trend for AF prevalence translates into approximately 3% of adults being affected with arrhythmia in the more recent report.[1,2]

AF confers a 5-fold elevated risk of stroke, characterized by prolonged hospitalizations, greater disability, and higher mortality when associated with arrhythmia, in comparison with patients without AF.[3] In real life, involvement of AF in stroke development seems to be even more profound; a substantial proportion of so-called cryptogenic stroke AF has been detected via prolonged electrocardiogram monitoring, as AF per se is often asymptomatic.[4]

Oral anticoagulation (OAC) is the recommended effective option for the prevention of stroke and other thromboembolic events in AF, with either dose-adjusted vitamin K antagonists (VKAs) (eg, warfarin) or non-VKA anticoagulants (eg, dabigatran, apixaban, rivaroxaban, or edoxaban).[5,6] Antithrombotic prophylaxis with adherence to guidelines has improved significantly during the last decade, but the rate of antiplatelet drug

This article originally appeared in Cardiology Clinics, Volume 32, Issue 4, November 2014.
Competing Interests: G.Y.H. Lip has served as a consultant for Bayer, Astellas, Merck, Sanofi, BMS/Pfizer, Biotronik, Medtronic, Portola, Boehringer Ingelheim, Microlife, and Daiichi-Sankyo, and has been on the speakers bureau for Bayer, BMS/Pfizer, Medtronic, Boehringer Ingelheim, Microlife, and Daiichi-Sankyo. M.S. Dzeshka has no competing interests.
[a] University of Birmingham Centre for Cardiovascular Sciences, City Hospital, Birmingham B18 7QH, UK;
[b] Grodno State Medical University, Grodno, Belarus
* Corresponding author.
E-mail address: g.y.h.lip@bham.ac.uk

http://dx.doi.org/10.1016/j.hfc.2015.08.021
1551-7136/16/$ – see front matter

administration instead of OAC remains significant, especially among the elderly and those at high risk of bleeding. In the EURObservational Research Programme Atrial Fibrillation General Pilot Survey (EORP-AF), for example, 95.6% of patients among those with the CHA_2DS_2-VASc score of 1 or higher, that is, with indications for OAC, received antithrombotic prophylaxis, with 80.5% of these taking OAC.[7] Another unfavorable trend found in the EORP-AF study was common administration of a combination of OAC with antiplatelet drugs in stable coronary artery disease (CAD).[7]

This article provides an overview of current evidence for antithrombotic therapy in patients with AF.

ASSESSMENT OF STROKE AND BLEEDING RISK

The risk for stroke is not homogeneous in AF patients. Thus, the decision to initiate OAC therapy has to be justified by the patient's individual risk assessment, and the net clinical benefit balancing stroke reduction against serious bleeding. A variety of risk factors for stroke development has been established, which subsequently formed the basis for various risk-stratification schemes for stroke.[8,9]

The CHA_2DS_2-VASc score[10] (see **Table 1** for expansion of the acronym) is recommended by the 2012 European Society of Cardiology and 2014 American Heart Association/American College of Cardiology/Heart Rhythm Society guidelines for the management of AF as the only risk-assessment tool for stroke in patients with nonvalvular AF.[5,6]

The annual rate of thromboembolic events (including ischemic stroke, pulmonary embolism, and peripheral artery embolism) increases gradually with increasing CHA_2DS_2-VASc score, ranging from 0.78 (95% confidence interval [CI] 0.58–1.04) per 100 person-years with CHA_2DS_2-VASc = 0, rising to 23.64 (95% CI 10.62–52.61) with CHA_2DS_2-VASc = 9.[11]

The major advantage of the CHA_2DS_2-VASc score in comparison with other risk-stratification schemes for stroke, including the older CHADS₂ score (heart failure, hypertension, age $\geq$75 years, diabetes, and stroke/transient ischemic attack)[12] is its ability to reliably distinguish the group of patients with a low risk of stroke, that is, a CHA_2DS_2-VASc score of 0 for males or 1 for females, which has been validated in several large real-world AF cohorts.[13–15] For example, in a retrospective analysis performed in the Danish nationwide cohort study involving 19,444 patients with CHADS₂

Table 1
Risk stratification for stroke and bleeding using the CHA_2DS_2-VASc and HAS-BLED scores

CHA_2DS_2-VASc	Score	HAS-BLED	Score
Congestive heart failure/LV dysfunction	1	Hypertension (systolic blood pressure >160 mm Hg)	1
Hypertension	1	Abnormal renal or liver function	1 or 2
Age $\geq$75 y	2	Stroke	1
Diabetes mellitus	1	Bleeding tendency or predisposition	1
Stroke/TIA/TE	2	Labile INR (if on warfarin)	1
Vascular disease (prior MI, PAD, or aortic plaque)	1	Age (eg, >65 y, frail condition)	1
Age 65–74 y	1	Drugs (eg, concomitant antiplatelet or NSAIDs) or alcohol excess/abuse	1 or 2
Sex category (ie, female gender)	1		
Maximum score	9		9

CHA_2DS_2-VASc: Heart failure (moderate to severe left ventricular systolic dysfunction referring to left ventricular ejection fraction $\leq$40% or recent decompensated heart failure requiring hospitalization), hypertension, age $\geq$75 years, diabetes, stroke/transient ischemic attack, vascular disease (specifically myocardial infarction, complex aortic plaque, and peripheral artery disease), age 65–74 years, female sex.

HAS-BLED: Uncontrolled hypertension, abnormal renal/liver function, stroke, bleeding history or predisposition, labile international normalized ratio, elderly (eg, age >65 years, frail condition), drugs (eg, antiplatelets, nonsteroidal anti-inflammatory drugs)/excessive alcohol.

Abbreviations: INR, international normalized ratio; LV, left ventricular; MI, myocardial infarction; NSAIDs, nonsteroidal anti-inflammatory drugs; PAD, peripheral artery disease; TIA/TE, transient ischemic attack/thromboembolism.

Data from Lip GY, Nieuwlaat R, Pisters R, et al. Refining clinical risk stratification for predicting stroke and thromboembolism in atrial fibrillation using a novel risk factor-based approach: the Euro Heart Survey on atrial fibrillation. Chest 2010;137(2):263–72; and Pisters R, Lane DA, Nieuwlaat R, et al. A novel user-friendly score (HAS-BLED) to assess 1-year risk of major bleeding in patients with atrial fibrillation: the Euro Heart Survey. Chest 2010;138(5):1093–100.

score = 0, annual stroke rates ranged from 0.84% (95% CI 0.65%–1.08%) in CHA_2DS_2-VASc score = 0 to 3.2% (95% CI 1.60%–6.40%) in CHA_2DS_2-VASc score = 3.[13]

Following the identification of these "truly low-risk" patients who do not need any antithrombotic therapy, effective stroke prevention (ie, OAC) can be offered to those with 1 or more risk factors for stroke given the positive net clinical benefit for these patients.[16–19] Of note, current American guidelines allow a choice between OAC, aspirin, or no antithrombotic therapy in patients with a CHA_2DS_2-VASc score = 1.[6] By contrast, European guidelines offer for consideration OAC only.[5] For AF patients with 1 or more risk factors for stroke, the net clinical benefit of OAC therapy is positive, meaning that risk reduction for stroke outweighs the potential increased risk of hemorrhage. Moreover, the net clinical benefit is greater in patients with the higher risk of bleeding; thus, a high risk of bleeding should not be considered a reason to avoid OAC.[16–18]

The HAS-BLED score (see **Table 1** for expansion of the acronym) is used for evaluation of individuals' risk of major bleeding.[20] This score performs well in comparison with other risk-stratification schemes for bleeding in different clinical settings: both AF and non-AF patients, patients on warfarin or other anticoagulants, and in cases of bridging therapy.[21–24] Moreover, it is able to predict intracerebral hemorrhage independently of other bleeding events.[22,23]

Risk stratification is a dynamic process, and the risk for both stroke and bleeding should be assessed each time a patient is followed up. Moreover, the HAS-BLED score includes risk factors that can be modified to thus reduce an individual's risk of bleeding and potentially make OAC therapy safer.[5,6]

ANTICOAGULATION THERAPY
Vitamin K Antagonists (eg, Warfarin)

Until recently, the VKAs (eg, warfarin) represented the only available OAC for the prevention of stroke and thromboembolism in AF patients. VKAs reduce stroke by 64% (95% CI 49%–74%), both in primary (2.7% annual absolute risk reduction) and secondary (8.4% annual absolute risk reduction) prevention, in addition to all-cause mortality, by 26% (95% CI 3%–43%).[25]

Warfarin inhibits the synthesis of the vitamin K–dependent coagulation factors (II, VII, IX, X) by reducing vitamin K in the liver from vitamin K epoxide (the inactive form that appears during oxidation of hydroquinone form) back to the active one with the enzyme, called vitamin K epoxide

reductase complex subunit 1 (VKORC1). Oxidation of the hydroquinone form is coupled with the posttranslational modification of vitamin K–dependent proteins, which includes carboxylation of glutamic acid residues and formation of the γ-carboxyl glutamic acid domains. These domains are capable of binding calcium ions (with positive charge), thereby making proteins attractable to injured cell surface, which carries a negative charge. Proteins lacking a sufficient amount of calcium-binding domain (partially carboxylated and decarboxylated) have significantly reduced coagulant activity.[26] Pharmacologic characteristics of warfarin are summarized in **Table 2**.

Despite high antithrombotic efficacy, warfarin has a range of disadvantages that make it inconvenient for use from both patients' and clinicians' points of view, specifically because of high intraindividual and interindividual variability of anticoagulant effect (patients can develop bleeding complications with the minimal dose or may have warfarin resistance), food and drug interaction, slow onset of action, long half-life, and so forth.[26] This drawback results in significant underuse of warfarin in patients with AF in the real world, particularly if the estimated risk of bleeding is high, in association with CAD and in the elderly.[7,30–32]

Genetic polymorphism of enzymes involved in warfarin metabolism (cytochromes CYP2C9, CYP3A4, CYP2C19, CYP1A2) and target enzyme for warfarin (VKORC1) is of particular importance in its pharmacology, and several attempts have been made to develop an algorithm for warfarin dosing based on a pharmacogenetic approach; however, genetic testing cannot be applied routinely given the growing population with AF who require OAC.[33–35]

To reach an optimal anticoagulation effect, slow titration at the beginning of therapy and regular monitoring of international normalized ratio (INR) is required because of the narrow therapeutic window for warfarin (INR 2.0–3.0). Time in therapeutic range (TTR) is used to evaluate the quality of anticoagulation with warfarin, and the average individual TTR has to be as high as greater than 70% to expect efficacious reduction in risk of stroke with a low risk of bleeding.[36] For example, in 27,458 patients taking warfarin from the United Kingdom General Practice Database, who spent at least 70% of time within the therapeutic range, significantly lower stroke and mortality rates were achieved in comparison with patients who spent less than 30% of time in the range.[37] While translating data on warfarin effectiveness from clinical trials, it is also important to keep in mind that TTR in the real-life population from everyday

Table 2
Pharmacologic characteristics of warfarin and non-VKA oral anticoagulants

Parameter	Warfarin	Dabigatran	Rivaroxaban	Apixaban	Edoxaban
Mechanism of action	Inhibition of VKORC1	Direct thrombin inhibitor (free or bound), reversible	Factor Xa inhibitor (free or bound), reversible	Factor Xa inhibitor (free or bound), reversible	Factor Xa inhibitor (free or bound), reversible
Onset of action	Slow, indirect inhibition of clotting factor synthesis	Fast	Fast	Fast	Fast
Offset of action	Long	Short	Short	Short	Short
Absorption	Rapid	Rapid, acid-dependent	Rapid	Rapid	Rapid
Bioavailability (%)	>95	6.5	>80	>50	62
T_{max} (h)	2.0–4.0	1.0–3.0	2.5–4.0	1.0–3.0	1.0–2.0
V_d (L)	10	60–70	50–55	21	>300
Protein binding (%)	99	35	95	87	40–59
$T_{1/2\beta}$ (h)	40	12–17	9–13	8–15	9–11
Renal clearance	None	80	35	27	50
Nonrenal clearance	None	20	65	73	50
CL/F (L/h)	0.35	70–140	10	5	30.2–33.7
Accumulation in plasma	Dependent on CYP2C9 metabolic efficiency	None	None	1.3–1.9	Negligible
Food effect	No effect on absorption; dietary vitamin K influence on pharmacodynamics	Delayed absorption with food with no influence on bioavailability	Delayed absorption with food with increased bioavailability	None	None
Age	Yes, lower CL/F as age increases	Yes, lower CL/F as age increases	None	Yes, lower CL/F as age increases	NR
Body weight	Yes, higher dose for increased weight	None	None	Yes, higher exposure with low body weight (<60 kg)	NR
Sex	Yes, lower CL/F in women	Yes, lower CL/F in women	None	Yes, higher exposure in women	NR

Ethnicity	Lower dose in Asian patients; higher dose in African American patients	None	Lower dose in Japanese patients	None	None
Drug transporter	None	P-gp	P-gp, BCRP	P-gp, BCRP	P-gp
CYP-mediated metabolism	CYP2C9, CYP3A4, CYP2C19, CYP1A2	None	CYP3A4/5, CYP2J2 (equal)	CYP3A4/5, CYP2J2 (minor), CYP1A2 (minor)	CYP3A4 (4%)
Drug-drug interactions[a]	Numerous	Potent P-gp inhibitors (verapamil: reduce dose; dronedarone: avoid) and inducers (avoid)	Potent CYP3A4 and P-gp inhibitors (avoid) and inducers (use with caution)	Potent CYP3A4 and P-gp inhibitors (avoid) and inducers (use with caution)	Potent P-gp inhibitors (reduce dose) and inducers (avoid)
Coagulation measurement	INR	TT, dTT, aPTT, ECA	PT, anti-FXa	Anti-FXa	PT, aPTT, anti-FXa
Reversal agents	Vitamin K (slow reversal, prolonged inhibition), FFP or PCCs (rapid reversal)	Activated charcoal or hemodialysis (overdose); PCCs or recombinant FVII (uncontrolled bleeding)	Activated charcoal, FFP, PCCs, activated FVII	Activated charcoal, FFP, PCCs, activated FVII	Activated charcoal, FFP, PCCs, activated FVII
Dosing for AF	Individualized for each patient according to INR response (0.5–16 mg qd)	150 mg bid or 110 mg bid in high risk of bleeding. Contraindicated if CrCl <30 mL/min	20 mg qd if CrCl >50 mL/min or 15 mg qd if CrCl 15–50 mL/min	5 mg bid or 2.5 mg bid if • CrCl 15–29 mL/min or • Any 2 of the following are present: o Age ≥80 y o body weight ≤60 kg o Serum creatinine ≥133 µmol/L	Awaiting EMA approval

Abbreviations: AF, atrial fibrillation; aPTT, activated partial thromboplastin test; BCRP, breast cancer resistance protein; bid, twice daily; Cl/F, apparent clearance; CrCl, creatinine clearance; CYP, cytochrome P450 isozymes; dTT, diluted thrombin test; ECT, ecarin chromogenic assay; EMA, European Medicines Agency; F, factor; FFP, fresh frozen plasma; INR, international normalized ratio; NR, not reported; P-gp, P-glycoprotein; PCC, prothrombin complex concentrate; PT, prothrombin time; qd, once daily; TT, thrombin time; T_{max}, time to maximum plasma concentration; $T_{1/2\beta}$, terminal half-life; V_d, volume of distribution; VKORC1, vitamin K epoxide reductase enzyme subunit 1.

[a] Potent inhibitors of CYP3A4 include antifungals (eg, ketoconazole, itraconazole, voriconazole, posaconazole), chloramphenicol, clarithromycin, and protease inhibitors (eg, ritonavir, atazanavir). P-gp inhibitors include verapamil, amiodarone, quinidine, and clarithromycin. P-gp inducers include rifampicin, St. John's wort (*Hypericum perforatum*), carbamazepine, and phenytoin. Potent CYP3A4 inducers include phenytoin, carbamazepine, phenobarbital, and St. John's wort.

Data from Refs.[27–29]

practice is usually lower. In their systematic review, van Walraven and colleagues[38] found significantly poorer control in the community practices than in either anticoagulation clinics or clinical trials (−12.2%; 95% CI −19.5% to −4.8%).

Non-VKA Oral Anticoagulants

Given the limitations of the VKAs, new classes of OAC have been developed that are capable of overcoming the challenges of warfarin therapy, as they selectively inhibit key factors in the coagulation cascade. These non-VKA oral anticoagulants (NOACs, previously referred to as new or novel OACs) include direct thrombin (factor II) inhibitors (eg, dabigatran) and factor Xa inhibitors (eg, apixaban, rivaroxaban, and, most recently, edoxaban).[27,39,40]

Direct thrombin inhibitors bind to the active catalytic site of thrombin, either free thrombin in plasma or clot (fibrin)-bound thrombin, thereby interfering with multiple effects realized with thrombin: fibrin production from fibrinogen and its stabilization; activation of coagulation factors V, VIII, XI, and XIII; platelet activation; inhibition of fibrinolysis; and proinflammatory changes.[41,42]

Factor X represents convergence of intrinsic and extrinsic coagulation pathways. One molecule of activated factor Xa as a result of a cascade of enzymatic reactions eventually leads to conversion of up to 1000 molecules of prothrombin to thrombin. Direct factor Xa inhibitors not only block free factor Xa via binding to its active site but also inactivate it within the prothrombinase complex bound to platelets.[41,42]

The principal differences that distinguish the NOACs from VKAs are the fixed dose administration and no necessity for intensive INR control, in addition to more rapid onset and shorter offset of action, fewer drug interactions, no food interactions, and kidney elimination.[27,39,40] Pharmacologic characteristics of the NOACs are summarized in **Table 2**.

Four large phase III prospective, randomized clinical trials on the safety and effectiveness of NOACs in comparison with warfarin have been completed (**Table 3**): RE-LY with dabigatran,[43] ROCKET AF with rivaroxaban,[44] ARISTOTLE with apixaban,[45] and ENGAGE AF-TIMI 48 with edoxaban[46] (see **Table 3** for expansion of acronyms). Trials on the oral direct factor Xa inhibitors were double-blind, whereas the trial on dabigatran was open-label between dabigatran and warfarin arms, but double-blind between 2 arms with different doses of dabigatran (150 mg vs 110 mg twice a day).

Patients in the ROCKET AF trial cohort were at higher risk of stroke (based on the CHADS$_2$ score),

with more patients with a history of stroke, transient ischemic attack (TIA), or systemic embolism, and a lower mean TTR (55%).[47]

All-cause (ischemic, hemorrhagic, or indeterminate) stroke and/or systemic embolism (non–central nervous system) thromboembolic events were analyzed as primary efficacy end points. Major bleeding (broadly defined as decrease of hemoglobin by at least 2 g/dL, transfusion of at least 2 units of red blood cells [within 24 hours in the ARISTOTLE trial], bleeding at a critical site, or resulting in death) was used as primary safety end point (clinically relevant nonmajor bleeding was also included in the ROCKET AF trial).[43–46]

In the effectiveness analyses, all NOACs appeared to be noninferior to warfarin in risk reduction with respect to the primary end point of stroke or systemic embolism. However, apixaban and dabigatran 150 mg were found to be superior to warfarin.[43,45] All NOACs appeared to be effective for secondary prophylaxis of stroke and/or TIA.[48–50]

In the safety analysis, the rate of major bleeding was found to be at least similar between NOACs and warfarin, or even significantly less with dabigatran 110 mg twice a day, apixaban, and edoxaban. Of note, a reduced risk of intracranial haemorrhage was apparent for all NOACs.[43–46]

A favorable trend in mortality was seen for all 3 NOACs in comparison with warfarin, which reached statistical significance when apixaban or edoxaban 60 mg was used.[43–46] A numerical but nonsignificant trend toward a higher rate of myocardial infarction was found for dabigatran, which was nonsignificant with inclusion of previously unidentified events[43,51] and low-dose edoxaban.[46]

Regarding long-term follow-up, dabigatran was further evaluated in the RELY-ABLE study, which included 5851 dabigatran-treated patients from the RE-LY study who were followed up for an additional 2.3 years, in addition to a "real-world" Danish nationwide cohort study, both of which showed results consistent with those of the original trial.[52,53]

In the meta-analysis of phase II and phase III randomized trials comparing NOACs with VKAs, the former were found to reduce total mortality (relative risk [RR] 0.89, 95% CI 0.83–0.96), cardiovascular mortality (RR 0.89, 95% CI 0.82–0.98), stroke/systemic embolism (RR 0.77, 95% CI, 0.70–0.86), and intracranial hemorrhage (RR 0.46, 95% CI 0.39–0.56).[54] These results are consistent with another systematic review using data from 3 pivotal studies (RE-LY, ROCKET AF, and ARISTOTLE): 8 (3–11) fewer deaths per 1000 patients (RR 0.88, 95% CI 0.82–0.96) and

Table 3
Summary of pivotal clinical trials of non-VKA oral anticoagulants in patients with nonvalvular AF

| | Clinical Trial | | | |
	RE-LY	ROCKET AF	ARISTOTLE	ENGAGE AF - TIMI 48
Non-VKA OAC examined	Dabigatran	Rivaroxaban	Apixaban	Edoxaban
Patients	18,113	14,264	18,201	21,105
Age (y)	71	73	70	72
Mean $CHADS_2$ score	2.1	3.5	2.1	2.8
Non-VKA OAC dosing arm	150 mg bid / 110 mg bid	20 (15[a]) mg qd	5 (2.5[b]) mg bid	60 mg qd / 30 mg qd
Prior vitamin K antagonist treatment (%)	50	62	57	58.8
Prior stroke or transient ischemic attack (%)	20 (including systemic embolism)	55	19 (including systemic embolism)	28.1 / 28.5
Mean TTR, warfarin arm (%)	64	55	62	68.4
Relative risk (95% CI) for non-VKA OAC vs warfarin				
Stroke or systemic embolism	0.65 (0.52–0.81) / 0.90 (0.74–1.10)	0.88 (0.75–1.03)	0.79 (0.66–0.96)	0.87 (0.73–1.04) / 1.13 (0.96–1.34)
Major bleeding	0.93 (0.81–1.07) / 0.80 (0.70–0.93)	1.04 (0.90–1.20)	0.69 (0.60–0.80)	0.80 (0.71–0.91) / 0.47 (0.41–0.55)
Intracranial hemorrhage	0.41 (0.28–0.60) / 0.30 (0.19–0.45)	0.67 (0.47–0.93)	0.42 (0.30–0.58)	0.47 (0.34–0.63) / 0.30 (0.21–0.43)
Gastrointestinal bleeding	1.49 (1.19–1.88) / 1.09 (0.85–1.39)	1.47 (1.20–1.81)	0.88 (0.67–1.14)	1.23 (1.02–1.50) / 0.67 (0.53–0.83)
Myocardial infarction	1.27 (0.94–1.71) / 1.29 (0.96–1.75)	0.81 (0.63–1.06)	0.88 (0.66–1.17)	0.94 (0.74–1.19) / 1.19 (0.95–1.49)
Death	0.88 (0.77–1.00) / 0.91 (0.80–1.03)	0.85 (0.70–1.02)	0.89 (0.80–0.99)	0.92 (0.83–1.01) / 0.87 (0.79–0.96)

Abbreviations: ARISTOTLE, Apixaban for Reduction In STroke and Other ThromboemboLic Events in atrial fibrillation; bid, twice daily; CHADS₂, congestive heart failure, hypertension, age >75 years, diabetes mellitus, stroke or transient ischemic attack (2 points); CI, confidence interval; ENGAGE AF - TIMI 48, Effective aNticoaGulation with factor Xa next GEneration in Atrial Fibrillation—Thrombolysis In Myocardial Infarction 48; OAC, oral anticoagulant; qd, once daily; RE-LY, Randomized Evaluation of Long-term anticoagulation therapY; ROCKET AF, Rivaroxaban Once daily oral direct factor Xa inhibition Compared with vitamin K antagonism for prevention of stroke and Embolism Trial in Atrial Fibrillation; TTR, time in therapeutic range.

[a] In patients with creatinine clearance of 30 to 49 mL/min.
[b] In patients with 2 or more of the following criteria: age greater than 80 years, body weight less than 60 kg, or serum creatinine greater than 133 µmol/L.
Data from Refs.[43–46]

4 (2–5 fewer) fewer hemorrhagic strokes per 1000 patients (RR 0.48, 95% CI 0.36–0.62), with an obvious trend toward reduced risk of ischemic stroke (RR 0.89, 95 CI% 0.78–1.02).[55] Administration of the NOACs appeared to be particularly advantageous in patients with a high risk for stroke and/or bleeding.[19] Considering the noninferiority of the NOACs for stroke/thromboembolism prevention and its better safety profile, NOACs are given preference over VKAs in current guidelines (**Fig. 1**).[5]

As no head-to-head studies have been conducted, there is no direct evidence of important differences in the efficacy and safety among the NOACs. Several indirect comparisons between dabigatran, rivaroxaban, and apixaban have been carried out, with broadly similar results obtained. These indirect comparisons found

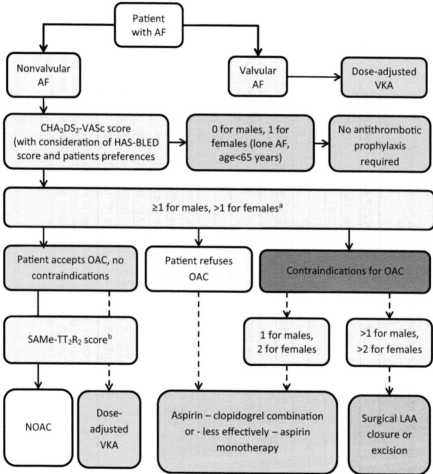

Fig. 1. Recommendations for prevention of thromboembolism in nonvalvular AF. [a] 2014 American Heart Association/American College of Cardiology/Heart Rhythm Society guideline for the management of patients with AF allows either OAC or aspirin or no antithrombotic therapy in patients with a CHA$_2$DS$_2$-VASc score = 1.[6] [b] Currently not in the guidelines. Solid line, best option; dashed line, alternative option. CHA$_2$DS$_2$-VASc: congestive heart failure, hypertension, age 75 years or older (doubled), diabetes mellitus, stroke or transient ischemic attack (doubled), vascular disease, age 65 to 74 years, sex category (female); HAS-BLED: hypertension, abnormal renal/liver function (1 point each), stroke, bleeding history or predisposition, labile international normalized ratio, elderly (≥65 years old), drugs/alcohol concomitantly (1 point each); SAMe-TT$_2$R$_2$: female sex, age less than 60 years, medical history (2 of the following: hypertension, diabetes, coronary artery disease/myocardial infarction, peripheral artery disease, heart failure, previous stroke, pulmonary, hepatic or renal disease), treatment with interacting drugs (eg, amiodarone), tobacco use (within 2 years, doubled), non-Caucasian race (doubled). LAA, left atrial appendage; OAC, oral anticoagulation; VKA, vitamin K antagonist. (*Data from* Camm AJ, Lip GY, De Caterina R, et al. 2012 focused update of the ESC guidelines for the management of atrial fibrillation: an update of the 2010 ESC guidelines for the management of atrial fibrillation. Europace 2012;14(10):1385–413.)

apixaban to be less causative of bleeding when compared with dabigatran 150 mg or rivaroxaban. Moreover, rivaroxaban seemed to be less effective than dabigatran 150 mg for stroke prevention. There were no compelling differences between the NOACs regarding reduction in ischemic strokes or mortality.[56,57]

In another comparison analysis performed separately for primary and secondary prevention of stroke, no significant differences in safety and efficacy end points between dabigatran 150 mg, rivaroxaban, and apixaban were found for secondary prevention, apart from a higher rate of myocardial infarction with dabigatran 150 mg. For the primary prevention of stroke, there were some differences between the agents; for example, apixaban was associated with more strokes in comparison with dabigatran 150 mg, but less major bleeding in comparison with both dabigatran 150 mg and rivaroxaban.[58]

In a recent indirect comparison of high-dose edoxaban with other NOACs, there were no significant differences in the efficacy end points (apart from higher rate of stroke, stroke or systemic embolism, and hemorrhagic stroke when compared with dabigatran 150 mg). A higher rate of major and clinically relevant nonmajor bleeding was observed when compared with apixaban, but a lower one when compared with rivaroxaban. There were higher bleeding rates with all NOACs in comparison with low-dose edoxaban while it was less effective for prevention of stroke/systemic embolism.[59]

Of importance, limitations of indirect comparisons (differences in study design, patient population, definitions of outcomes) have been acknowledged in all analyses.

The advantages of NOACs in particular clinical situations may become disadvantageous. No need for anticoagulation monitoring may result in decreased patient adherence to treatment, given that the short half-lives of the NOACs place patients at higher risk of adverse events. Moreover, there are no routine anticoagulation tests to evaluate reliably the effect of NOACs, which is essential in acute settings (eg, acute ischemic or hemorrhagic stroke). Those available in everyday practice supply physicians only with tentative qualitative information.[27,60]

Furthermore, there are no specific antidotes for the NOACs. Prothrombin complex concentrates (either activated or nonactivated) appear to be standard for the management of bleeding with NOACs.[27] Other reversal agents (antidabigatran antibody fragments, recombinant factor VIIa, factor Xa missing Gla [carboxyglutamic acid] residues in Gla domains, and so forth) are mostly investigational thus far, although early results seem promising.[61]

Finally, the NOACs are currently approved for nonvalvular AF and are contraindicated in patients with severe kidney dysfunction (ie, creatinine clearance <30 mL/min).[5,6]

Defining nonvalvular AF in clinical practice is a subject of controversy, as no universal definition of nonvalvular AF is available thus far. European guidelines refer nonvalvular AF to AF in the absence of rheumatic valvular disease (predominantly mitral stenosis) or prosthetic heart valves.[5] American guidelines define nonvalvular AF as AF in the absence of rheumatic mitral stenosis, a mechanical or bioprosthetic heart valve, or mitral valve repair.[6] Patient populations in pivotal trials of NOACs can also be taken into account. Patients with moderate or severe mitral stenosis or prosthetic mechanical heart valves were excluded in all trials.[43–46] However, in the RE-LY trial patients with any hemodynamically relevant valve disease were excluded.[43] The ROCKET AF cohort included patients with annuloplasty with or without prosthetic ring, commissurotomy, and/or valvuloplasty,[44] and the ENGAGE AF-TIMI 48 trial included those with bioprosthetic heart valves and/or valve repair.[46]

Given the lack of compelling evidence for superiority of the NOACs over well-controlled VKAs (ie, high TTRs, >70%) and limited data on the performance of NOACs in the real-world population, attempts have been made to reliably identify the proportion of AF patients who will reach a high TTR while on VKAs. The SAMe-TT$_2$R$_2$ score (**Table 4**) is a decision tool that may help to discriminate patients with anticipated high TTR (ie, suitable for warfarin therapy) from those with anticipated low TTR (ie, suitable for NOACs).[62,63]

ANTITHROMBOTIC THERAPY

Aspirin (acetylsalicylic acid) has previously been considered as an alternative to OAC, particularly in patients with a moderate risk of stroke development[64]; that is, up to 60% of the AF population classified with the CHADS$_2$ score (congestive heart failure, hypertension, age ≥75, diabetes mellitus, stroke/TIA).[65]

Aspirin use was supported by the results of a few older trials, which together showed a nonsignificant relative reduction in the risk of stroke of 19% (95% CI −1% to 35%) for aspirin versus placebo/control, with no effect on all-cause mortality.

The nonsignificant 19% reduction was driven by the results of only one single positive trial for aspirin, the SPAF-I trial (Stroke Prevention in Atrial Fibrillation), which used aspirin 325 mg once daily

Table 4
Quality of anticoagulation control assessment with the SAMe-TT$_2$R$_2$ score

Risk Factor	Score
Sex category (ie, female gender)	1
Age <60 y	1
Medical history (≥2 of the following: hypertension, DM, CAD/MI, PAD, CHF, previous stroke, pulmonary, hepatic or renal disease)	1
Treatment with interacting drugs (eg, amiodarone)	1
Tobacco use (within 2 y)	2
Race (ie, non-Caucasian)	2
Maximum score	8

Abbreviations: CAD, coronary artery disease; CHF, congestive heart failure; DM, diabetes mellitus; MI, myocardial infarction; PAD, peripheral artery disease.

Data from Apostolakis S, Sullivan RM, Olshansky B, et al. Factors affecting quality of anticoagulation control among patients with atrial fibrillation on warfarin: the SAMe-TT$_2$R$_2$ score. Chest 2013;144(5):1555–63.

and found a 42% reduction in the risk of stroke in comparison with controls, but with marked internal heterogeneity for its effect in the OAC-eligible and OAC-ineligible arms of SPAF-I.[25] In SPAF-I, aspirin did not have any benefit in those older than 75 years nor did it prevent severe strokes. Moreover, no significant reduction in stroke (either all stroke, ischemic, disabling, or fatal) or all-cause mortality was found in the Cochrane review.[66]

More contemporary trials do not support aspirin use. Aspirin was found to be noneffective for stroke prevention in low-risk patients with AF in the Japan Atrial Fibrillation Stroke Trial.[67] Aspirin did not benefit the elderly in the BAFTA trial (the Birmingham Atrial Fibrillation Treatment of the Aged Study) where warfarin was superior to aspirin, and, importantly, warfarin and aspirin had similar risks of major bleeding and intracranial hemorrhage.[31]

Aspirin was also clearly inferior to apixaban in the AVERROES trial (Apixaban VERsus acetylsalicylic acid to prevent stroke in atrial fibrillation patiEntS who have failed or are unsuitable for vitamin K antagonist treatment), in which apixaban therapy resulted in 55% relative risk reduction in the stroke rate (particularly ischemic and disabling strokes) with no difference between aspirin and apixaban for major bleeding or intracranial hemorrhage.[68,69]

Dual antiplatelet therapy with aspirin and clopidogrel may be marginally better than aspirin monotherapy: an 11% (95% CI 2%–19%) risk reduction for major vascular events (stroke, systemic embolism, myocardial infarction, death from vascular causes) and a 28% (95% CI 17%–38%) risk reduction of stroke development was seen in the ACTIVE (Atrial fibrillation Clopidogrel Trial with Irbesartan for prevention of Vascular Events) trial for aspirin-clopidogrel combination therapy, but at cost of increased major bleeding.[70] However, the combination of aspirin and clopidogrel still remained inferior to OAC.[71] Considering the aforementioned assertions, antiplatelet therapy as a means of stroke prophylaxis is only recommended for AF patients who are unsuitable for or with contraindications to any form of OAC (see **Fig. 1**).[5]

ANTIPLATELET AGENTS IN AF PATIENTS UNDERGOING PERCUTANEOUS CORONARY INTERVENTION/STENTING

The lesser ability of antiplatelet drugs to prevent stroke and systemic embolism can perhaps be explained from a pathophysiologic point of view. Thrombi in AF are fibrin-rich, and activation of coagulation factors plays greater role in their development than platelet activation. By contrast, platelet activation and development of platelet-rich thrombi is the hallmark of thrombotic complications in CAD (acute coronary syndrome [ACS], stent thrombosis, and so forth).[72–74]

Given the high prevalence of AF associated with CAD[75] and the need to undergo percutaneous intervention, often with stent implantation, these patients therefore require a combination of OAC and antiplatelet agents (triple therapy) to cover both pathways and reduce the risk of complications.[76]

Obviously, triple therapy is associated with a higher risk of bleeding complications, and its duration of use depends on several factors including initial risk of bleeding, type of stent (bare metal or drug-eluting stent and its generation), and clinical setting (ACS or elective procedure) to balance the risk of bleeding and thrombotic/thromboembolic complications (**Table 5**).[76]

Table 5
Recommended antithrombotic strategies following coronary artery stenting in patients with atrial fibrillation at moderate to high thromboembolic risk

			Recommendations in Timeline		
Hemorrhagic Risk	Clinical Setting	Stent Implanted	Triple Therapy of Warfarin (INR 2.0–2.5) + Aspirin ≤100 mg/d + Clopidogrel 75 mg/d	Dual Therapy of Warfarin (INR 2.0–2.5) + Clopidogrel 75 mg/d (or Aspirin 100 mg/d)	Monotherapy of Warfarin (INR 2.0–3.0)
Low or moderate	Elective	Bare metal	1 mo	—	Lifelong
		Drug-eluting	3–6 mo	12 mo	
	ACS	Bare metal/ drug-eluting	6 mo	12 mo	
High	Elective	Bare metal[a]	2–4 wk	—	Lifelong
	ACS		4 wk	12 mo	

Abbreviations: ACS, acute coronary syndrome; INR, international normalized ratio.
  [a] Drug-eluting stents should be avoided.
  Adapted from Lip GY, Huber K, Andreotti F, et al. Management of antithrombotic therapy in atrial fibrillation patients presenting with acute coronary syndrome and/or undergoing percutaneous coronary intervention/stenting. Thromb Haemost 2010;103(1):22; with permission.

Considering the increased risk of major bleeding in triple therapy[77–79] and the low adherence to it (specifically, underuse of OAC),[80] several studies attempted to compare the effectiveness and safety of different prophylactic regimens against triple therapy.

Broadly similar effectiveness and safety for triple therapy, dual antiplatelet therapy, and warfarin plus single antiplatelet agent was observed in the AFCAS registry (Atrial Fibrillation Undergoing Coronary Artery Stenting) and Danish nationwide registries.[81,82] In the WOEST study (What is the Optimal antiplatElet and anticoagulant therapy in patients with oral anticoagulation and coronary StenTing) there was a significantly lower bleeding rate and mortality was lower in the warfarin plus clopidogrel arm in comparison with triple therapy (hazard ratio [HR] 0.36, 95% CI 0.26–0.50 and HR 0.39, 95% CI 0.16–0.93, respectively), with no significant differences in the rate of thrombotic events.[83]

However, these studies cannot change current practice, as the data are inconclusive (small sample, heterogeneity in design, combinations and doses of antithrombotic agents, and so forth). Larger, prospective, randomized trials are required to prove the efficacy and safety of the various combinations of oral anticoagulants (including NOACs) and antiplatelet drugs (including the newer P_2Y_{12}-receptor inhibitors prasugrel and ticagrelor).

In patients with stable coronary heart disease and AF, treated chronically with OAC, antiplatelet medications bring no significant benefits with respect to reduction in strokes, acute coronary events, or mortality, but are associated with an increased risk of serious bleeding (HR 1.5, 95% CI 1.23–1.82 for aspirin or HR 1.84, 95% CI 1.11–3.06 for clopidogrel), particularly ICH.[84]

PREVENTION OF NONPHARMACOLOGIC STROKE AND THROMBOEMBOLISM

A range of comorbidities may make patients with AF ineligible for chronic OAC (eg, hepatic and/or kidney dysfunction, mechanical valve prostheses, hereditary coagulation disorders).

Because the left atrial appendage (LAA) is known to be the major source of stroke-causing thrombi in AF because of loss of coordinated contraction, dilation, and blood stasis, LAA exclusion offers an alternative to OAC for stroke prevention in AF.

This goal can be achieved via percutaneous access (with closure devices) or during open heart surgery for any other reason (by ligating, stapling, or amputation).[85] Overall, LAA devices were found to be noninferior to warfarin, for example, the WATCHMAN device (Boston Scientific, Natick, MA, USA) in the PROTECT AF study (LAA System for Embolic Protection in Patients with Atrial Fibrillation).[86]

However, LAA occlusion may not completely eliminate the risk of stroke because of sources of thrombi other than the LAA,[87] which taken together with the risk of procedural complications and scarce data allows this option to be applied only for patients at high risk of stroke who are unable to tolerate OAC (see **Fig. 1**).[5] Surgical excision of the LAA may be considered in patients undergoing cardiac surgery.[6]

SUMMARY

Optimal prevention of thromboembolic events in most occurrences of AF requires oral anticoagulation. When the NOACs became available, antithrombotic prophylaxis seemed to overcome the range of inconveniences associated with warfarin treatment. The role of antiplatelet agents for stroke prevention in AF has diminished significantly, but may still be required for the prevention of thrombotic complications in coronary disease, which appear to be common in AF. An informed assessment of the risk of stroke (using CHA_2DS_2-VASc) and bleeding (using HAS-BLED) is of importance when balancing risks and considering the net clinical benefit of thromboprophylaxis.

REFERENCES

1. Go AS, Hylek EM, Phillips KA, et al. Prevalence of diagnosed atrial fibrillation in adults: national implications for rhythm management and stroke prevention: the AnTicoagulation and Risk Factors in Atrial Fibrillation (ATRIA) Study. JAMA 2001;285(18): 2370–5.
2. Björck S, Palaszewski B, Friberg L, et al. Atrial fibrillation, stroke risk, and warfarin therapy revisited: a population-based study. Stroke 2013; 44(11):3103–8.
3. Lamassa M, Di Carlo A, Pracucci G, et al. Characteristics, outcome, and care of stroke associated with atrial fibrillation in Europe: data from a multicenter multinational hospital-based registry (The European Community Stroke Project). Stroke 2001;32(2):392–8.
4. Cotter PE, Martin PJ, Ring L, et al. Incidence of atrial fibrillation detected by implantable loop recorders in unexplained stroke. Neurology 2013; 80(17):1546–50.
5. Camm AJ, Lip GY, De Caterina R, et al. 2012 focused update of the ESC guidelines for the management of atrial fibrillation: an update of the 2010 ESC guidelines for the management of atrial fibrillation. Europace 2012;14(10):1385–413.
6. January CT, Wann LS, Alpert JS, et al. 2014 AHA/ ACC/HRS Guideline for the management of patients with atrial fibrillation: a report of the American College of Cardiology/American Heart Association Task Force on Practice Guidelines and the Heart Rhythm Society. Circulation 2014. [Epub ahead of print].
7. Lip GY, Laroche C, Dan GA, et al. 'Real-world' antithrombotic treatment in atrial fibrillation: the EURObservational Research Programme Atrial Fibrillation General Pilot survey. Am J Med 2014. http://dx.doi.org/10.1016/j.amjmed.2013.12.022.
8. Stroke Risk in Atrial Fibrillation Working Group. Independent predictors of stroke in patients with atrial fibrillation: a systematic review. Neurology 2007;69(6):546–54.
9. Pisters R, Lane DA, Marin F, et al. Stroke and thromboembolism in atrial fibrillation. Circ J 2012; 76(10):2289–304.
10. Lip GY, Nieuwlaat R, Pisters R, et al. Refining clinical risk stratification for predicting stroke and thromboembolism in atrial fibrillation using a novel risk factor-based approach: the Euro Heart Survey on atrial fibrillation. Chest 2010;137(2):263–72.
11. Olesen JB, Lip GY, Hansen ML, et al. Validation of risk stratification schemes for predicting stroke and thromboembolism in patients with atrial fibrillation: nationwide cohort study. BMJ 2011;342:d124. http://dx.doi.org/10.1136/bmj.d124.
12. Gage BF, Waterman AD, Shannon W, et al. Validation of clinical classification schemes for predicting stroke: results from the national registry of atrial fibrillation. JAMA 2001;285(22):2864–70.
13. Olesen JB, Torp-Pedersen C, Hansen ML, et al. The value of the CHA2DS2-VASc score for refining stroke risk stratification in patients with atrial fibrillation with a CHADS2 score 0–1: a nationwide cohort study. Thromb Haemost 2012;107(6):1172–9.
14. Van Staa TP, Setakis E, Di Tanna GL, et al. A comparison of risk stratification schema for stroke in 79884 atrial fibrillation patients in general practice. J Thromb Haemost 2011;9(1):39–48.
15. Potpara TS, Polovina MM, Licina MM, et al. Reliable identification of 'truly low' thromboembolic risk in patients initially diagnosed with 'lone' atrial fibrillation: the Belgrade Atrial Fibrillation Study. Circ Arrhythm Electrophysiol 2012;5(2):319–26.
16. Singer DE, Chang Y, Fang MC, et al. The net clinical benefit of warfarin anticoagulation in atrial fibrillation. Ann Intern Med 2009;151(5):297–305.
17. Olesen JB, Lip GY, Lindhardsen J, et al. Risks of thromboembolism and bleeding with thromboprophylaxis in patients with atrial fibrillation: a net clinical benefit analysis using a 'real world' nationwide cohort study. Thromb Haemost 2011;106(4): 739–49.
18. Friberg L, Rosenqvist M, Lip G. Net clinical benefit of warfarin in patients with atrial fibrillation: a report from the Swedish Atrial Fibrillation Cohort Study. Circulation 2012;125(19):2298–307.
19. Banerjee A, Lane DA, Torp-Pedersen C, et al. Net clinical benefit of new oral anticoagulants (dabigatran, rivaroxaban, apixaban) versus no treatment in a 'real world' atrial fibrillation population: a

modeling analysis based on a nationwide cohort study. Thromb Haemost 2012;107(3):584–9.

20. Pisters R, Lane DA, Nieuwlaat R, et al. A novel user-friendly score (HAS-BLED) to assess 1-year risk of major bleeding in patients with atrial fibrillation: the Euro Heart Survey. Chest 2010;138(5):1093–100.

21. Apostolakis S, Lane DA, Guo Y, et al. Performance of the Hemorr(2)hages, ATRIA, and HAS-BLED bleeding risk-prediction scores in patients with atrial fibrillation undergoing anticoagulation: the AMADEUS (evaluating the use of sr34006 compared to warfarin or acenocoumarol in patients with atrial fibrillation) Study. J Am Coll Cardiol 2012; 60(9):861–7.

22. Overvad TF, Larsen TB, Albertsen IE, et al. Balancing bleeding and thrombotic risk with new oral anticoagulants in patients with atrial fibrillation. Expert Rev Cardiovasc Ther 2013;11(12):1619–29.

23. Lip GY, Lin HJ, Hsu HC, et al. Comparative assessment of the HAS-BLED score with other published bleeding risk scoring schemes, for intracranial haemorrhage risk in a non-atrial fibrillation population: the Chi-Shan Community Cohort Study. Int J Cardiol 2013;168(3):1832–6.

24. Omran H, Bauersachs R, Rubenacker S, et al. The HAS-BLED score predicts bleedings during bridging of chronic oral anticoagulation. Results from the National Multicentre BNK Online Bridging Registry (BORDER). Thromb Haemost 2012; 108(1):65–73.

25. Hart RG, Pearce LA, Aguilar MI. Meta-analysis: antithrombotic therapy to prevent stroke in patients who have nonvalvular atrial fibrillation. Ann Intern Med 2007;146(12):857–67.

26. De Caterina R, Husted S, Wallentin L, et al. Vitamin K antagonists in heart disease: current status and perspectives (Section III). Position paper of the ESC Working Group on Thrombosis–Task Force on Anticoagulants in Heart Disease. Thromb Haemost 2013;110(6):1087–107.

27. Heidbuchel H, Verhamme P, Alings M, et al. European Heart Rhythm Association Practical Guide on the use of new oral anticoagulants in patients with non-valvular atrial fibrillation. Europace 2013; 15(5):625–51.

28. Gong IY, Kim RB. Importance of pharmacokinetic profile and variability as determinants of dose and response to dabigatran, rivaroxaban, and apixaban. Can J Cardiol 2013;29(7 Suppl):S24–33.

29. Camm AJ, Bounameaux H. Edoxaban: a new oral direct factor Xa inhibitor. Drugs 2011;71(12): 1513–26.

30. Ogilvie IM, Newton N, Welner SA, et al. Underuse of oral anticoagulants in atrial fibrillation: a systematic review. Am J Med 2010;123:638–45.

31. Mant J, Hobbs FD, Fletcher K, et al. Warfarin versus aspirin for stroke prevention in an elderly community population with atrial fibrillation (the Birmingham Atrial Fibrillation Treatment of the Aged study, BAFTA): a randomised controlled trial. Lancet 2007;370:493–503.

32. Wang C, Yang Z, Wang C, et al. Significant underuse of warfarin in patients with nonvalvular atrial fibrillation: results from the China National Stroke Registry. J Stroke Cerebrovasc Dis 2013. http://dx.doi.org/10. 1016/j.jstrokecerebrovasdis.2013.10.006.

33. Horne BD, Lenzini PA, Wadelius M, et al. Pharmacogenetic warfarin dose refinements remain significantly influenced by genetic factors after one week of therapy. Thromb Haemost 2012;107(2):232–40.

34. Kurnik D, Qasim H, Sominsky S, et al. Effect of the VKORC1 D36Y variant on warfarin dose requirement and pharmacogenetic dose prediction. Thromb Haemost 2012;108(4):781–8.

35. Xu Q, Xu B, Zhang Y, et al. Estimation of the warfarin dose with a pharmacogenetic refinement algorithm in Chinese patients mainly under low-intensity warfarin anticoagulation. Thromb Haemost 2012;108(6):1132–40.

36. Morgan CL, McEwan P, Tukiendorf A, et al. Warfarin treatment in patients with atrial fibrillation: observing outcomes associated with varying levels of INR control. Thromb Res 2009;124(1):37–41.

37. Gallagher AM, Setakis E, Plumb JM, et al. Risks of stroke and mortality associated with suboptimal anticoagulation in atrial fibrillation patients. Thromb Haemost 2011;106(5):968–77.

38. van Walraven C, Jennings A, Oake N, et al. Effect of study setting on anticoagulation control: a systematic review and metaregression. Chest 2006; 129(5):1155–66.

39. Ahrens I, Lip GY, Peter K. New oral anticoagulant drugs in cardiovascular disease. Thromb Haemost 2010;104(1):49–60.

40. Potpara TS, Lip GY. Novel oral anticoagulants in non-valvular atrial fibrillation. Best Pract Res Clin Haematol 2013;26(2):115–29.

41. De Caterina R, Husted S, Wallentin L, et al. General mechanisms of coagulation and targets of anticoagulants (Section I). Position Paper of the ESC Working Group on Thrombosis - Task Force on Anticoagulants in Heart Disease. Thromb Haemost 2013;109(4):569–79.

42. Weitz JI. Factor Xa and thrombin as targets for new oral anticoagulants. Thromb Res 2011;127(Suppl 2):S5–12.

43. Connolly SJ, Ezekowitz MD, Yusuf S, et al, RE-LY Steering Committee and Investigators. Dabigatran versus warfarin in patients with atrial fibrillation. N Engl J Med 2009;361(12):1139–51.

44. Patel MR, Mahaffey KW, Garg J, et al, ROCKET AF Investigators. Rivaroxaban versus warfarin in non-valvular atrial fibrillation. N Engl J Med 2011; 365(10):883–91.

45. Granger CB, Alexander JH, McMurray JJ, et al, ARISTOTLE Committees and Investigators. Apixaban versus warfarin in patients with atrial fibrillation. N Engl J Med 2011;365(11):981–92.

46. Giugliano RP, Ruff CT, Braunwald E, et al, ENGAGE AF-TIMI 48 Investigators. Edoxaban versus warfarin in patients with atrial fibrillation. N Engl J Med 2013;369(22):2093–104.

47. Lee S, Monz BU, Clemens A, et al. Representativeness of the dabigatran, apixaban and rivaroxaban clinical trial populations to real-world atrial fibrillation patients in the United Kingdom: a cross-sectional analysis using the General Practice Research Database. BMJ Open 2012;2(6). http://dx.doi.org/10.1136/bmjopen-2012-001768.

48. Diener HC, Connolly SJ, Ezekowitz MD, et al, RE-LY Study Group. Dabigatran compared with warfarin in patients with atrial fibrillation and previous transient ischaemic attack or stroke: a subgroup analysis of the RE-LY trial. Lancet Neurol 2010;9(12):1157–63.

49. Hankey GJ, Patel MR, Stevens SR, et al, ROCKET AF Steering Committee Investigators. Rivaroxaban compared with warfarin in patients with atrial fibrillation and previous stroke or transient ischaemic attack: a subgroup analysis of ROCKET AF. Lancet Neurol 2012;11(4):315–22.

50. Easton JD, Lopes RD, Bahit MC, et al, ARISTOTLE Committees and Investigators. Apixaban compared with warfarin in patients with atrial fibrillation and previous stroke or transient ischaemic attack: a subgroup analysis of the ARISTOTLE trial. Lancet Neurol 2012;11(6):503–11.

51. Connolly SJ, Ezekowitz MD, Yusuf S, et al, Randomized Evaluation of Long-Term Anticoagulation Therapy Investigators. Newly identified events in the RE-LY trial. N Engl J Med 2010;363(19):1875–6.

52. Connolly SJ, Wallentin L, Ezekowitz MD, et al. The long-term multicenter observational study of dabigatran treatment in patients with atrial fibrillation (RELY-ABLE) Study. Circulation 2013;128(3):237–43.

53. Larsen TB, Rasmussen LH, Skjøth F, et al. Efficacy and safety of dabigatran etexilate and warfarin in "real-world" patients with atrial fibrillation: a prospective nationwide cohort study. J Am Coll Cardiol 2013;61(22):2264–73.

54. Dentali F, Riva N, Crowther M, et al. Efficacy and safety of the novel oral anticoagulants in atrial fibrillation. Circulation 2012;126(20):2381–91.

55. Adam SS, McDuffie JR, Ortel TL, et al. Comparative effectiveness of warfarin and new oral anticoagulants for the management of atrial fibrillation and venous thromboembolism. Ann Intern Med 2012;157(11):796–807.

56. Lip GY, Larsen TB, Skjøth F, et al. Indirect comparisons of new oral anticoagulants for efficacy and safety when used for stroke prevention in atrial fibrillation. J Am Coll Cardiol 2012;60(8):738–46.

57. Mantha S, Ansell J. An indirect comparison of dabigatran, rivaroxaban, and apixaban for atrial fibrillation. Thromb Haemost 2012;108(3):476–84.

58. Rasmussen LH, Larsen TB, Graungaard T, et al. Primary and secondary prevention with new oral anticoagulant drugs for stroke prevention in atrial fibrillation: indirect comparison analysis. BMJ 2012;345:e7097. http://dx.doi.org/10.1136/bmj.e7097.

59. Skjøth F, Larsen TB, Rasmussen LH, et al. Efficacy and safety of edoxaban in comparison with dabigatran, rivaroxaban and apixaban for stroke prevention in atrial fibrillation. An indirect comparison analysis. Thromb Haemost 2014;111(5). http://dx.doi.org/10.1160/TH14-02-0118.

60. Douxfils J, Mullier F, Robert S, et al. Impact of dabigatran on a large panel of routine or specific coagulation assays. Thromb Haemost 2012;107(5):985–97.

61. Capodannoa D, Giacchia G, Tamburinoa C. Current status and ongoing development of reversing agents for novel oral anticoagulants. Recent Pat Cardiovasc Drug Discov 2013;8:2–9.

62. Apostolakis S, Sullivan RM, Olshansky B, et al. Factors affecting quality of anticoagulation control among patients with atrial fibrillation on warfarin: the SAMe-TT2R2 score. Chest 2013;144(5):1555–63.

63. Lip GY, Haguenoer K, Saint-Etienne C, et al. Relationship of the SAMe-TT$_2$R$_2$ score to poor quality anticoagulation, stroke, clinically relevant bleeding and mortality in patients with atrial fibrillation. Chest 2014. [Epub ahead of print].

64. Fuster V, Ryden LE, Cannom DS, et al. ACC/AHA/ESC 2006 guidelines for the management of patients with atrial fibrillation: full text: a report of the American College of Cardiology/American Heart Association Task Force on practice guidelines and the European Society of Cardiology Committee for practice guidelines (writing committee to revise the 2001 guidelines for the management of patients with atrial fibrillation) developed in collaboration with the European Heart Rhythm Association and the Heart Rhythm Society. Europace 2006;8(9):651–745.

65. Fang MC, Go AS, Chang Y, et al, ATRIA Study Group. Comparison of risk stratification schemes to predict thromboembolism in people with non-valvular atrial fibrillation. J Am Coll Cardiol 2008;51(8):810–5.

66. Aguilar M, Hart R. Antiplatelet therapy for preventing stroke in patients with non-valvular atrial fibrillation and no previous history of stroke or transient ischemic attacks. Cochrane Database Syst Rev 2005;(4). CD001925. Available at: http://onlinelibrary.wiley.com/doi/10.1002/14651858.CD001925.pub2/pdf.

67. Sato H, Ishikawa K, Kitabatake A, et al, Japan Atrial Fibrillation Stroke Trial Group. Low-dose aspirin for prevention of stroke in low-risk patients with atrial fibrillation: Japan Atrial Fibrillation Stroke Trial. Stroke 2006;37(2):447–51.

68. Connolly SJ, Eikelboom J, Joyner C, et al, AVER-ROES Steering Committee and Investigators. Apixaban in patients with atrial fibrillation. N Engl J Med 2011;364(9):806–17.

69. Diener HC, Eikelboom J, Connolly SJ, et al, AVER-ROES Steering Committee and Investigators. Apixaban versus aspirin in patients with atrial fibrillation and previous stroke or transient ischaemic attack: a predefined subgroup analysis from AVERROES, a randomised trial. Lancet Neurol 2012;11(3):225–31.

70. ACTIVE Investigators, Connolly SJ, Pogue J, et al. Effect of clopidogrel added to aspirin in patients with atrial fibrillation. N Engl J Med 2009;360(20): 2066–78.

71. ACTIVE Writing Group of the ACTIVE Investigators, Connolly S, Pogue J, et al. Clopidogrel plus aspirin versus oral anticoagulation for atrial fibrillation in the Atrial fibrillation Clopidogrel Trial with Irbesartan for prevention of Vascular Events (ACTIVE W): a randomised controlled trial. Lancet 2006;367(9526): 1903–12.

72. Depta JP, Bhatt DL. Atherothrombosis and atrial fibrillation: important and often overlapping clinical syndromes. Thromb Haemost 2010;104(4):657–63.

73. Watson T, Shantsila E, Lip GY. Mechanisms of thrombogenesis in atrial fibrillation: Virchow's triad revisited. Lancet 2009;373(9658):155–66.

74. Wysokinski WE, Owen WG, Fass DN, et al. Atrial fibrillation and thrombosis: immunohistochemical differences between in situ and embolized thrombi. J Thromb Haemost 2004;2(9):1637–44.

75. Nieuwlaat R, Capucci A, Camm AJ, et al, European Heart Survey Investigators. Atrial fibrillation management: a prospective survey in ESC member countries: the Euro Heart Survey on Atrial Fibrillation. Eur Heart J 2005;26:2422–34.

76. Lip GY, Huber K, Andreotti F, et al. Management of antithrombotic therapy in atrial fibrillation patients presenting with acute coronary syndrome and/or undergoing percutaneous coronary intervention/stenting. Thromb Haemost 2010;103(1):13–28.

77. Lamberts M, Olesen JB, Ruwald MH, et al. Bleeding after initiation of multiple antithrombotic drugs, including triple therapy, in atrial fibrillation patients following myocardial infarction and coronary intervention: a nationwide cohort study. Circulation 2012;126(10):1185–93.

78. Manzano-Fernandez S, Pastor FJ, Marín F, et al. Increased major bleeding complications related to triple antithrombotic therapy usage in patients with atrial fibrillation undergoing percutaneous coronary artery stenting. Chest 2008;134(3):559–67.

79. Azoulay L, Dell'Aniello S, Simon T, et al. The concurrent use of antithrombotic therapies and the risk of bleeding in patients with atrial fibrillation. Thromb Haemost 2013;109(3):431–9.

80. Bernard A, Fauchier L, Pellegrin C, et al. Anticoagulation in patients with atrial fibrillation undergoing coronary stent implantation. Thromb Haemost 2013;110(3):560–8.

81. Rubboli A, Schlitt A, Kiviniemi T, et al. One-year outcome of patients with atrial fibrillation undergoing coronary artery stenting: an analysis of the AFCAS registry. Clin Cardiol 2014. http://dx.doi.org/10.1002/clc.22254.

82. Lamberts M, Gislason GH, Olesen JB, et al. Oral anticoagulation and antiplatelets in atrial fibrillation patients after myocardial infarction and coronary intervention. J Am Coll Cardiol 2013;62(11): 981–9.

83. Dewilde WJ, Oirbans T, Verheugt F, et al. Use of clopidogrel with or without aspirin in patients taking oral anticoagulant therapy and undergoing percutaneous coronary intervention: an open-label, randomized, controlled trial. Lancet 2013;381(9872): 1107–15.

84. Lamberts M, Gislason GH, Lip GY, et al. Antiplatelet therapy in stable coronary artery disease in atrial fibrillation patients on oral anticoagulant: a nationwide cohort study. Circulation 2014. http://dx.doi.org/10.1161/CIRCULATIONAHA.113.004834.

85. Shemin RJ, Cox JL, Gillinov AM, et al, Workforce on Evidence-Based Surgery of the Society of Thoracic Surgeons. Guidelines for reporting data and outcomes for the surgical treatment of atrial fibrillation. Ann Thorac Surg 2007;83:1225–30.

86. Holmes DR, Reddy VY, Turi ZG, et al, PROTECT AF Investigators. Percutaneous closure of the left atrial appendage versus warfarin therapy for prevention of stroke in patients with atrial fibrillation: a randomised non-inferiority trial. Lancet 2009;374(9689): 534–42.

87. Whitlock RP, Healey JS, Connolly SJ. Left atrial appendage occlusion does not eliminate the need for warfarin. Circulation 2009;120(19):1927–32.

Left Atrial Appendage Exclusion for Atrial Fibrillation

 CrossMark

Faisal F. Syed, MBChB, MRCP[a], Christopher V. DeSimone, MD, PhD[a],
Paul A. Friedman, MD, FHRS[a], Samuel J. Asirvatham, MD, FHRS[a,b],*

KEYWORDS

- Left atrial appendage • Percutaneous appendage closure • Stroke prevention • Atrial fibrillation

KEY POINTS

- Given that the left atrial appendage is the predominant site of thrombus formation in patients with nonvalvular atrial fibrillation, resecting or closing it is an attractive alternative strategy to prevent strokes in patients who cannot tolerate anticoagulation therapy.
- Current approaches to left atrial appendage closure are surgical or percutaneous.
- Percutaneous approaches can be classified as endocardial occlusion, epicardial ligation, or hybrid epiendocardial ligation, with an increasing number of devices becoming available for clinical use.
- Percutaneous endovascular occlusion of the left atrial appendage has been shown to be equivalent to warfarin in preventing stroke in atrial fibrillation and is associated with a lower bleeding risk.

INTRODUCTION

Patients with atrial fibrillation (AF) may have left atrial appendage (LAA)-dependent (LAA thromboembolism)[1,2] and LAA-independent (aortic arch, carotid, and intracerebral artery disease) stroke mechanisms (**Fig. 1**).[3,4] Most strokes in AF are associated with left atrial thrombi, found in approximately 15% of patients with nonvalvular AF, with 90% located in the LAA (**Figs. 2** and **3**).[2,5] Given that warfarin does not significantly affect atheroembolic or arterial occlusive disease, and yet it dramatically reduces stroke in AF, it is reasonable to expect that an LAA occlusion strategy prevents most warfarin-sensitive strokes in AF.[6,7] Evidence of the noninferiority of LAA exclusion compared with warfarin therapy in the PROTECT-AF (Percutaneous Closure of the Left Atrial Appendage versus Warfarin Therapy for Prevention of Stroke in Patients with Atrial Fibrillation) randomized controlled trial[8] provides proof for this concept. Further evidence comes from a randomized trial[9] reporting similar event rates after electrical cardioversion when transesophageal echocardiography (TEE) was used to exclude LAA thrombus compared with conventional anticoagulation.

Several techniques at obliterating the LAA have emerged[10,11] as a strategy to simultaneously reduce stroke risk, the need for anticoagulation, and hemorrhagic complications.[12,13] In this article, the published studies on surgical and percutaneous approaches to LAA closure are reviewed, focusing on stroke mechanisms in AF, LAA structure and function relevant to stroke prevention, practical differences in procedural approach, and clinical considerations surrounding management.

This article originally appeared in Cardiology Clinics, Volume 32, Issue 4, November 2014.
Disclosures: None.
[a] Division of Cardiovascular Diseases, Department of Internal Medicine, Mayo Clinic, 200 First Street Southwest, Rochester, MN 55905, USA; [b] Department of Pediatrics and Adolescent Medicine, Mayo Clinic, 200 First Street Southwest, Rochester, MN 55905, USA
* Corresponding author. Division of Cardiovascular Diseases, 200 First Street Southwest, Rochester, MN 55905.
E-mail address: asirvatham.samuel@mayo.edu

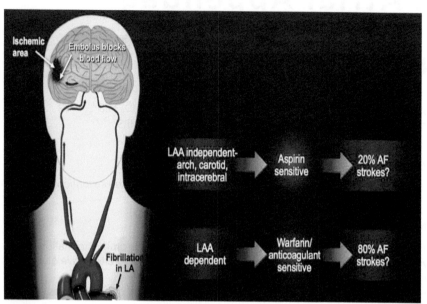

Fig. 1. Left atrial appendage (LAA)-dependent and LAA-independent stroke in AF. (*From* Syed FF, Friedman PA. Left atrial appendage closure for stroke prevention emerging technologies. Cardiac Electrophysiol Clin 2014;6(1): 141–60; with permission.)

LAA STRUCTURE AND FUNCTION
Morphology

The LAA is the remnant of the embryonic left atrium, which forms during the third week of gestation and derives a blood supply from the left circumflex and right coronary arteries at the atrioventricular groove.[14,15] In postnatal life, it is an irregular, tubular diverticulum, which continues to grow until the end of the second decade of life, with an ostium, which is wider in taller individuals. It is differentiated from the pulmonary vein-derived smooth-walled cavity of the remaining left atrium by rich endocardial trabeculations (see **Fig. 3**) formed by parallel-running muscle bars, termed pectinate muscles.[15] The LAA ostium is separated from the left superior pulmonary vein by a narrow tissue invagination (the left lateral ridge),[16] in which lies the ligament of Marshall, a developmental remnant of the left-sided vena cava of importance in AF arrhythmogenesis.[17,18] The left lateral ridge is seen as a q-tip on echocardiography (see **Fig. 2**) and clearly defines the superoposterior border of the LAA ostium endocardially, with the other borders being less well defined.[19] The ostial

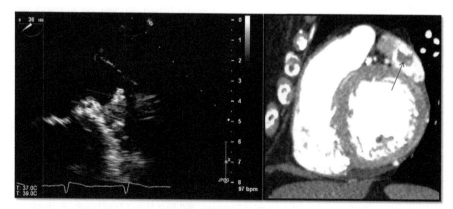

Fig. 2. Appearance of LAA thrombus on TEE (*left, slim arrow*) and CT imaging with intravenous radiopaque contrast (*right, arrow*). Red asterisk marks the left lateral ridge, which separates the left superior pulmonary vein above and the appendage below. Thick arrow marks left circumflex artery.

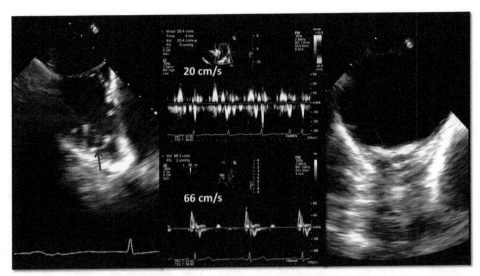

Fig. 3. Correlates of LAA thrombus and stroke in AF. (*Left*) TEE image of dense echocardiographic spontaneous contrast in LAA adjacent to pectinate ridges (*thick arrow*), which then drifts toward the main left atrium (*slim arrow*). (*Mid top*) Pulse waved Doppler signal at LAA ostium in same patient, showing discoordinated and reduced LAA emptying velocities (maximum 20 cm/s) in AF. (*Mid bottom*) Sinus rhythm in another patient with normal LAA emptying pattern and velocity (66 cm/s). (*Right*) Calcified aortic atheroma in descending thoracic aorta (*arrow*) in first patient with AF and dense spontaneous LAA contrast.

rim is smooth, and the atrial tissue immediately surrounding the outside of the ostium may be pitted and focally thin.[19] In approximately 30% of individuals, muscular trabeculations can be found extending inferiorly from the appendage to the vestibule of the mitral valve.[16] The muscular architecture of the LAA is complex, with overlapping cardiomyocytes of different orientations, and is invested by extensions of the Bachmann bundle, which bifurcate around the LAA neck, with contributions from the septopulmonary and septoatrial bundles.[16,20] In dogs, the epicardial LAA tip is the last to activate,[21] although similar human data are lacking.[22–25]

Regional Anatomy

The LAA arises from the free wall of the left atrium and extends superiorly to rest above the left ventricular free wall, with the main pulmonary artery positioned immediately superior (**Fig. 4**).[15,16,19] It rests freely within the confines of the pericardial sac, with the left phrenic nerve having a variable superimposed course as part of the pericardiophrenic neurovascular bundle.[26,27] The ostium shares important relationships with the left superior pulmonary vein endocardially and the coronary vessels epicardially, with the left aortic sinus and main coronary artery lying posterior and medial, and the great cardiac vein and circumflex artery lying inferior.[19] The circumflex artery is usually

less than 2 mm from the LAA ostium.[28] The left anterior descending artery runs underneath the body, emerging at a point immediately below the LAA tip, although the position of the tip can vary.[16] In a few patients, the sinus node artery arising from the circumflex artery runs nearby[19] and can assume an S-shape as it courses between the LAA and left superior pulmonary vein.[16]

Morphologic Variation

The LAA has marked variation in size and shape between individuals,[19,29–32] including the degree of curvilinearity, size and number of pectinate muscles, and the amount of branches and twigs formed by outpouchings and lobes.[19,29,30] The number of lobes also varies (see **Fig. 4**), with 20% to 70% of individuals having a single lobe, 16% to 54% having 2, and the remainder having up to 4 lobes.[30,33,34] The ostium is oval in most (70%) but can be ovaloid (18%), triangular (8%), or round (6%) (**Fig. 5**).[33] In AF, it has been reported to be more elliptical compared with age-matched controls.[35] It lies horizontal to the left superior pulmonary vein in most but can assume a position superior or inferior to it.[28] The left lateral ridge usually extends from the upper border of the left superior to the lower border of the left inferior pulmonary vein, whereas in a few, it terminates at the junction between the 2 left pulmonary veins.[28] Congenital anomalies include LAA aneurysm,[36,37] absence,[38]

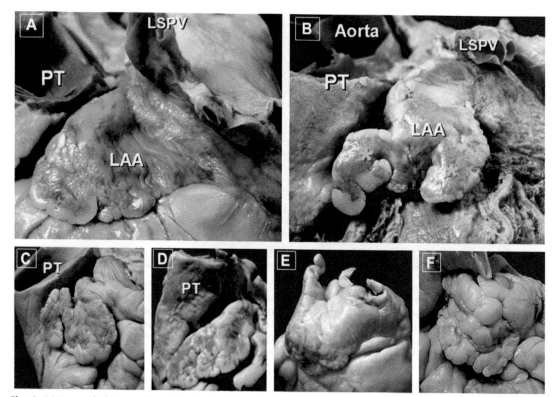

Fig. 4. LAA morphology and spatial relationships. (*A*) Relation to pulmonary trunk and left superior pulmonary vein. (*B*) Multilobed LAA (*asterisk*) in relation to left superior pulmonary vein, pulmonary trunk, and aorta. (*C–F*) Variations of LAA morphology: chicken wing (*C*), windsock (*D*), cactus (*E*), and cauliflower (*F*) shapes. LSPV, left superior pulmonary vein; PT, pulmonary trunk. (*From* Cabrera JA, Saremi F, Sánchez-Quintana D. Left atrial appendage: anatomy and imaging landmarks pertinent to percutaneous transcatheter occlusion. Heart 2014. http://dx.doi.org/10.1136/heartjnl-2013-304464; with permission.)

juxtaposition,[39] inversion,[40] and obstructive membrane at the LAA ostium.[40] Rarely, the appendage can be closely adherent to the underlying left ventricular wall.

Function

The LAA is ideally positioned to act as an adaptive chamber in conditions of volume overload.[15] In dogs, its compliance exceeds that of the remaining left atrium,[41,42] and its contractility obeys a Frank-Starling mechanism,[43,44] with ejection velocity increasing from tip to ostium.[45] It is the main source of atrial natriuretic peptide at supranormal levels of wall stress,[46–49] thus mediating major adaptive responses, which reduce circulating blood volume. The LAA is a rich source of cardiac progenitor cells.[50] In humans, LAA relaxation declines with age,[51] as does the thickness of pectinate muscles.[30]

Dog studies of LAA exclusion show acute reduction in atrial reservoir function and increased restrictive physiology, in keeping with loss of the atrial compliance chamber,[52,53] findings that are also reflected in patients undergoing surgical LAA closure,[54,55] and with a reduction in atrial booster function by up to a third when the appendage is removed.[56,57] Patients with AF undergoing percutaneous LAA ligation (detailed later) have a marked reduction in circulating renin, aldosterone, and noradrenaline levels.[58]

STROKE MECHANISMS IN ATRIAL FIBRILLATION
Systemic Factors, Clinical Risk Prediction, and Ventricular-Vascular Interactions

In patients with AF, the best validated methods of identifying patients at increased risk of stroke, are the $CHADS_2$[59,60] and CHA_2DS_2-VASc score,[61,62] the constitutive components of which are mainly risk factors for vascular disease. A complex interaction exists between these scores, the presence of atherosclerotic arterial (especially aortic, mainly descending thoracic aorta) disease, increasing AF

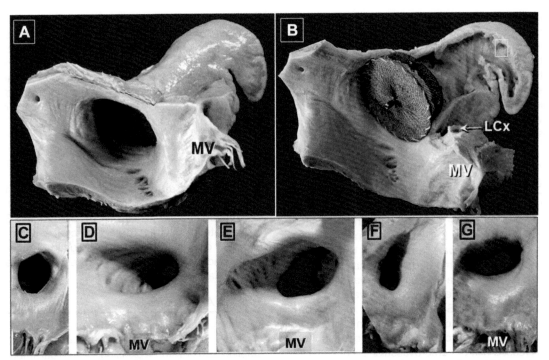

Fig. 5. LAA ostial variations. (A) and (B) show gross anatomic specimen of the LAA with a chicken-wing morphology without (A) and with (B) ACP. (C–G) show the various ostial morphologies that can be associated with LAAs: round (C), elliptical (D), triangular (E), and ovaloid (F, water drop–like; G, footlike). (*From* Cabrera JA, Saremi F, Sánchez-Quintana D. Left atrial appendage: anatomy and imaging landmarks pertinent to percutaneous transcatheter occlusion. Heart 2014. http://dx.doi.org/10.1136/heartjnl-2013-304464; with permission.)

burden, progressive left atrial dysfunction, and LAA thrombus formation (see **Fig. 2**).[63–77] One possible unifying mechanism is reduced aortic compliance, resulting in ventricular diastolic dysfunction from abnormal ventricular-vascular interactions.[78]

LAA Dysfunction and Myopathy

Studies of LAA function have provided increasing insight into the importance of blood stasis within the LAA. The Stroke Prevention in Atrial Fibrillation III trial reported a 2.5-fold increase in stroke risk if appendage thrombi were visualized on TEE,[79] with an association between reduced peak LAA emptying velocity of less than 20 cm/s, the presence of dense spontaneous echocardiographic contrast, believed to reflect blood stasis and red cell clumping, and appendage thrombi (see **Fig. 2**).[80] The close association between the presence of LAA thrombus and mitral E/e' (an estimate of increased left ventricular filling pressures)[71,81] and B-type natriuretic peptide,[70] independently of the CHADS$_2$ score, is further evidence that increased diastolic ventricular pressure transmitted to the atrium is important in LAA

thrombogenesis. There may be a lack of correlation between AF and LAA thrombus,[82] because LAA mechanical function may be relatively preserved during fibrillatory activity and significantly reduced in others that are in sinus rhythm with left ventricular diastolic dysfunction.[83] AF may in addition increase thrombogenesis through irregular or reduced time for ventricular filling, resulting in acutely decreased LAA emptying,[84] whereas left ventricular diastolic dysfunction sensitizes LAA emptying velocity to changes in atrioventricular synchrony.[85]

Atrial tissue changes that accompany AF include cardiomyocyte hypertrophy, interstitial fibrosis, and molecular changes of oxidative stress.[86] The degree of atrial fibrosis as assessed by late gadolinium enhancement on magnetic resonance imaging (MRI) has been associated with the presence of LAA thrombi and spontaneous contrast,[87] as has left atrial dysfunction identified by strain imaging, which identifies abnormalities in myocardial deformation.[88,89] Bipolar voltage mapping of the left atrium in AF has correlated the extent of myopathic low-voltage electrograms ($\leq$0.5 mV) with reduced LAA emptying velocity.[90] These tissue changes have been proposed to contribute to increased local thrombogenicity at the blood-endocardium interface.[91] However, a recent small study comparing markers of endothelial damage and inflammatory-hemostatic cascade activation between right atrial (which has a lower incidence of thrombi in AF) and left atrial blood found no differences.[92] In contrast, the acute, transient decline in LAA function that accompanies electrical cardioversion from AF is accompanied by an increase in spontaneous contrast.[93]

LAA Morphology and Microstructure Complexity

Increased complexity of appendage morphology and microstructure is associated with risk of stroke independent of clinical risk scores. In a study of 932 patients with nonvalvular AF in the United States and Europe, LAA morphology as characterized by computed tomography (CT) or MRI was significantly associated with cerebrovascular event risk, independent of $CHADS_2$ score, age, and AF subtype.[94] The morphologies described varied in degree of trabeculations and complexity, and a corresponding increased risk of cerebrovascular events: chicken wing (48%, event rate 4.4% [20/451]); windsock (19%, event rate 10.6% [19/179]); cactus (30%, event rate 12.6% [35/278]); and cauliflower (3%, event rate 16.7% [4/24]) (see Fig. 4). The least complex chicken wing morphology was found to confer significantly less event risk than the others (odds ratio [OR] 0.21, $P = .036$), with OR for stroke increasing from 4.1 to 8.0 with increasing morphologic complexity.[94] A substudy of 348 patients with MRI-detected silent cerebral ischemia[95] noted an 85% cerebral event rate with a repeat of these risk profile findings. In a Japanese study[96] of 30 patients with stroke with AF matched to 50 controls with AF and no stroke, although the distribution in these morphologies was different (chicken wing 17.5%, windsock 37.5%, cactus 5%, cauliflower 40%), the cauliflower morphology was associated with increased stroke risk independent to CHA_2DS_2-VASc score (OR 3.4, $P = .017$). In a study of 678 patients from the United States, with a similar distribution of morphologies (45% chicken wing, 26% windsock, 18% cactus, and 10% cauliflower), the presence of extensive trabeculations (ie, if seen throughout the LAA wall), reflecting pectinate muscles, was independently associated with risk of stroke (OR 3.1; $P = .012$).[97] No independent effect of morphology classification on stroke risk was shown, although the cauliflower morphology was associated with increased trabeculations and present in 11 of 65 (17%) of patients with stroke compared with 57 of 613 (9%) without. In a Japanese study of 564 patients with three-dimensional (3D) TEE,[98] left atrial volume and

number of LAA lobes were independently associated with LAA thrombus, with 94% (32/34) of those with thrombus having 3 or more lobes. In contrast, LAA ostial size has been associated with both an increased[32] and decreased[97] risk with larger ostial size. Dimensional changes need to interpreted with caution, because AF is associated with larger atrial and LAA dimensions.[30,99]

LAA CLOSURE FOR CARDIOEMBOLIC RISK REDUCTION

LAA closure as a strategy for stroke prevention can be performed surgically or percutaneously. Percutaneous approaches can be divided into 3 broad categories: transseptally placed endocardial plug devices, epicardial LAA ligation procedures, and hybrid ligation approaches, which use transseptal and epicardial access.[10]

Surgical Approaches

Techniques for surgical LAA closure are suture closure from an endocardial or epicardial aspect, stapling with or without excision, or surgical amputation and oversewing.[100] A significant factor determining success is incomplete closure, affecting 35% to 50% of patients,[101,102] because both residual leak from incomplete ligation and residual stump with stapled excisions have been associated with subsequent atrial thrombus,[101–106] with recurrent thrombus formation in up to 50% and thromboembolic clinical events in 15% to 20% of patients with incomplete closure.[101,102,104] Surgical amputation with oversewing seems to be the most successful approach.[100,101,104] A recent, large retrospective propensity matched case-control study[107] reported significant stroke risk reduction with surgical LAA closure in patients with AF undergoing cardiac surgery. Prospective randomized data are in the form of 2 small, inconclusive trials (LAAOS [the Left Atrial Appendage Occlusion Study], n = 77[103] and LAAOS II, n = 51[108]), which have set the scene for the LAAOS III randomized trial of a planned 4700 patients with AF with CHA_2DS_2-VASc score of 2 or higher.[109] Until the results of this trial become available, the effects on stroke reduction from the current literature are difficult to determine, because most studies are retrospective, successful closure rates vary, and overall benefit is variable.[110] In addition, it is difficult to justify the risks of an open surgical procedure specifically to target LAA in patients who are not undergoing cardiac surgery for other reasons. Surgical closure currently has a class IIb recommendation (ie, may be considered, although overall efficacy is less well established) by the 2014 American College of Cardiology (ACC)/American

Heart Association (AHA)/Heart Rhythm Society Atrial Fibrillation Guidelines,[111] the 2014 ACC/AHA Valvular Heart Disease Guidelines (which specify its use for mitral stenosis surgery patients with recurrent embolic events despite therapeutic anticoagulation),[112] and the 2012 European Society of Cardiology (ESC) focused update of AF guidelines.[113]

Minimally Invasive and Hybrid Surgical Approaches

Clinical experience has been reported with video-assisted thoracoscopy using either Endoloop or staple exclusion[1,114,115] or excision,[116] with good outcome and low rates of subsequent thromboembolism. Minimally invasive approaches have also been used in conjunction with treatment of AF, with bilateral video-assisted thoracoscopic pulmonary vein isolation, atrial ganglia ablation, ligament of Marshall division, and LAA staple excision, with a reported success rate of 50% to 90% in maintaining sinus rhythm for paroxysmal AF, 30% to 85% for persistent AF, and 30% to 75% for long-standing persistent AF,[117–119] and up to 90% if followed by a touch-up catheter ablation procedure.[120] The effects on stroke risk reduction of these hybrid approaches are unknown.

Percutaneous LAA Closure

Percutaneous LAA closure offers a less invasive strategy than surgical closure, which may be better tolerated in an often frail and elderly population,[121] and typically uses concomitant confirmation of closure at the time of procedure. However, as with surgical strategies, the evidence showing stroke prevention remains limited, and significant complications may occur. The 2012 ESC guidelines have given a class IIb recommendation (ie, may be considered, although overall efficacy is less well established) for percutaneous LAA closure for patients with a high stroke risk and contraindications for long-term oral anticoagulation.[113] The UK 2006 NICE (National Institute for Health and Clinical Excellence) guidelines recommend percutaneous LAA occlusion as an efficacious strategy for reducing the risk of thromboembolic complications associated with nonvalvular AF.[122] Although several devices have been developed, only the LARIAT[123,124] (SentreHEART, Redwood City, CA) suture delivery device LAA occlusion system has approval from the US Food and Drug Administration (FDA) and commercial availability in the United States. It also has CE (Conformitè Européene) mark approval for commercial use in Europe. The AMPLATZER[125,126] (St Jude Medical, Saint Paul, MN) cardiac plug (ACP) received CE mark approval

in December, 2008 with a trial planned toward attaining FDA approval.[11] A second-generation ACP, the Amplatzer Amulet Left Atrial Appendage Occluder (St Jude Medical, St Paul, MN), received European CE mark approval in 2013. The WATCHMAN[8,127–129] (Boston Scientific, Natick, MA) LAA occluder has received a CE mark, whereas use in the United States is restricted to clinical trials, with the PREVAIL (Prospective Randomized Evaluation of the Watchman Left Atrial Appendage Closure Device in Patients with Atrial Fibrillation versus Long-Term Warfarin Therapy) trial (clinicaltrials.gov: NCT01182441) and ensuing Continued Access to PREVAIL (CAP2) registry (clinicaltrials.gov: NCT01760291) having recently stopped recruiting. The newer WaveCrest[130] Left Atrial Appendage Occlusion System (Coherex Medical, Salt Lake City, UT) received a CE mark in 2013.

TRANSSEPTAL APPROACH
Percutaneous Left Atrial Appendage Transcatheter Occlusion

The Percutaneous Left Atrial Appendage Transcatheter Occlusion (PLAATO) system (eV3, Sunnyvale, CA, intellectual property since acquired by Atritech/Boston Scientific) was the first device designed specifically for LAA occlusion. It consisted of a self-expanding nitinol cage covered with a blood impermeable material, which sealed the LAA. It is no longer available, because the manufacturer discontinued production for financial reasons, despite initially promising clinical results.[131–134] The intellectual property rights for PLAATO were acquired by Atritech in 2007 during their development of the WATCHMAN program.[135]

ACP

The ACP is a nitinol device composed of a lobe designed to prevent migration and a proximal disk that occludes the LAA orifice, with an interconnecting articulating waist to facilitate adequate positioning in variable ostial configurations (see Fig. 5; Fig. 6).[136] It is available in sizes 16 to 30 mm, and oversizing by least 2 mm to the diameter of the LAA landing zone is necessary for secure placement. After ACP implantation, dual antiplatelet therapy with aspirin and clopidogrel for 1 month and aspirin monotherapy thereafter is recommended.[122,137]

There has been increasing clinical experience published of using this device in patients with contraindications to oral anticoagulant therapies. In a European registry,[126] successful deployment was reported in 132 of 137 patients. Complications were seen in 7% and included 3 ischemic stroke,

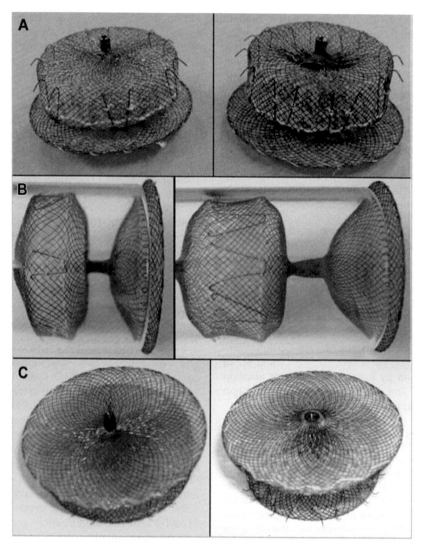

Fig. 6. ACP (*left*) and the newer AMPLATZER Amulet Left Atrial Appendage Occluder (*right*) indicating the greater distal lobe length of the Amulet (ie, thickness reaching into LAA) (*A*), waist (*B*), and inversion of the disk and screw (*C*). (*From* Freixa X, Chan JL, Tzikas A, et al. The Amplatzer™ Cardiac Plug 2 for left atrial appendage occlusion: novel features and first-in-man experience. EuroIntervention 2013;8(9):1094–8; with permission.)

3 device embolization, and 5 clinically significant pericardial effusions. One center in Germany,[138] which also contributed to the initial report, recently published its 10-year experience with endovascular LAA occlusion. A total of 152 patients had attempted LAA closure, and the investigators used nondedicated devices in 32 (patent foramen ovale [PFO], atrial septal defect, and ventricular septal defect occluders) and the ACP in the remaining 120. Procedure-related complications (pericardial effusion, device embolization, and procedure-related stroke) and major bleeds were seen in 8 (6.7%) with cardiac plug and 7 (22%) with nondedicated devices ($P = .0061$), the major difference being caused by difference in device embolization

rates (2 [1.6%] vs 5 [12%], $P = .0048$). Thus, in successfully treated patients, the annual incidence of stroke and major bleeding was 0.8% after a mean follow-up period of 2.6 years.

In the Belgian registry[139] of 90 consecutive patients across 7 centers at high stroke risk (mean CHA_2DS_2-VASc 4.4) and bleeding risk (mean HAS-BLED score 3.3), acute procedural success was 95%, with 3 patients developing tamponade, of whom 1 died. Minor complications were reported to be 3 insignificant pericardial effusions, 2 transient myocardial ischemia caused by air embolism, and 1 femoral pseudoaneurysm. At 1 year, the observed stroke rate was lower than the expected annual stroke rate estimated by the CHA_2DS_2-VASc score

(2.1% vs 5.1%). There were 4 deaths, 2 minor strokes, 1 tamponade, and 1 myocardial infarction.

Cumulated experience has also been reported from 7 centers in Canada, which reported on 52 patients with 98.1% acute procedural success, with serious adverse effects of device embolization (1.9%) and pericardial effusion (1.9%).[140] At a mean follow-up of 20 months, the rates of death, stroke, systemic embolism, pericardial effusion, and major bleeding were 5.8%, 1.9%, 0%, 1.9%, and 1.9%, respectively. The presence of mild peri-device leak was observed in 16.2% of patients at the 6-month follow-up, as evaluated by TEE. There were no cases of device thrombosis.

Data from other published series globally[141–146] reported similar success rates of between 92% and 100% acute success rate and complications of tamponade, coronary air embolism, catheter-related thrombosis, acute pulmonary edema, and pulmonary artery tear, with complications on follow-up being mainly thrombus formation on device or thromboembolism.

Unlike WATCHMAN, there are no randomized trial data on AMPLATZER. A small, prospective 1:1 comparison with WATCHMAN reported no significant differences in procedural times or outcome. In the United States, a randomized open-label noninferiority trial comparing ACP with optimal medical therapy with either warfarin or dabigatran is on hold given limited enrollment (clinicaltrials.gov: NCT01118299). In Europe, the ELIGIBLE (Efficacy of Left Atrial Appendage Closure after Gastrointestinal Bleeding) randomized trial is randomizing patients with history of gastrointestinal bleeding and high embolic risk to LAA closure or usual oral anticoagulant therapy (clinicaltrials.gov: NCT01628068).

The second-generation AMPLATZER Amulet (see **Fig. 6**) has a similarly designed lobe-disk structure, but the lobe is deeper, with more wires for stability, the left atrial disk is larger to better cover the ostium, and an end screw sits flush with the disk to ensure a smoother surface facing the left atrium.[147] Having larger available sizes (31 and 34 mm), it is better suited for closure of larger LAA.[148]

WATCHMAN

The WATCHMAN device is made of a self-expanding nitinol frame, with fixation barbs and a permeable polyester fabric cover, and is available in sizes between 21 and 33 mm in diameter (**Fig. 7**). Proper positioning and stability of the device are verified by TEE and angiography before device release (**Fig. 8**).[11] The WATCHMAN is the only percutaneous LAA closure device with randomized prospective trial–based data guiding its

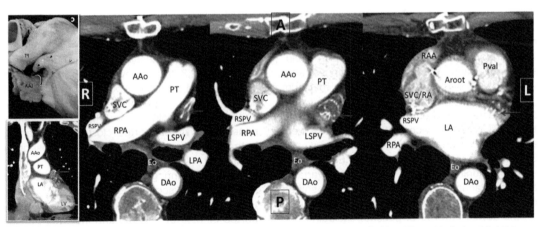

Fig. 7. LAA with a WATCHMAN in situ showing regional anatomy. Superior (*left*), mid, and inferior (*right*) transverse CT sections (with intravenous contrast) through the LAA. Arrows point to WATCHMAN device within the LAA. Note the relationship to the main pulmonary trunk, which serves as an excellent site to visualize the LAA using intracardiac echocardiography, left coronary artery (*asterisk*). (*Inset top*) Cadaveric dissection oriented appropriately to reflect the CT images; the arc identifies the site of the ostium and the appendage is deflected up to show its undersurface. Arrows track the course of the left anterior descending artery and the letters *V* track the great cardiac vein. (*Inset bottom*) Coronal CT section to correlate with the sagittal images. Pacemaker lead artifact can be seen in the superior vena cava (SVC) and right atrial appendage (RAA). A, anterior; AAo, ascending aorta; Aroot, aortic root; DAo, descending aorta; Eo, esophagus; L, left; LA, left atrium; LPA, left pulmonary artery; LSPV, left superior pulmonary vein; P, posterior; PT, pulmonary trunk; Pval, pulmonary valve; R, right; RA, right atrium; RAA, right atrial appendage; RPA, right pulmonary artery; RSPV, right superior pulmonary vein; SVC, superior vena cava. (*From* Su P, McCarthy KP, Ho SY. Occluding the left atrial appendage: anatomical considerations. Heart 2008;94(9):1166–70; with permission.)

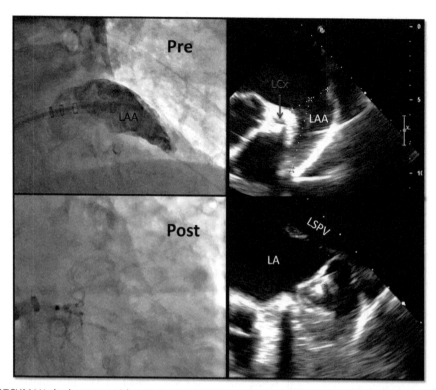

Fig. 8. WATCHMAN deployment with LAA imaged on fluoroscopy (*left*) and TEE (*right*) before (Pre) and after (Post) deployment (*asterisk* points to WATCHMAN). Dotted lines represent points at which appendage dimensions were measured. Multiple planes of view are necessary for accurate assessment. LA, left atrium; LCx, left circumflex artery; LSPV, left superior pulmonary vein.

use. In the PROTECT-AF trial,[149] 707 patients with nonvalvular AF and a CHADS$_2$ score of 1 or more were randomized 2:1 to percutaneous LAA occlusion or warfarin. Warfarin was continued after WATCHMAN placement for 45 days minimum (longer if TEE showed residual leak 5 mm or wider) and thereafter switched to long-term aspirin. With the WATCHMAN device, 86% of patients were able to stop warfarin therapy at 45 days, and 93% were off warfarin at 12 months. Early results reported noninferiority of closure to warfarin, although placement of a device in the LAA shifted the stroke mechanisms. Thrombus was identified on the device in 3.7% of patients, including one in whom it was detected 6 days after an ischemic stroke. During the trial, ischemic stroke was more common in the device group (3.0% vs 2.0% for control) and tended to occur early. Approximately 5% of patients developed a periprocedural pericardial effusion, and although this did not affect the clinical end points, it did increase hospital stay.[150] However, the hemorrhagic risk was significantly lower in the device group (relative risk 0.009, 0.00–0.45). With extended follow-up, the benefits of reduced hemorrhagic risk accrued with time, such that after a mean 3.8-year follow-

up, there was superiority of closure over warfarin with a reduction in the primary end point of the trial of stroke, cardiovascular death, and systemic embolism (2.3 vs 3.8 events per 100 patient-years, hazard ratio 0.61, confidence interval [CI] 0.38–0.97, $P = .03$), and a 34% relative reduction in all-cause mortality ($P = .04$).[150] A net clinical benefit analysis supported closure over warfarin both in the trial (1.73%/y) and the subsequent Continued Access Protocol (CAP) registry (4.97%/y), having greater benefit in those with higher CHADS$_2$ scores.[151]

Significant procedural complications were reported in 12% of patients and included pericardial effusion requiring drainage, embolic stroke, device migration, and device sepsis. Incomplete endothelialization at 10 months in a patient requiring device explantation as a result of thromboembolism is also described.[152] With increased procedural experience and device redesign, the complication rate has significantly decreased by more than 50%, with periprocedural stroke decreasing from 0.9% to 0% in a subsequent report[128] of 542 patients in the PROTECT-AF and 460 patients in the CAP registry ($P = .04$).

Major criticisms of PROTECT-AF include small sample size, low CHADS$_2$ score, and contribution of the initial 45-day warfarin period in the device group to enhanced outcome.[150] Whether a similar success can be achieved in a higher-risk population (CHADS$_2$ score ≥2) is being tested by the PREVAIL study, the formal results of which are awaited (ClinicalTrials.gov identifier NCT00129545). Although the trial protocol still mandates the use of warfarin in the United States, the ASA-Plavix feasibility study performed in Europe prospectively evaluated 150 patients undergoing WATCHMAN implantation with 6 months of clopidogrel or ticlopidine, and lifelong aspirin, with only a 1.7%/y ischemic stroke risk, approximately 70% to 80% lower than expected given the CHADS$_2$ score.[153]

The interplay with the novel oral anticoagulants is uncertain, because they confer lower bleeding risk to warfarin.[154–157] Compared with the favorable comparisons of closure versus warfarin, predicted 10-year performance of closure was only marginally better than against dabigatran 150 mg, because bleeding, especially hemorrhagic stroke, was less than with warfarin (all-cause mortality 29% vs 30%; ischemic stroke 12% vs 8%, hemorrhagic stroke 3% vs 1%, major bleeding 12% vs 27%).[158] There are no head-to-head comparisons of device closure against the novel anticoagulants. How the next-generation WATCHMAN, which is under development, influences this situation is uncertain, and an initial European nonrandomized evaluation is planned (EVOLVE (Evaluation of the Next Generation WATCHMAN LAA Closure Technology in Non-Valvular AF Patients), clinicaltrials.gov: NCT01196897).

WaveCrest

The WaveCrest Left Atrial Appendage Occlusion System is designed to be positioned at the LAA ostium, with an impermeable, less thrombogenic material facing the left atrium to minimize thrombosis and leaks, and independently deployable distal anchors, which allows the device to be use in a range of appendage depths (**Fig. 9**).[159] It is available in 3 sizes (22 mm, 27 mm, 32 mm). The WaveCrest I trial[130] (multicenter, prospective, nonrandomized registry) recruited 73 patients from Europe, Australia, and New Zealand, with mean CHADS$_2$ score of 2.5, previous cerebral embolism in 34%, and a warfarin contraindication in 49%. After TEE-guided deployment, dual antiplatelet therapy was administered for 90 days and then aspirin continued long-term. Successful deployment with acute closure was seen in 68 of 73 (93%), with 3 mm or less peridevice flow at 6 weeks in 65 of 68 (96%). Acute tamponade occurred in 2 of 73 (3%), and there was no procedural stroke, device embolization, or device-related thrombosis. The pivotal US WaveCrest II trial is anticipated in 2014.[159]

Other Transeptal Devices

The Transcatheter Patch (Custom Medical Devices, Athens, Greece)[160] is a frameless bioabsorbable device deployed by balloon inflation, with adherence of the patch to cardiac tissues over 48 hours via fibrin formation. The Cardia Ultrasept LAA Occluder (Cardia, Eagan, MN) consists of a distal cylindrical bulb anchoring into the LAA and a separately articulated sail unfolding over the ostium.[161] The Lifetech LAmbre (Lifetech Scientific, Shenzhen, China) (clinicaltrials.gov: NCT01920412) also incorporates an articulation at the waist between the LAA plug and ostial lip, allowing self-orientation, and is fully repositionable after deployment. The Occlutech LAA Occluder (Occlutech International, Helsingborg, Sweden) has a conical shape designed for improved expansile force and wire loops at the side to anchor to the LAA trabeculae.[159]

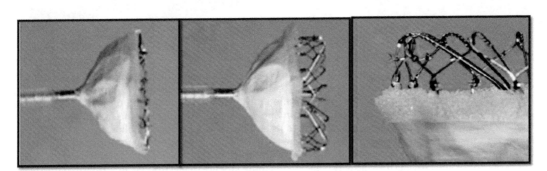

Fig. 9. The WaveCrest Left Atrial Appendage Occlusion System. Expanded polytetrafluoroethylene (ePTFE) lines the surface facing the left atrium to minimize thrombus formation, whereas the distal anchors are independently deployable. (*Courtesy of* Coherex Medical, Salt Lake City, UT; with permission.)

EPICARDIAL APPROACH

Epicardial approaches (**Fig. 10**) offer advantages of avoiding the need for transseptal puncture, risk of acute procedure-related thromboembolism, device embolism, erosion, infection, and necessary anticoagulation therapy.[10] Such an approach was first reported with video-assisted thoracoscopy and subsequent left lung collapse with surgical pericardiotomy to access the LAA.[1]

The Aegis system (Aegis Medical, Vancouver, Canada, Epitek, Minneapolis, MN)[21,162] introduces an appendage grabber, via percutaneous sub-xiphoid pericardial access, with embedded electrodes within the jaws, permitting electrical navigation onto the appendage via bipolar electrograms that identify the electrical activity of the tissue captured by the jaws. A hollow suture preloaded with a support wire to permit remote suture loop manipulation and fluoroscopic visualization is advanced to the appendage base and looped around the appendage. The loop can be variably sized to accommodate multiple LAA lobes and shapes. After loop closure, the wire is removed, leaving only suture behind, which is remotely locked with a clip to maintain closure. A loop may be opened and repositioned if the initial closure is unsatisfactory, or additional loops may be placed for multilobed LAAs that are not fully closed with the first loop, using the suture tails from the first loop as a rail. A firm closure is confirmed by the elimination of LAA electrical activity, which occurs within seconds and is accompanied by shortening of the surface electrocardiographic P wave in dogs.[21] Chronically, the LAA involutes and becomes atretic.[162] Whether LAA elimination by this means will affect rhythm control (by eliminating a mass of fibrillating atrial tissue) is not known. A small series[163] has shown feasibility in humans. Major limitations for the use of this approach are previous cardiac surgery or adhesions from previous pericarditis.

The EPITEK (Epitek, Medford, NJ) is a fiber-optic endoscope system that uses a grabber deployed under direct vision, but in early human testing there were technical difficulties with pericardial access and device positioning.[164]

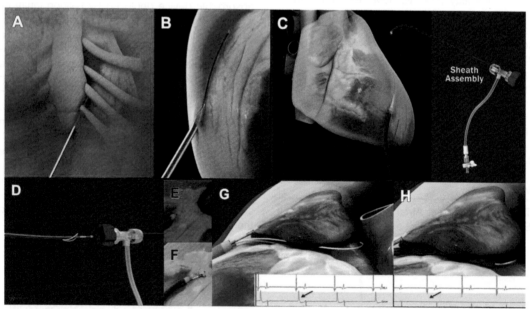

Fig. 10. Epicardial system for percutaneous LAA closure. (*A, B*) Percutaneous puncture to gain access to the pericardial space. (*C*) Placement of sheath in pericardial space using Seldinger technique. (*D*) Introduction of multielectrode LAA grabber with a preloaded looped suture into sheath. (*E, F*) Positioning of grabber toward LAA using electrograms from the electrodes embedded in and immediately proximal to the grabber jaws. (*G*) The grabber is used to identify the appendage and record its electrograms, whereas the hollow suture loop delivery tool is used to place the loop around the base of the LAA. (*H*) On tightening of the suture, the LAA ostium is closed. The arrows show the LAA electrogram obtained from electrodes embedded in the grabber jaws. Within seconds of closure, the LAA electrical activity is eliminated (note absence of electrogram at *arrow*) and the surface P wave becomes shorter because the LAA no longer contributes to the P wave (*not shown*). Simultaneous TEE is used to confirm placement at the LAA ostium and its complete closure. (*Courtesy of* Mayo Clinic Foundation, Rochester, MN; with permission.)

HYBRID APPROACH

The LARIAT system (SentreHEART, Palo Alto, CA)[7,123] uses percutaneous epicardial LAA ligation guided by an endocardial magnet-tipped wire placed in the LAA via the transseptal approach, with a second magnet-tipped wire placed epicardially in union to form a rail, over which an epicardial suture loop is advanced and then closed (**Fig. 11**). An endocardial balloon at the LAA ostium defines where the epicardial suture needs to be placed. Specific advantages include ability to reposition the snare and ease of deployment over a stable loop. Limitations include the combined risks of both transseptal and epicardial approaches, limited usefulness in appendages superiorly directed, greater than 40 mm diameter (limit of snare on first-generation devices) or with multiple lobes; and difficult use in patients with pectus excavatum.[7,10] It is estimated that 90% of LAAs have morphologies amenable to closure via this system. After initial human reports,[123] experience in a series of 89 patients has been reported, with successful closure in 85 (96%).[118] Three patients had a 2 mm or less residual leak, and 1 had a leak less than 3 mm. There were 2

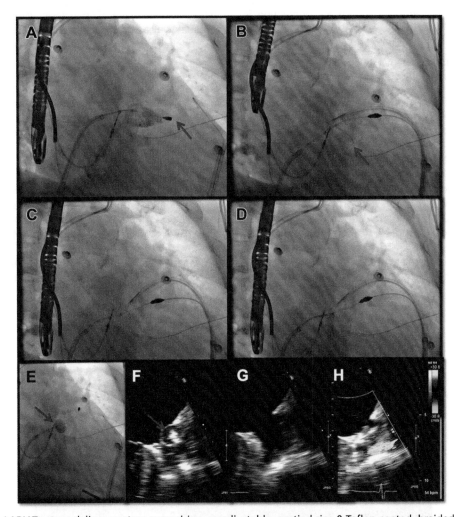

Fig. 11. LARIAT suture delivery system comprising an adjustable, pretied size 0 Teflon-coated, braided polyester suture and radiopaque closure snare. (*A*) Contrast injection identifies the LAA and the magnet-tipped 0.025-inch endocardial wire (transseptal access), which is advanced carefully to the LAA tip (*arrow*). (*B*) End to end connection of the magnet tip of the 0.035-inch epicardial (percutaneous pericardial access) to that of the endocardial wires is used for alignment and stability, with snare positioned at the LAA base (*arrow*). (*C*) Tightening of snare for closure. (*D*) Contrast injection after closure. (*E, F*) Arrow points to balloon, which is inflated during the procedure to identify the ostium and guide snare positioning. (*G*) LAA before closure. (*H*) LAA after closure with color flow imaging, showing no flow into LAA.

complications related to percutaneous epicardial access and 1 related to transseptal puncture. Adverse events include severe pericarditis post-operatively (n = 2), late pericardial effusion (n = 1), late strokes (n = 2), and unexplained death (n = 2). In a subsequent report[165] of 27 patients with AF and high stroke risk unable to take antico-agulants, acute success was seen in 25, with TEE-confirmed persistent closure at 4 months in 22. Complications included LAA perforation (**Fig. 12**) (n = 1), pericarditis (n = 3), transseptal sheath thrombus causing stroke (n = 1), and late cerebro-vascular accident (n = 1).[165] Although promising, there are no controlled data, and even although the acute closure rate is high, the clinical relevance of this as a surrogate for stroke prevention is unproved.[150]

PREVENTION AND MANAGEMENT OF COMPLICATIONS

Data from the WATCHMAN studies show the importance of procedural experience in preventing complications, such that rate of serious pericardial effusions was 7% starting PROTECT-AF and declined to 2% during CAP.[8,128] Appropriate selection of procedural approach (**Table 1**), preprocedural anatomic definition toward proce-dure planning (**Box 1**), and procedural technique (**Table 2**) are all important in optimizing chances of successful closure and avoiding complications. Imaging with CT or TEE before implantation has complementary roles, with CT better able to image LAA morphologic features, LAA tip orientation, and the coronary vasculature, and TEE better suited to identify thrombus and differentiate it from pectinate muscles.[11] Therefore, for a planned LARIAT proce-dure, a preprocedural CT scan identifies patients with unsuitable appendage morphology, size, or orientation, whereas TEE confirms absence of mo-bile left atrial thrombus. Another example is con-firming a minimum LAA depth of 10 mm for the AMPLATZER, checking in multiple planes. With certain shapes, such as the oval LAA ostium, two-dimensional TEE tends to underestimate area and 3D TEE or CT may be better.[166] It is important to have familiarity with the anatomy of the interatrial septum[16] and techniques of transseptal[167] and epicardial puncture.[168] Intraprocedural imaging, either with TEE or ICE,[169] can assist with these fea-tures, as well as monitoring for complications after LAA occlusion, including checking that patency of the left superior pulmonary vein and left circumflex coronary artery is maintained. The left circumflex coronary arteries are vulnerable to injury during both endovascular and epicardial suture closure, and epicardial devices can in addition risk injury to vessels near the LAA tip, including the left ante-rior descending artery, venous grafts to obtuse marginal or diagonal arteries, or the S-shaped sinus node artery.

The most common long-term complication after device closure is thromboembolism and de novo thrombus formation at the site of closure (**Fig. 13**). A study of 34 patients with AMPLATZER screened systematically for up to a year with TEE[170] identified CHA_2DS_2-VASc, lower left ven-tricular ejection fraction, and higher platelet count

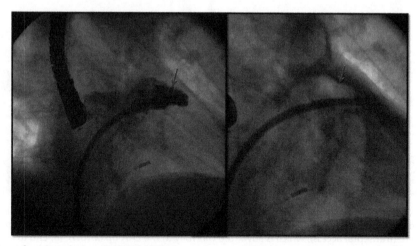

Fig. 12. LAA perforation during WATCHMAN placement resulting in acute tamponade. (*Left*) LAA identified by contrast injection before perforation (*arrow*). (*Right*) LAA silhouetted against contrast (*arrow*) in the peri-cardial cavity after perforation. Immediate administration of intravenous fluid and pericardiocentesis stabi-lized the patient. The pericardial effusion did not recur on careful observation for 24 hours and the patient had full recovery.

Table 1
Appropriate selection of percutaneous approaches for LAA closure

Device/Method	Advantages	Limitations
Transseptal device placement	Transseptal technique widely available Available in the setting of previous cardiac surgery Validated as noninferior to warfarin for stroke prevention (WATCHMAN)	Need for procedural and short-term anticoagulation or antithrombotic regimen until endothelialization occurs Foreign body left in central circulation (small risk of embolization, erosion, dislodgement) Device must be sized to match LAA Previous atrial septal defect closure may preclude transseptal delivery
Epicardial	No foreign body left behind No need for procedural anticoagulation because no contact with central circulation and no transseptal puncture (which exposes blood to tissue factor) Adjustable size loop to accommodate variable LAA shape/morphology without need for sizing Pericardial control facilitates management of effusion should one develop	Human experience not yet reported Previous cardiac surgery limits pericardial access and maneuverability Epicardial access techniques less widely available than transseptal puncture
Hybrid	No foreign body left behind Pericardial control facilitates management of effusion should one develop	Need for both transseptal and epicardial access with risks of both, and delivery failure if cannot achieve both Superiorly directed LAA, multiple lobes, and pectus excavatum may preclude use

From Friedman PA, Holmes DR. Non-surgical left atrial appendage closure for stroke prevention in atrial fibrillation. J Cardiovasc Electrophysiol 2011;22(10):1190; with permission.

as risk factors for thrombus development, seen in 3 of 34 (9%) patients. The significance of AF recurrence or endothelial damage from the procedure is unknown. Anecdotally, flush coverage of the ostium may be important to obliterate remnant cul-de-sacs, which act as a nidus for thrombus formation.[136] Unlike in surgical closure, persistent leaks after endovascular occlusion, which are commonly seen (30%–60%) as a result of mismatch between the oval LAA ostium and circular device profiles, do not seem to increase risk of thromboembolism.[127,132,134,146] Whether this is also the case for epicardial ligation is unknown **(Fig. 14)**.[171,172] The velocity of the leak, the degree of residual exposed LAA anatomic complexity, and the ability of the leak to accommodate a thrombus may be different between patients with a surgical leak, epicardial ligation leak, and peridevice leak. In addition, an important unknown is how to determine when the appendage is adequately closed, and whether the definition should be anatomic, electrical, or functional[7,10] and whether transesophageal or intracardiac echocardiography, CT, or MRI is the optimal imaging study.[140,141,166,173–176] All closure devices and techniques leave a small beak, where tissues are approximated or adjacent to a device; whether these beaks affect stroke prevention is not known. In addition, accessory lobes, pectinate muscles, or other structures may exist proximal to a device or closure; their impact is uncertain.

UNANSWERED QUESTIONS

There is a need for randomized trial data in patients not treated with anticoagulants.[150] There are also limited data against the novel oral anticoagulants, which may demand an increased safety profile from device closure to show net clinical benefit. In addition, optimal adjunctive pharmacology both early and late after LAA device closure has varied in clinical trials and warrants

---

Box 1
Anatomic and imaging determinant for LAA occlusion

Left atrium (LA)

Dimensions of the LA: for all devices

Myocardial thickness: anterior wall and venoatrial junctions may be very thin

Distance from the OF to the LAA ostium: for all devices

Accessory LAA: mainly anterior wall and mitral isthmus

Webs and septa

Interatrial septum: should be a low posterior transseptal puncture. OF dimensions, rim thickness, proximity to the aortic root, PFO, patches, occluder devices, and septal aneurysm

LAA

Morphologic variants: LAA apex directed behind the pulmonary trunk (exclusion criteria for LARIAT)

Ostial diameters/circumference: 17–31 mm (WATCHMAN) and 12.6–28.5 mm (ACP)

LAA length: LAA width greater than 40 mm (LARIAT), should exceed the maximal ostial diameter (WATCHMAN)

LAA angulation: for all devices, less able to be angled a special concern for the WATCHMAN

Maximal length of dominant lobe: for all devices

Multilobular LAA: multilobed LAA oriented in different planes greater than 40 mm (exclusion criteria for LARIAT)

Distance from the ostium to the first bend of the LAA: landing zone that exceeds the maximal ostial diameter for the WATCHMAN, landing zone 10 mm or greater for the ACP

Trabeculations (pectinate muscle): should not be mistaken for thrombus

Myocardial thickness: thinner posterior wall and risk of cardiac perforation for all devices

Extra-appendicular trabeculations: risk of cardiac perforation and periprosthetic leaks

Ostial diameters of LSPV

Relation of LSPV and LAA orifices: usually at the same level

Lateral ridge orientation and width: poor definition of the orifice limits in ellipsoid LAA

Thrombus: contraindication for ablation

Neighboring structures

Left circumflex artery: risk for artery compression between the anchoring lobe and the disk for the ACP

Left sinus node artery

Great cardiac vein and obtuse marginal vein

Persistent left superior vena cava

Post-CABG venous grafts

Pericardial adhesions: of special concern for the LARIAT

Left phrenic nerve: of special concern for the LARIAT

Abbreviations: CABG, coronary artery bypass graft; LA, left atrium; LSPV, left superior pulmonary vein; OF, oval fossa.
  From Cabrera JA, Saremi F, Sánchez-Quintana D. Left atrial appendage: anatomy and imaging landmarks pertinent to percutaneous transcatheter occlusion. Heart 2014. http://dx.doi.org/10.1136/heartjnl-2013-304464; with permission.

---

additional investigation. However, not all devices are created equal, and it remains to be seen whether epicardial suture ligation provides similar clinical benefit to endovascular occlusion strategies, noting that there is no strong evidence that complete LAA closure is a surrogate for clinical efficacy,[150] and if they are as sensitive to incomplete closure[177] as surgical ligation strategies seem to be. The role of LAA morphology in clinical risk stratification remains undefined, and the same

Table 2
Major procedural complications of percutaneous LAA closure devices

Complication	Cause	Preventative Strategy
Pericardial effusion	Initial transseptal puncture	TEE guidance (eg, X-plane) Avoid severe tenting of the interatrial septum (increases the risk of free-wall puncture): alternative strategies (eg, application of radiofrequency energy) Puncturing at the fossa ovalis
	Guidewire or catheter into LAA after initial transseptal puncture	Advance dilator into LAA under fluoroscopy over 0.32-in wire with distal curve or coronary wire
	Manipulation of delivery sheath/system into and within LAA	Advance delivery sheath into LAA over pigtail catheter rather than guidewire Posterior-inferior puncture to optimize coaxial approach to LAA; avoid using PFO, which guides entry superiorly and suboptimally to work within LAA
	LARIAT endocardial wire pulls epicardial wire into the LAA	Recognize tension on LARIAT endocardial wire when connected to epicardial wire including when balloon being placed at ostium
	Device deployment and retrieval	Maintain delivery sheath position; minimize retrievals and reimplantations if possible
Procedural stroke	Preexisting thrombus in LAA	Careful baseline TEE
	Insufficient anticoagulation	Monitor anticoagulation, if possible; consider anticoagulation before transseptal puncture
	Air embolus from delivery sheath/system	Flush sheath only after entering LAA, and after device exchange, if performed
Device embolization	Inappropriate size	Tug test; confirm device compression (WATCHMAN should be 8%–20% compressed) or appropriate fluoroscopic appearance
	Inappropriate position	Confirm device position and seal by TEE and fluoroscopy
Vascular (hematoma, arteriovenous fistula, pseudoaneurysm, bleeding)	Venous access	Careful technique; consider ultrasound guidance as needed
Pericardial pain	Common after LARIAT closure? Pericardial inflammation/LAA necrosis	Anecdotal: prophylactic nonsteroidal antiinflammatory drugs, oral colchicine course, intrapericardial therapy (eg, local anesthetic flushes)

Modified from Price MP. Prevention and management of complications of left atrial appendage closure devices. Intervent Cardiol Clin 2014;3:303; with permission.

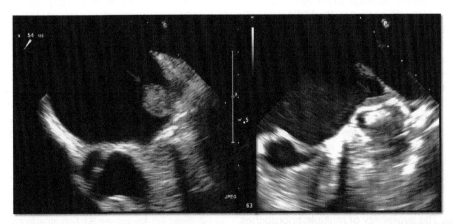

Fig. 13. Thrombus formation after LAA closure identified by TEE. (*Left*) TEE showing thrombus on WATCHMAN (*arrow*). (*Right*) Another patient with a layer on atrial surface of WATCHMAN concerning for laminated thrombus (*arrow*).

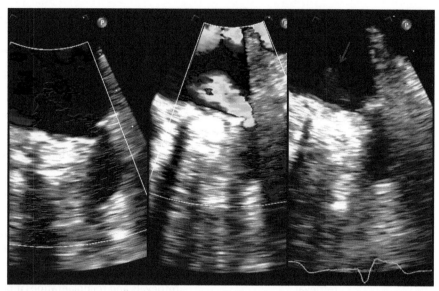

Fig. 14. Incomplete LARIAT closure with blood flow into (*left*) and out of (*mid*) the appendage on color flow imaging (*left*), with extrusion of echocardiographic spontaneous contrast into the left atrium associated with blood outflow (*right, arrow*). It is unknown whether incomplete LARIAT closure is associated with increased thromboembolic risk.

microstructural elements that act as potential nidus for stroke are also believed to increase arrhythmia. Given the emerging role for LAA occlusion as a treatment strategy for refractory appendage arrhythmia,[178] the strategy of combined LAA closure with AF ablation requires further study to define the predicted reduction in stroke risk and recurrent AF. In addition to any arrhythmic effects, the clinical hemodynamic and humeral effects of LAA closure remain poorly defined and are the area of ongoing study.

SUMMARY

Percutaneous epicardial closure is increasingly used as a treatment strategy to prevent thromboembolism in high-risk patients with AF treated with warfarin. With the advent of emerging devices, increasing procedural and clinical experience and clinical trial data, LAA closure has the potential for becoming an attractive option for stroke prevention in those at greatest risk of both stroke and bleeding. For patients with previous cardiac surgery, recurrent pericarditis, or thoracic radiation, endovascular strategies will be attractive, because pericardial access and manipulation may be limited. For patients with a strict contraindication to anticoagulation or with a high infection risk, epicardial/nondevice strategies are appealing, because entry to the central circulation is avoided. The availability of multiple approaches allows the physician to select the optimal

approach for a given patient based on physiologic, anatomic, and clinical considerations.

REFERENCES

1. Blackshear JL, Johnson WD, Odell JA, et al. Thoracoscopic extracardiac obliteration of the left atrial appendage for stroke risk reduction in atrial fibrillation. J Am Coll Cardiol 2003;42(7):1249–52.
2. Blackshear JL, Odell JA. Appendage obliteration to reduce stroke in cardiac surgical patients with atrial fibrillation. Ann Thorac Surg 1996;61(2):755–9.
3. Hart RG, Pearce LA, Miller VT, et al. Cardioembolic vs. noncardioembolic strokes in atrial fibrillation: frequency and effect of antithrombotic agents in the stroke prevention in atrial fibrillation studies. Cerebrovasc Dis 2000;10(1):39–43.
4. Naya T, Yukiiri K, Hosomi N, et al. Brain natriuretic peptide as a surrogate marker for cardioembolic stroke with paroxysmal atrial fibrillation. Cerebrovasc Dis 2008;26(4):434–40.
5. Mahajan R, Brooks AG, Sullivan T, et al. Importance of the underlying substrate in determining thrombus location in atrial fibrillation: implications for left atrial appendage closure. Heart 2012; 98(15):1120–6.
6. Chimowitz MI, Lynn MJ, Howlett-Smith H, et al. Comparison of warfarin and aspirin for symptomatic intracranial arterial stenosis. N Engl J Med 2005;352(13):1305–16.
7. Syed FF, Asirvatham SJ. Left atrial appendage as a target for reducing strokes: justifiable rationale?

Safe and effective approaches? Heart Rhythm 2011;8(2):194–8.

8. Holmes DR Jr, Fountain R. Stroke prevention in atrial fibrillation: WATCHMAN versus warfarin. Expert Rev Cardiovasc Ther 2009;7(7):727–9.

9. Klein AL, Grimm RA, Murray RD, et al. Use of transesophageal echocardiography to guide cardioversion in patients with atrial fibrillation. N Engl J Med 2001;344(19):1411–20.

10. Friedman PA, Holmes DR. Non-surgical left atrial appendage closure for stroke prevention in atrial fibrillation. J Cardiovasc Electrophysiol 2011;22(10):1184–91.

11. Yu CM, Khattab AA, Bertog SC, et al. Mechanical antithrombotic intervention by LAA occlusion in atrial fibrillation. Nat Rev Cardiol 2013;10(12):707–22.

12. Brass LM, Krumholz HM, Scinto JM, et al. Warfarin use among patients with atrial fibrillation. Stroke 1997;28(12):2382–9.

13. Onalan O, Lashevsky I, Hamad A, et al. Nonpharmacologic stroke prevention in atrial fibrillation. Expert Rev Cardiovasc Ther 2005;3(4):619–33.

14. James TN. Small arteries of the heart. Circulation 1977;56(1):2–14.

15. Al-Saady NM, Obel OA, Camm AJ. Left atrial appendage: structure, function, and role in thromboembolism. Heart 1999;82(5):547–54.

16. Cabrera JA, Saremi F, Sanchez-Quintana D. Left atrial appendage: anatomy and imaging landmarks pertinent to percutaneous transcatheter occlusion. Heart 2014. http://dx.doi.org/10.1136/heartjnl-2013-304464.

17. De Simone CV, Noheria A, Lachman N, et al. Myocardium of the superior vena cava, coronary sinus, vein of Marshall, and the pulmonary vein ostia: gross anatomic studies in 620 hearts. J Cardiovasc Electrophysiol 2012;23(12):1304–9.

18. Macedo PG, Kapa S, Mears JA, et al. Correlative anatomy for the electrophysiologist: ablation for atrial fibrillation. Part I: pulmonary vein ostia, superior vena cava, vein of Marshall. J Cardiovasc Electrophysiol 2010;21(6):721–30.

19. Su P, McCarthy KP, Ho SY. Occluding the left atrial appendage: anatomical considerations. Heart 2008;94(9):1166–70.

20. Lemery R, Guiraudon G, Veinot JP. Anatomic description of Bachmann's bundle and its relation to the atrial septum. Am J Cardiol 2003;91(12):1482–5, A1488.

21. Friedman PA, Asirvatham SJ, Dalegrave C, et al. Percutaneous epicardial left atrial appendage closure: preliminary results of an electrogram guided approach. J Cardiovasc Electrophysiol 2009;20(8):908–15.

22. De Ponti P, Ho SY, Salerno-Uriarte JA, et al. Electro-anatomic analysis of sinus impulse propagation in normal human atria. J Cardiovasc Electrophysiol 2002;13(1):1–10.

23. Markides V, Schilling RJ, Ho SY, et al. Characterization of left atrial activation in the intact human heart. Circulation 2003;107(5):733–9.

24. Cosio FG, Martin-Penato A, Pastor A, et al. Atrial activation mapping in sinus rhythm in the clinical electrophysiology laboratory: observations during Bachmann's bundle block. J Cardiovasc Electrophysiol 2004;15(5):524–31.

25. Lemery R, Birnie D, Tang AS, et al. Normal atrial activation and voltage during sinus rhythm in the human heart: an endocardial and epicardial mapping study in patients with a history of atrial fibrillation. J Cardiovasc Electrophysiol 2007;18(4):402–8.

26. Matsumoto Y, Krishnan S, Fowler SJ, et al. Detection of phrenic nerves and their relation to cardiac anatomy using 64-slice multidetector computed tomography. Am J Cardiol 2007;100(1):133–7.

27. Lachman N, Syed FF, Habib A, et al. Correlative anatomy for the electrophysiologist, part II: cardiac ganglia, phrenic nerve, coronary venous system. J Cardiovasc Electrophysiol 2011;22(1):104–10.

28. Wongcharoen W, Tsao HM, Wu MH, et al. Morphologic characteristics of the left atrial appendage, roof, and septum: implications for the ablation of atrial fibrillation. J Cardiovasc Electrophysiol 2006;17(9):951–6.

29. Ernst G, Stollberger C, Abzieher F, et al. Morphology of the left atrial appendage. Anat Rec 1995;242(4):553–61.

30. Veinot JP, Harrity PJ, Gentile F, et al. Anatomy of the normal left atrial appendage: a quantitative study of age-related changes in 500 autopsy hearts: implications for echocardiographic examination. Circulation 1997;96(9):3112–5.

31. Ramaswamy P, Lytrivi ID, Srivastava S, et al. Left atrial appendage: variations in morphology and position causing pitfalls in pediatric echocardiographic diagnosis. J Am Soc Echocardiogr 2007;20(8):1011–6.

32. Beinart R, Heist EK, Newell JB, et al. Left atrial appendage dimensions predict the risk of stroke/TIA in patients with atrial fibrillation. J Cardiovasc Electrophysiol 2011;22(1):10–5.

33. Wang Y, Di Biase L, Horton RP, et al. Left atrial appendage studied by computed tomography to help planning for appendage closure device placement. J Cardiovasc Electrophysiol 2010;21(9):973–82.

34. Heist EK, Refaat M, Danik SB, et al. Analysis of the left atrial appendage by magnetic resonance angiography in patients with atrial fibrillation. Heart Rhythm 2006;3(11):1313–8.

35. O'Brien J, Al-Hassan D, Ng J, et al. Three-dimensional assessment of left atrial appendage orifice geometry and potential implications for device closure. Int J Cardiovasc Imaging 2014;30(4):819–23.

36. Chowdhury UK, Seth S, Govindappa R, et al. Congenital left atrial appendage aneurysm: a case report and brief review of literature. Heart Lung Circ 2009;18(6):412–6.

37. Bramlet DA, Edwards JE. Congenital aneurysm of left atrial appendage. Br Heart J 1981;45(1):97–100.

38. Collier P, Cavalcante JL, Phelan D, et al. Congenital absence of the left atrial appendage. Circ Cardiovasc Imaging 2012;5(4):549–50.

39. Frescura C, Thiene G. Juxtaposition of the atrial appendages. Cardiovasc Pathol 2012;21(3):169–79.

40. Zhang H, Sun JP, Zhao Y, et al. Inverted left atrial appendage. Int J Cardiol 2014;170(3):e57–8.

41. Davis CA 3rd, Rembert JC, Greenfield JC Jr. Compliance of left atrium with and without left atrium appendage. Am J Phys 1990;259(4 Pt 2):H1006–8.

42. Hoit BD, Walsh RA. Regional atrial distensibility. Am J Phys 1992;262(5 Pt 2):H1356–60.

43. Hondo T, Okamoto M, Yamane T, et al. The role of the left atrial appendage. A volume loading study in open-chest dogs. Jpn Heart J 1995;36(2):225–34.

44. Killeen RP, Ryan R, MacErlane A, et al. Accessory left atrial diverticulae: contractile properties depicted with 64-slice cine-cardiac CT. Int J Cardiovasc Imaging 2010;26(2):241–8.

45. Goldberg YH, Gordon SC, Spevack DM, et al. Disparities in emptying velocity within the left atrial appendage. Eur J Echocardiogr 2010; 11(3):290–5.

46. Moe GW, Grima EA, Angus C, et al. Response of atrial natriuretic factor to acute and chronic increases of atrial pressures in experimental heart failure in dogs. Role of changes in heart rate, atrial dimension, and cardiac tissue concentration. Circulation 1991;83(5):1780–7.

47. Stewart JM, Dean R, Brown M, et al. Bilateral atrial appendectomy abolishes increased plasma atrial natriuretic peptide release and blunts sodium and water excretion during volume loading in conscious dogs. Circ Res 1992;70(4):724–32.

48. Stewart JM, O'Dea DJ, Shapiro GC, et al. Atrial compliance determines the nature of passive atrial stretch and plasma atrial natriuretic factor in the conscious dog. Cardiovasc Res 1991;25(9):784–92.

49. Tabata T, Oki T, Yamada H, et al. Relationship between left atrial appendage function and plasma concentration of atrial natriuretic peptide. Eur J Echocardiogr 2000;1(2):130–7.

50. Winter EM, van Oorschot AA, Hogers B, et al. A new direction for cardiac regeneration therapy: application of synergistically acting epicardium-derived cells and cardiomyocyte progenitor cells. Circ Heart Fail 2009;2(6):643–53.

51. Yoshida N, Okamoto M, Nanba K, et al. Transthoracic tissue Doppler assessment of left atrial appendage contraction and relaxation: their changes with aging. Echocardiography 2010;27(7):839–46.

52. Hoit BD, Shao Y, Tsai LM, et al. Altered left atrial compliance after atrial appendectomy. Influence on left atrial and ventricular filling. Circ Res 1993;72(1):167–75.

53. Kamohara K, Popovic ZB, Daimon M, et al. Impact of left atrial appendage exclusion on left atrial function. J Thorac Cardiovasc Surg 2007;133(1): 174–81.

54. Tabata T, Oki T, Yamada H, et al. Role of left atrial appendage in left atrial reservoir function as evaluated by left atrial appendage clamping during cardiac surgery. Am J Cardiol 1998;81(3):327–32.

55. Melduni R, Wiggins M, Suri R, et al. Physiological significance of left atrial appendage closure: implication for postoperative atrial fibrillation. J Am Coll Cardiol 2013;61(10_S).

56. Lee CH, Kim JB, Jung SH, et al. Left atrial appendage resection versus preservation during the surgical ablation of atrial fibrillation. Ann Thorac Surg 2014; 97(1):124–32.

57. Bois JP, Sheldon S, Stulak J, et al. Surgical therapy for atrial fibrillation: impact of left atrial appendage exclusion or amputation on atrial mechanical function. J Am Coll Cardiol 2014;63(12_S).

58. Lakkireddy D. Left atrial appendage exclusion as adjunct strategy for AF ablation. Paper presented at: Heart Rhythm Society Annual Sessions. San Francisco, May 9, 2014.

59. Gage BF, Waterman AD, Shannon W, et al. Validation of clinical classification schemes for predicting stroke: results from the National Registry of Atrial Fibrillation. JAMA 2001;285(22):2864–70.

60. Rietbrock S, Heeley E, Plumb J, et al. Chronic atrial fibrillation: incidence, prevalence, and prediction of stroke using the congestive heart failure, Hypertension, age >75, diabetes mellitus, and prior stroke or transient ischemic attack (CHADS2) risk stratification scheme. Am Heart J 2008;156(1):57–64.

61. Lip GY, Nieuwlaat R, Pisters R, et al. Refining clinical risk stratification for predicting stroke and thromboembolism in atrial fibrillation using a novel risk factor-based approach: the Euro heart survey on atrial fibrillation. Chest 2010;137(2):263–72.

62. Lip GY, Frison L, Halperin JL, et al. Identifying patients at high risk for stroke despite anticoagulation: a comparison of contemporary stroke risk stratification schemes in an anticoagulated atrial fibrillation cohort. Stroke 2010;41(12):2731–8.

63. Blackshear JL, Pearce LA, Hart RG, et al. Aortic plaque in atrial fibrillation: prevalence, predictors, and thromboembolic implications. Stroke 1999; 30(4):834–40.

64. Asinger RW, Koehler J, Pearce LA, et al. Pathophysiologic correlates of thromboembolism in nonvalvular atrial fibrillation: II. Dense spontaneous echocardiographic contrast (The Stroke Prevention in Atrial Fibrillation [SPAF-III] study). J Am Soc Echocardiogr 1999;12(12):1088–96.

65. Welles CC, Whooley MA, Na B, et al. The CHADS2 score predicts ischemic stroke in the absence of atrial fibrillation among subjects with coronary heart disease: data from the Heart and Soul Study. Am Heart J 2011;162(3):555–61.

66. Wang YC, Lin JL, Hwang JJ, et al. Left atrial dysfunction in patients with atrial fibrillation after successful rhythm control for >3 months. Chest 2005;128(4): 2551–6.

67. Azarbal F, Welles CC, Wong JM, et al. Association of CHADS2, CHA2DS2-VASc, and R2CHADS2 scores with left atrial dysfunction in patients with coronary heart disease (from the Heart and Soul study). Am J Cardiol 2014;113(7):1166–72.

68. Puwanant S, Varr BC, Shrestha K, et al. Role of the CHADS2 score in the evaluation of thromboembolic risk in patients with atrial fibrillation undergoing transesophageal echocardiography before pulmonary vein isolation. J Am Coll Cardiol 2009; 54(22):2032–9.

69. Fukuda S, Watanabe H, Shimada K, et al. Left atrial thrombus and prognosis after anticoagulation therapy in patients with atrial fibrillation. J Cardiol 2011; 58(3):266–77.

70. Doukky R, Gage H, Nagarajan V, et al. B-type natriuretic peptide predicts left atrial appendage thrombus in patients with nonvalvular atrial fibrillation. Echocardiography 2013;30(8):889–95.

71. Doukky R, Garcia-Sayan E, Gage H, et al. The value of diastolic function parameters in the prediction of left atrial appendage thrombus in patients with nonvalvular atrial fibrillation. Cardiovasc Ultrasound 2014;12(1):10.

72. Di Angelantonio E, Ederhy S, Benyounes N, et al. Comparison of transesophageal echocardiographic identification of embolic risk markers in patients with lone versus non-lone atrial fibrillation. Am J Cardiol 2005;95(5):592–6.

73. Glotzer TV, Daoud EG, Wyse DG, et al. The relationship between daily atrial tachyarrhythmia burden from implantable device diagnostics and stroke risk: the TRENDS study. Circulation 2009; 2(5):474–80.

74. Healey JS, Connolly SJ, Gold MR, et al. Subclinical atrial fibrillation and the risk of stroke. N Engl J Med 2012;366(2):120–9.

75. Boriani G, Glotzer TV, Santini M, et al. Device-detected atrial fibrillation and risk for stroke: an analysis of >10,000 patients from the SOS AF project (Stroke prevention strategies based on atrial fibrillation information from implanted devices). Eur Heart J 2014;35(8):508–16.

76. Boriani G, Botto GL, Padeletti L, et al. Improving stroke risk stratification using the CHADS2 and CHA2DS2-VASc risk scores in patients with paroxysmal atrial fibrillation by continuous arrhythmia burden monitoring. Stroke 2011;42(6):1768–70.

77. Daoud EG, Glotzer TV, Wyse DG, et al. Temporal relationship of atrial tachyarrhythmias, cerebrovascular events, and systemic emboli based on stored device data: a subgroup analysis of TRENDS. Heart Rhythm 2011;8(9):1416–23.

78. Coutinho T, Borlaug BA, Pellikka PA, et al. Sex differences in arterial stiffness and ventricular-arterial interactions. J Am Coll Cardiol 2013;61(1):96–103.

79. Zabalgoitia M, Halperin JL, Pearce LA, et al. Transesophageal echocardiographic correlates of clinical risk of thromboembolism in nonvalvular atrial fibrillation. Stroke Prevention in Atrial Fibrillation III Investigators. J Am Coll Cardiol 1998;31(7):1622–6.

80. Goldman ME, Pearce LA, Hart RG, et al. Pathophysiologic correlates of thromboembolism in nonvalvular atrial fibrillation: I. Reduced flow velocity in the left atrial appendage (The Stroke Prevention in Atrial Fibrillation [SPAF-III] study). J Am Soc Echocardiogr 1999;12(12):1080–7.

81. Iwakura K, Okamura A, Koyama Y, et al. Effect of elevated left ventricular diastolic filling pressure on the frequency of left atrial appendage thrombus in patients with nonvalvular atrial fibrillation. Am J Cardiol 2011;107(3):417–22.

82. Pollick C, Taylor D. Assessment of left atrial appendage function by transesophageal echocardiography. Implications for the development of thrombus. Circulation 1991;84(1):223–31.

83. Fatkin D, Feneley MP. Patterns of Doppler-measured blood flow velocity in the normal and fibrillating human left atrial appendage. Am Heart J 1996;132(5):995–1003.

84. Obel OA, Luddington L, Maarouf N, et al. Effects of ventricular rate and regularity on the velocity and magnitude of left atrial appendage flow in atrial fibrillation. Heart 2005;91(6):764–8.

85. Kanadasi M, Cayli M, Sahin DY, et al. The effect of different atrioventricular delays on left atrium and left atrial appendage function in patients with DDD pacemaker. Echocardiography 2011;28(6): 626–32.

86. Corradi D, Callegari S, Manotti L, et al. Persistent lone atrial fibrillation: clinicopathologic study of 19 cases. Heart Rhythm 2014;11(7):1250–8.

87. Akoum N, Fernandez G, Wilson B, et al. Association of atrial fibrosis quantified using LGE-MRI with atrial appendage thrombus and spontaneous contrast on transesophageal echocardiography in patients with atrial fibrillation. J Cardiovasc Electrophysiol 2013;24(10):1104–9.

88. Karabay CY, Zehir R, Guler A, et al. Left atrial deformation parameters predict left atrial appendage function and thrombus in patients in sinus rhythm with suspected cardioembolic stroke: a speckle tracking and transesophageal echocardiography study. Echocardiography 2013;30(5): 572–81.

89. Leong DP, Penhall A, Perry R, et al. Speckle-tracking strain of the left atrium: a transoesophageal echocardiographic validation study. Eur Heart J Cardiovasc Imaging 2013;14(9):898–905.

90. Sung SH, Chang SL, Hsu TL, et al. Do the left atrial substrate properties correlate with the left atrial mechanical function? A novel insight from the electromechanical study in patients with atrial fibrillation. J Cardiovasc Electrophysiol 2008; 19(2):165–71.

91. Watson T, Shantsila E, Lip GY. Mechanisms of thrombogenesis in atrial fibrillation: Virchow's triad revisited. Lancet 2009;373(9658):155–66.

92. Jesel L, Arentz T, Herrera-Siklody C, et al. Do atrial differences in endothelial damage, leukocyte and platelet activation, or tissue factor activity contribute to chamber-specific thrombogenic status in patients with atrial fibrillation? J Cardiovasc Electrophysiol 2014;25(3):266–70.

93. Grimm RA, Stewart WJ, Maloney JD, et al. Impact of electrical cardioversion for atrial fibrillation on left atrial appendage function and spontaneous echo contrast: characterization by simultaneous transesophageal echocardiography. J Am Coll Cardiol 1993;22(5):1359–66.

94. Di Biase L, Santangeli P, Anselmino M, et al. Does the left atrial appendage morphology correlate with the risk of stroke in patients with atrial fibrillation? Results from a multicenter study. J Am Coll Cardiol 2012;60(6):531–8.

95. Anselmino M, Scaglione M, Di Biase L, et al. Left atrial appendage morphology and silent cerebral ischemia in patients with atrial fibrillation. Heart Rhythm 2014;11(1):2–7.

96. Kimura T, Takatsuki S, Fukuda K. The left atrial appendage: can anatomical characteristics be used to predict strokes in nonvalvular atrial fibrillation patients? Future Cardiol 2013;9(4):451–3.

97. Khurram IM, Dewire J, Mager M, et al. Relationship between left atrial appendage morphology and stroke in patients with atrial fibrillation. Heart Rhythm 2013;10(12):1843–9.

98. Yamamoto M, Seo Y, Kawamatsu N, et al. Complex left atrial appendage morphology and left atrial appendage thrombus formation in patients with atrial fibrillation. Circ Cardiovasc Imaging 2014; 7(2):337–43.

99. Shirani J, Alaeddini J. Structural remodeling of the left atrial appendage in patients with chronic non-valvular atrial fibrillation: implications for thrombus formation, systemic embolism, and assessment by transesophageal echocardiography. Cardiovasc Pathol 2000;9(2):95–101.

100. Chatterjee S, Alexander JC, Pearson PJ, et al. Left atrial appendage occlusion: lessons learned from surgical and transcatheter experiences. Ann Thorac Surg 2011;92(6):2283–92.

101. Kanderian AS, Gillinov AM, Pettersson GB, et al. Success of surgical left atrial appendage closure: assessment by transesophageal echocardiography. J Am Coll Cardiol 2008;52(11):924–9.

102. Katz ES, Tsiamtsiouris T, Applebaum RM, et al. Surgical left atrial appendage ligation is frequently incomplete: a transesophageal echocardiographic study. J Am Coll Cardiol 2000;36(2):468–71.

103. Healey JS, Crystal E, Lamy A, et al. Left Atrial Appendage Occlusion Study (LAAOS): results of a randomized controlled pilot study of left atrial appendage occlusion during coronary bypass surgery in patients at risk for stroke. Am Heart J 2005; 150(2):288–93.

104. Cullen MW, Stulak J, Li Z, et al. Value of transesophageal echocardiography to guide cardioversion in patients with atrial fibrillation after cardiac surgery. J Am Coll Cardiol 2013;61(10_S).

105. Klemm HU, Steven D, Johnsen C, et al. Catheter motion during atrial ablation due to the beating heart and respiration: impact on accuracy and spatial referencing in three-dimensional mapping. Heart Rhythm 2007;4(5):587–92.

106. Stergiopoulos K, Seifert F, Brown DL. Thrombus formation after successful stapler exclusion of the left atrial appendage. J Am Coll Cardiol 2010;55(4): 379.

107. Kim R, Baumgartner N, Clements J. Routine left atrial appendage ligation during cardiac surgery may prevent postoperative atrial fibrillation-related cerebrovascular accident. J Thorac Cardiovasc Surg 2013;145(2):582–9 [discussion: 589].

108. Whitlock RP, Vincent J, Blackall MH, et al. Left atrial appendage occlusion study II (LAAOS II). Can J Cardiol 2013;29(11):1443–7.

109. Whitlock R, Healey J, Vincent J, et al. Rationale and design of the Left Atrial Appendage Occlusion Study (LAAOS) III. Ann Cardiothorac Surg 2014; 3(1):45–54.

110. Dawson AG, Asopa S, Dunning J. Should patients undergoing cardiac surgery with atrial fibrillation have left atrial appendage exclusion? Interact Cardiovasc Thorac Surg 2010;10(2):306–11.

111. January CT, Wann LS, Alpert JS, et al. 2014 AHA/ACC/HRS Guideline for the management of patients with atrial fibrillation: a report of the American College of Cardiology/American Heart Association Task Force on Practice Guidelines and the Heart Rhythm Society. Circulation 2014. [Epub ahead of print].

112. Nishimura RA, Otto CM, Bonow RO, et al. 2014 AHA/ACC guideline for the management of patients with valvular heart disease: a report of the American College of Cardiology/American Heart Association Task Force on Practice Guidelines. Circulation 2014;129(23):e521–643.

113. Camm AJ, Lip GY, De Caterina R, et al. 2012 focused update of the ESC Guidelines for the

management of atrial fibrillation: an update of the 2010 ESC Guidelines for the management of atrial fibrillation. Developed with the special contribution of the European Heart Rhythm Association. Eur Heart J 2012;33(21):2719–47.

114. Yilmaz A, Van Putte BP, Van Boven WJ. Completely thoracoscopic bilateral pulmonary vein isolation and left atrial appendage exclusion for atrial fibrillation. J Thorac Cardiovasc Surg 2008;136(2):521–2.

115. Muhammad MI. Role of video-assisted thoracoscopy in the management of stroke. Asian Cardiovasc Thorac Ann 2014;22(2):155–9.

116. Ohtsuka T, Ninomiya M, Nonaka T, et al. Thoracoscopic stand-alone left atrial appendectomy for thromboembolism prevention in nonvalvular atrial fibrillation. J Am Coll Cardiol 2013;62(2):103–7.

117. Santini M, Loiaconi V, Tocco MP, et al. Feasibility and efficacy of minimally invasive stand-alone surgical ablation of atrial fibrillation. A single-center experience. J Interv Card Electrophysiol 2012; 34(1):79–87.

118. Wolf RK. Treatment of lone atrial fibrillation: minimally invasive pulmonary vein isolation, partial cardiac denervation and excision of the left atrial appendage. Ann Cardiothorac Surg 2014;3(1):98–104.

119. Zheng S, Li Y, Han J, et al. Long-term results of a minimally invasive surgical pulmonary vein isolation and ganglionic plexi ablation for atrial fibrillation. PLoS One 2013;8(11):e79755.

120. Kurfirst V, Mokracek A, Bulava A, et al. Two-staged hybrid treatment of persistent atrial fibrillation: short-term single-centre results. Interact Cardiovasc Thorac Surg 2014;18(4):451–6.

121. Gafoor S, Franke J, Bertog S, et al. Left atrial appendage occlusion in octogenarians: short-term and 1-year follow-up. Catheter Cardiovasc Interv 2014;83(5):805–10.

122. National Institute for Health and Clinical Excellence: Percutaneous occlusion of the left atrial appendage for atrial fibrillation. 2006. Available at: http://www.nice.org.uk/nicemedia/pdf/IPG181guidance.pdf. Accessed May 12, 2014.

123. Bartus K, Bednarek J, Myc J, et al. Feasibility of closed-chest ligation of the left atrial appendage in humans. Heart Rhythm 2011;8(2):188–93.

124. Bartus K, Han FT, Bednarek J, et al. Percutaneous left atrial appendage suture ligation using the LARIAT device in patients with atrial fibrillation: initial clinical experience. J Am Coll Cardiol 2013; 62(2):108–18.

125. Meier B, Palacios I, Windecker S, et al. Transcatheter left atrial appendage occlusion with Amplatzer devices to obviate anticoagulation in patients with atrial fibrillation. Catheter Cardiovasc Interv 2003; 60(3):417–22.

126. Park JW, Bethencourt A, Sievert H, et al. Left atrial appendage closure with Amplatzer cardiac plug in atrial fibrillation: initial European experience. Catheter Cardiovasc Interv 2011;77(5):700–6.

127. Bai R, Horton RP, DI Biase L, et al. Intraprocedural and long-term incomplete occlusion of the left atrial appendage following placement of the WATCHMAN device: a single center experience. J Cardiovasc Electrophysiol 2012;23(5):455–61.

128. Reddy VY, Holmes D, Doshi SK, et al. Safety of percutaneous left atrial appendage closure: results from the Watchman Left Atrial Appendage System for Embolic Protection in Patients with AF (PROTECT AF) clinical trial and the Continued Access Registry. Circulation 2011;123(4):417–24.

129. Viles-Gonzalez JF, Kar S, Douglas P, et al. The clinical impact of incomplete left atrial appendage closure with the Watchman Device in patients with atrial fibrillation: a PROTECT AF (Percutaneous Closure of the Left Atrial Appendage Versus Warfarin Therapy for Prevention of Stroke in Patients With Atrial Fibrillation) substudy. J Am Coll Cardiol 2012;59(10):923–9.

130. Reddy VY, Franzen O, Worthley S, et al. Clinical experience with the Wavecrest LA appendage occlusion device for stroke prevention in AF: acute results of the WAVECREST I trial. The Heart Rhythm Society's 35th Annual Scientific Sessions. San Francisco, May 7–10, 2014. p. PO01–112.

131. Sousa JE, Costa MA, Tuzcu EM, et al. New frontiers in interventional cardiology. Circulation 2005; 111(5):671–81.

132. Ostermayer SH, Reisman M, Kramer PH, et al. Percutaneous left atrial appendage transcatheter occlusion (PLAATO system) to prevent stroke in high-risk patients with non-rheumatic atrial fibrillation: results from the international multi-center feasibility trials. J Am Coll Cardiol 2005;46(1):9–14.

133. Block PC, Burstein S, Casale PN, et al. Percutaneous left atrial appendage occlusion for patients in atrial fibrillation suboptimal for warfarin therapy: 5-year results of the PLAATO (Percutaneous Left Atrial Appendage Transcatheter Occlusion) Study. J Am Coll Cardiol 2009;2(7):594–600.

134. Bayard YL, Omran H, Neuzil P, et al. PLAATO (Percutaneous Left Atrial Appendage Transcatheter Occlusion) for prevention of cardioembolic stroke in non-anticoagulation eligible atrial fibrillation patients: results from the European PLAATO study. Eurointervention 2010;6(2):220–6.

135. Supreme Court Proceedings of the State of Delaware. Filing ID 54541646. Case Number 515, 2013. 2013.

136. Berti S, Santoro G, Palmieri C, et al. Tools and techniques clinical: transcatheter closure of left atrial appendage using the Amplatzer Cardiac Plug. Eurointervention 2013;9(4):524–6.

137. Jain AK, Gallagher S. Percutaneous occlusion of the left atrial appendage in non-valvular atrial

fibrillation for the prevention of thromboembolism: NICE guidance. Heart 2011;97(9):762–5.

138. Cruz-Gonzalez I, Martin Moreiras J, Garcia E. Thrombus formation after left atrial appendage exclusion using an Amplatzer cardiac plug device. Catheter Cardiovasc Interv 2011;78(6):970–3.

139. Kefer J, Vermeersch P, Budts W, et al. Transcatheter left atrial appendage closure for stroke prevention in atrial fibrillation with Amplatzer cardiac plug: the Belgian Registry. Acta Cardiol 2013; 68(6):551–8.

140. Mohrs OK, Wunderlich N, Petersen SE, et al. Contrast-enhanced CMR in patients after percutaneous closure of the left atrial appendage: a pilot study. J Cardiovasc Magn Reson 2011;13:33.

141. Lockwood SM, Alison JF, Obeyesekere MN, et al. Imaging the left atrial appendage prior to, during, and after occlusion. J Am Coll Cardiol 2011;4(3):303–6.

142. Guerios EE, Schmid M, Gloekler S, et al. Left atrial appendage closure with the Amplatzer Cardiac Plug in patients with atrial fibrillation. Arq Bras Cardiol 2012;98(6):528–36.

143. Lopez-Minguez JR, Eldoayen-Gragera J, Gonzalez-Fernandez R, et al. Immediate and one-year results in 35 consecutive patients after closure of left atrial appendage with the Amplatzer cardiac plug. Rev Esp Cardiol 2013;66(2):90–7.

144. Lam YY, Yip GW, Yu CM, et al. Left atrial appendage closure with AMPLATZER cardiac plug for stroke prevention in atrial fibrillation: initial Asia-Pacific experience. Catheter Cardiovasc Interv 2012;79(5): 794–800.

145. Versaci F, Sacca S, Mugnolo A, et al. Simultaneous patent foramen ovale and left atrial appendage closure. J Cardiovasc Med (Hagerstown) 2012; 13(10):663–4.

146. Viles-Gonzalez JF, Reddy VY, Petru J, et al. Incomplete occlusion of the left atrial appendage with the percutaneous left atrial appendage transcatheter occlusion device is not associated with increased risk of stroke. J Interv Card Electrophysiol 2012; 33(1):69–75.

147. Freixa X, Chan JL, Tzikas A, et al. The Amplatzer Cardiac Plug 2 for left atrial appendage occlusion: novel features and first-in-man experience. Eurointervention 2013;8(9):1094–8.

148. Freixa X, Kwai Chan JL, Tzikas A, et al. Percutaneous closure of a very large left atrial appendage using the Amplatzer amulet. Can J Cardiol 2013; 29(10):1329.e9–11.

149. Holmes DR, Reddy VY, Turi ZG, et al. Percutaneous closure of the left atrial appendage versus warfarin therapy for prevention of stroke in patients with atrial fibrillation: a randomised non-inferiority trial. Lancet 2009;374(9689):534–42.

150. Holmes DR Jr, Lakkireddy DR, Whitlock RP, et al. Left atrial appendage occlusion: opportunities

and challenges. J Am Coll Cardiol 2014;63(4): 291–8.

151. Gangireddy SR, Halperin JL, Fuster V, et al. Percutaneous left atrial appendage closure for stroke prevention in patients with atrial fibrillation: an assessment of net clinical benefit. Eur Heart J 2012;33(21):2700–8.

152. Massarenti L, Yilmaz A. Incomplete endothelialization of left atrial appendage occlusion device 10 months after implantation. J Cardiovasc Electrophysiol 2012;23(12):1384–5.

153. Reddy VY, Mobius-Winkler S, Miller MA, et al. Left atrial appendage closure with the Watchman device in patients with a contraindication for oral anticoagulation: the ASAP study (ASA Plavix Feasibility Study With Watchman Left Atrial Appendage Closure Technology). J Am Coll Cardiol 2013; 61(25):2551–6.

154. Albers GW, Diener HC, Frison L, et al. Ximelagatran vs warfarin for stroke prevention in patients with nonvalvular atrial fibrillation: a randomized trial. JAMA 2005;293(6):690–8.

155. Connolly SJ, Ezekowitz MD, Yusuf S, et al. Dabigatran versus warfarin in patients with atrial fibrillation. N Engl J Med 2009;361(12):1139–51.

156. Patel MR, Mahaffey KW, Garg J, et al. Rivaroxaban versus warfarin in nonvalvular atrial fibrillation. N Engl J Med 2011;365(10):883–91.

157. Granger CB, Alexander JH, McMurray JJ, et al. Apixaban versus warfarin in patients with atrial fibrillation. N Engl J Med 2011;365(11):981–92.

158. Amorosi SL, Armstrong S, Da Deppo L, et al. The budget impact of left atrial appendage closure compared with adjusted-dose warfarin and dabigatran etexilate for stroke prevention in atrial fibrillation. Europace 2014;16(8):1131–6.

159. Whisenant B, Weiss B. Left atrial appendage closure with transcatheter-delivered devices. Intervent Cardiol Clin 2014;3(2):209–18.

160. Toumanides S, Sideris EB, Agricola T, et al. Transcatheter patch occlusion of the left atrial appendage using surgical adhesives in high-risk patients with atrial fibrillation. J Am Coll Cardiol 2011;58(21): 2236–40.

161. Cheng Y, Conditt G, Yi G, et al. TCT-765 first in-vivo evaluation of the Ultrasept left atrial appendage closure device. J Am Coll Cardiol 2012;60(17_S).

162. Bruce CJ, Stanton CM, Asirvatham SJ, et al. Percutaneous epicardial left atrial appendage closure: intermediate-term results. J Cardiovasc Electrophysiol 2011;22(1):64–70.

163. Bruce CJ, Asirvatham SJ, McCaw T, et al. Novel percutaneous left atrial appendage closure. Cardiovasc Revasc Med 2013;14(3):164–7.

164. Santoro F, Di Biase L, Santangeli P, et al. Catheter-based epicardial closure of the left atrial appendage. Intervent Cardiol Clin 2014;3(2):219–27.

165. Stone D, Byrne T, Pershad A. Early results with the LARIAT device for left atrial appendage exclusion in patients with atrial fibrillation at high risk for stroke and anticoagulation. Catheter Cardiovasc Interv 2013. [Epub ahead of print].

166. Nucifora G, Faletra FF, Regoli F, et al. Evaluation of the left atrial appendage with real-time 3-dimensional transesophageal echocardiography: implications for catheter-based left atrial appendage closure. Circ Cardiovasc Imaging 2011;4(5):514–23.

167. Earley MJ. How to perform a transseptal puncture. Heart 2009;95(1):85–92.

168. Syed F, Lachman N, Christensen K, et al. The pericardial space: obtaining access and an approach to fluoroscopic anatomy. Card Electrophysiol Clin 2010;2(1):9–23.

169. Baran J, Stec S, Pilichowska-Paszkiet E, et al. Intracardiac echocardiography for detection of thrombus in the left atrial appendage: comparison with transesophageal echocardiography in patients undergoing ablation for atrial fibrillation: the Action-Ice I Study. Circulation 2013;6(6):1074–81.

170. Plicht B, Konorza TF, Kahlert P, et al. Risk factors for thrombus formation on the Amplatzer Cardiac Plug after left atrial appendage occlusion. J Am Coll Cardiol 2013;6(6):606–13.

171. Baker MS, Paul Mounsey J, Gehi AK, et al. Left atrial thrombus after appendage ligation with LARIAT. Heart Rhythm 2013;11(8):1489.

172. Giedrimas E, Lin AC, Knight BP. Left atrial thrombus after appendage closure using LARIAT. Circulation 2013;6(4):e52–3.

173. Krishnaswamy A, Patel NS, Ozkan A, et al. Planning left atrial appendage occlusion using cardiac multidetector computed tomography. Int J Cardiol 2012;158(2):313–7.

174. Chue CD, de Giovanni J, Steeds RP. The role of echocardiography in percutaneous left atrial appendage occlusion. Eur J Echocardiogr 2011; 12(10):i3–10.

175. MacDonald ST, Newton JD, Ormerod OJ. Intracardiac echocardiography off piste? Closure of the left atrial appendage using ICE and local anesthesia. Catheter Cardiovasc Interv 2011;77(1):124–7.

176. Budge LP, Shaffer KM, Moorman JR, et al. Analysis of in vivo left atrial appendage morphology in patients with atrial fibrillation: a direct comparison of transesophageal echocardiography, planar cardiac CT, and segmented three-dimensional cardiac CT. J Interv Card Electrophysiol 2008;23(2):87–93.

177. Briceno DF, Fernando RR, Laing ST. Left atrial appendage thrombus post LARIAT closure device. Heart Rhythm 2013;11(1):17–25.

178. Guo XG, Zhang JL, Ma J, et al. Management of focal atrial tachycardias originating from the atrial appendage with the combination of radiofrequency catheter ablation and minimally invasive atrial appendectomy. Heart Rhythm 2014;11(1):17–25.

Postoperative Atrial Fibrillation
Incidence, Mechanisms, and Clinical Correlates

Mrinal Yadava, MD[a,b], Andrew B. Hughey, MD[c],
Thomas Christopher Crawford, MD[a,*]

KEYWORDS

- Atrial fibrillation • Postoperative atrial fibrillation • Beta-blockers • Coronary artery bypass grafting

KEY POINTS

- Atrial fibrillation is often encountered after cardiac and noncardiac surgical procedures.
- Atrial fibrillation is associated with an increased hospital stay and stroke risk, and a reduced in-hospital and long-term survival.
- Understanding the underlying pathophysiology of POAF remains elusive; however, numerous risk factors predisposing to its development have been identified, including advanced age, structural damage to the heart, left ventricular dysfunction, hypertension, and valve surgery.
- Further investigation into the mechanisms underlying POAF, and the effects of various therapeutic modalities, will enable a better understanding of this phenomenon.
- Risk stratification, and targeted interventions for high-risk patients, may hold the key to mitigating the morbidity and financial burden associated with this arrhythmia.

INTRODUCTION

Atrial fibrillation (AF) is a commonly encountered arrhythmia in clinical practice, and is a well-recognized complication of cardiac surgery. The occurrence of postoperative AF (POAF) is associated with an increased length of stay, stroke risk, health care costs, and mortality.[1–14] The incidence of POAF varies from 15% to 60%,[3,5–11,15–19] with the highest rates observed in patients undergoing valve surgery (37%–60%).[5,7,17] POAF has also been known to complicate noncardiac surgery, especially esophagectomy, lung surgery, and large colorectal surgery.[13,20–22] The onset of POAF peaks on the second day after surgery and declines to 2% at discharge.[16,23] Although usually self-limiting in nature, the risks of hemodynamic compromise and thromboembolism exist.[4,5,24]

MECHANISM

Although the exact pathophysiology of POAF remains incompletely understood, it is likely multifactorial in cause. Patient-related factors known to contribute include atrial dilatation, age-related fibrosis, structural damage to the heart, hypertension, and other comorbid conditions.[6,18,25] The concept of (structural) predisposition for AF seems

This article originally appeared in Cardiology Clinics, Volume 32, Issue 4, November 2014.
Conflicts of Interest: None reported.
Disclosures: None reported.
[a] Division of Cardiology, Department of Medicine, University of Michigan, 1500 East Medical Center Drive, SPC 5856, Ann Arbor, MI 48109, USA; [b] Department of Medicine, Michigan State University, 788 Service Road, Rm B301, East Lansing, MI 48824, USA; [c] Division of Cardiology, Department of Medicine, University of Michigan, 3116 Taubman Center, SPC 5368, Ann Arbor, MI 48109, USA
* Corresponding author.
E-mail address: thomcraw@med.umich.edu

to be true for vulnerability of certain patients to AF after cardiac surgery.[26] The electrophysiologic substrate may be pre-existing or may develop because of heterogeneity of refractoriness after surgery. Furthermore, the role of ectopic beats from the pulmonary veins in the development of POAF, as in nonsurgical patients, is yet to be delineated. This represents an area of significant interest, because such sites may be amenable to isolation at the time of surgery.

Several factors related to the surgical procedure also potentially contribute to the development of AF. These include operative trauma from surgical dissection and manipulation, pericardial lesions (pericarditis), atrial dilatation (caused by left ventricular dysfunction and intraoperative volume overload), perioperative use of catecholamines, parasympathetic activation, and electrolyte imbalances.[3,5,6,16,25,27,28] Current cardioplegia techniques and inadequate atrial cooling may be responsible for atrial ischemia. This has led some to postulate that ischemic injury and subsequent oxidative stress on reperfusion are potential triggers for POAF.[6,29,30] However, there have been conflicting reports regarding the effect of cardiopulmonary bypass time and aortic cross-clamp time on the incidence of the arrhythmia.[5,6,28,31,32]

The time course of development of POAF corresponds with the activation of the complement system, as evidenced by the release of proinflammatory cytokines and an increase in inflammatory markers.[14,33–37] This suggests an inflammatory component to the development of POAF. Inflammation is often related to the development of varying degrees of pericarditis. In support of this theory, some studies have demonstrated a benefit of drugs with anti-inflammatory action, including corticosteroids and statins, in decreasing the incidence of POAF.[38–41]

There seems to be a significant increase in sympathetic tone postoperatively in patients that subsequently develop POAF.[42–45] Withdrawal of preoperative β-blockers and nonuse of perioperative β-blockers are associated with a higher rate of AF,[7,18,46–48] thereby reinforcing the hypothesis of increased sympathetic tone being a facilitating factor in the development of POAF.

EPIDEMIOLOGY

The reported incidence of POAF varies depending on the type of surgery, definition of arrhythmia used, and method of arrhythmia surveillance.[16,17,49] Highest rates have been observed with combined valve surgery and coronary artery bypass grafting (CABG; 62%).[3,26,50] A lower incidence has been observed in patients undergoing isolated CABG (15%–40%),[5,7,50] cardiac transplantation (11%–24%),[5,17,51] and noncardiac surgery (0.3%–13.7%).[13,20–22] The different modalities used to monitor for arrhythmias after surgery also contribute to the variation in reported incidence. When intermittent 12-lead electrocardiograms are used for detection, a rate of 11% has been reported, compared with greater than 40% when diagnosis is based on continuous Holter monitoring.[15,31]

Advanced age has consistently been described as the most significant predictor of developing AF after cardiac and noncardiac surgery.[3,5–7,9,18,28,52,53] Structural changes of the heart with age, such as atrial fibrosis and dilatation, and age-related comorbidities, are likely responsible for this increase in incidence with age.[54,55] Villareal and colleagues[3] found age greater than 65 years to be an independent risk factor for developing POAF after revascularization (odds ratio [OR], 2.4; 95% confidence interval [CI], 2.06–2.74; $P<.0001$). In another study done on 2588 patients, the incidence of POAF in patients undergoing thoracic surgery increased with age as follows: age 50 to 59 years (relative risk [RR], 1.70; 95% CI, 1.01–2.88), age 60 to 69 years (RR, 4.49; 95% CI, 2.79–7.22), age 70 years or greater (RR, 5.30; 95% CI, 3.28–8.59).[53]

Patient-related risk factors for developing POAF also include left ventricular dysfunction and presence of congestive heart failure (CHF), obesity, hypertension, chronic obstructive airways disease, and severe underlying coronary artery disease.[3,6,56,57] The $CHADS_2$ and CHA_2DS_2-VASc scores were also found to be predictive of AF after cardiac surgery.[58]

Several studies have also described a difference in the incidence of POAF based on geographic region and race.[8,49] Higher rates were observed in the Middle East (41.6%), Canada (36.6%), Europe (34%), and United States (33.7%), with relatively lower rates being reported in South America (17.4%) and Asia (15.7%).[8] Whether this divergence represents a racial predisposition of whites toward the development of POAF, comorbid conditions, or a disparity in arrhythmia surveillance and reporting remains unknown. However, racial differences in POAF incidence have previously been described, with white race/ethnicity found to be an independent risk factor for POAF (OR, 1.8; 95% CI, 1.5–2.0; $P<.0001$).[49]

Because structural factors, such as fibrosis, scarring, and dilatation of the atria, predispose to the development of POAF, it has been hypothesized that electrophysiologic measurements before surgery may help predict the development of AF after surgery. The measurement of prolonged atrial conduction time has shown promise in this context.[59,60] Signal-averaged P-wave duration of greater than 140 milliseconds has been identified as a risk factor for POAF with a positive predictive value of 37%, and a negative predictive value of 87%.[60]

Identifying risk factors, and developing accurate prediction models, represents an important aspect of POAF management. Risk stratification helps identify patients who are most likely to benefit from prophylactic therapy, thereby potentially mitigating the morbidity and economic burden of this arrhythmia.

PROGNOSIS

AF after cardiac surgery had historically been considered a "benign," self-limiting arrhythmia. Despite its usually transient nature, it is now known to have a significant bearing on patient morbidity, mortality, and resource use. Numerous studies have looked at the stroke risk associated with POAF, with most observing between a two- and four-fold increase in risk at 30 days.[3,5,25,61] It has also been associated with a prolongation in the length of hospital stay by 4 to 5 days,[3,6] and an additional cost of $10,000 to $11,500 per patient.[6]

Numerous postoperative complications have been correlated with POAF. These include CHF, perioperative myocardial infarction, renal insufficiency, infection, ventricular arrhythmias, increased need for pacing and inotropic support, use of intra-aortic balloon pump, re-exploration of the chest for bleeding or cardiac tamponade, prolonged ventilation, reintubation, and readmission to the intensive care unit.[3,5,7,18,62] A direct causal relationship between POAF and these complications is, however, yet to be determined. It is likely that patients who develop AF after surgery are generally older and have more structural damage of the heart, with a higher propensity to develop other postoperative complications. It is logical to infer that the morbidity and economic burden associated with POAF might, at least in part, be contributed to by the associated adverse surgical outcomes. In this context, it is interesting that Villareal and colleagues[3] observed an increase in early and late mortality that persisted after adjustment for confounders, such as myocardial infarction, CHF, prior stroke, peripheral vascular disease, chronic obstructive pulmonary disease, diabetes, and advanced age, suggesting that AF in itself carries a risk for adverse outcomes. However, the question of whether prophylactic and therapeutic interventions directed at decreasing the incidence of POAF also decrease the associated morbidity and financial burden is

one that warrants further investigation in "real-world" settings.

MANAGEMENT GOALS

The clinical significance AF depends on the underlying cardiac function, duration, ventricular response rate, and comorbidities. POAF is usually self-limiting, with up to 30% of patients converting within 2 hours, and 25% to 80% of patients converting within 24 hours with either digoxin alone or no medication.[63,64] The essential goals of management are freedom from symptoms, maintaining hemodynamic stability, prevention of thromboembolism, and managing recurrence.

For patients requiring treatments, the strategies used are either rate or rhythm control, as in nonsurgical patients, with anticoagulation, if appropriate. Rate control is often preferred initially, because most patients usually convert within the first few weeks on rate-controlling medications alone. This strategy seems to be as effective as rhythm control, and is associated with early discharge.[65,66] Anticoagulation should be considered with a rate-control strategy, after thorough evaluation of the individual ischemic and hemorrhagic risks. In patients with persistent symptoms, hemodynamic instability, or contraindications to anticoagulation, rhythm control may be necessary.

PHARMACOLOGIC STRATEGIES
β-Blockers

β-Adrenergic blockade helps offset the effect of increased sympathetic tone, which is believed to be a significant contributor to the development of AF in the postoperative period.[15,28,67,68] The initiation of β-blockers preoperatively has been demonstrated to be more effective than postoperative initiation.[15] In a meta-analysis of 33 studies including 4698 participants, β-blocker administration demonstrated a reduction in POAF in the treatment group (16.3%) compared with the control group (31.7%; OR, 0.33; 95% CI, 0.26–0.43).[69] β-Blockers were initiated in the postoperative period in most (81.8%) studies. There are insufficient data to comment on the effect of β-blockade in reducing the incidence of postoperative stroke. β-Blockers have the added benefit of controlling the ventricular rate in the event of AF. In light of the extensive evidence demonstrating benefit from β-blockers, the 2006 American College of Cardiology/American Heart Association (ACC/AHA) guidelines gave a class I recommendation to preoperative or early postoperative β-blocker therapy in patients undergoing cardiac surgery without a contraindication.[70]

Antiarrhythmic Drugs

Amiodarone

Amiodarone is the most widely studied antiarrhythmic agent for POAF. Several trials have demonstrated a benefit of prophylactic amiodarone in preventing the onset of AF after surgery.[69,72–78] In a large randomized, controlled trial, oral amiodarone (10 mg/kg) started 6 days before surgery decreased the incidence of atrial tachyarrhythmias compared with placebo (hazard ratio, 0.52; 95% CI, 0.34–0.69; $P<.001$).[74] A 2013 meta-analysis demonstrated a borderline significant reduction in the postoperative cerebrovascular event rate in the amiodarone treatment group (1.6%) compared with the control group (2.8%) (OR, 0.60; CI, 0.35–1.02).[69] Both oral and intravenous regimes have been found to be effective. In light of the low risk of proarrhythmia, and relative safety, it is the antiarrhythmic drug (AAD) most frequently used for POAF prophylaxis. However, the additional benefit of amiodarone over β-blockade alone is yet to be established. The 2006 AHA/ACC guidelines recommend preoperative administration of amiodarone in high-risk patients undergoing cardiac surgery (class IIa).[70]

Sotalol

Sotalol, a class III AAD with additional β-blocking activity, has been found to decrease the incidence of POAF compared with placebo.[51,79,80] Data comparing it with conventional β-blockers are currently lacking. Sotalol is effective when started 24 to 48 hours before surgery or within 4 hours after surgery.[79,81] Prophylactic administration of sotalol has a IIb recommendation for high-risk patients undergoing cardiac surgery in the 2006 AHA/ACC guidelines.[70]

Ibutilide and dofetilide

The class III agents ibutilide and dofetilide have been reported to convert 40% to 44% of patients when administered intravenously.[82–84] However, only the oral formulation of dofetilide is available in the United States, the efficacy of which has not been studied in this setting. In addition, dofetilide carries a significant risk of torsades de pointes (0.3%–10.5%) even with careful in-hospital monitoring and requires dose adjustments in patients with renal insufficiency.[85]

Class I AADs

Data are inconclusive regarding the use of class I AADs in surgical patients. Some studies demonstrate efficacy of intravenous administration in converting post-CABG AF.[83,86] Data regarding the prophylactic use of procainamide (class IA)[87,88] and propafenone (class IC)[89] have not shown any significant benefit. Additionally, the proarrhythmic risk of class IC AADs in patients with coronary artery disease precludes their use in this population.

Calcium Channel Blockers and Digoxin

Calcium channel blockers and digoxin have not been shown to prevent the onset of POAF.[15,68,90] Their use in this setting is currently limited to controlling ventricular rates in patients with AF, in whom a rate-control strategy is deemed appropriate.

Magnesium

Magnesium supplementation has demonstrated benefit in mitigating the risk of POAF in some[91,92] but not all studies.[93] In a meta-analysis of 2988 participants, magnesium demonstrated a significant reduction in AF in the treatment group (16.5%) compared with the control group (26.2%; OR, 0.55; 95% CI, 0.41–0.73; $I^2 = 51\%$).[69] In light of the low cost and safety of administration, most would favor the repletion of magnesium before surgery.

Miscellaneous Agents

Considering the inflammatory component of POAF, there has been some interest in the use of medications with anti-inflammatory and antioxidant effects. Statins, angiotensin-converting enzyme inhibitors, acetylcysteine, and glucocorticoids have shown promise[38–41,94,95]; however, data are currently insufficient to recommend regular use of these agents. Further work in this area will likely help identify the specific roles of these drugs in patients undergoing surgery.

NONPHARMACOLOGIC STRATEGIES
Prophylactic Atrial Pacing

Dispersion of atrial refractoriness and atrial premature beats are known to facilitate the onset of AF after cardiac surgery.[60] Suppressing these triggers forms the basis for using overdrive atrial pacing in preventing the onset of POAF. Numerous algorithms for atrial pacing have been studied, including left atrial, right atrial, biatrial, and Bachman bundle pacing protocols.[96–100] Although single-site left atrial pacing alone has failed to

The European Society of Cardiothoracic Surgery 2006 guidelines also recommend β-blockers as the first choice in all patients undergoing cardiac surgery, unless otherwise contraindicated.[71] Future investigation will help delineate preferred agents, optimal dosage, and routes of administration.

show any significant benefit,[96,100] the results with right atrial and biatrial pacing have been more promising, with studies observing a benefit in reducing the incidence of POAF and hospital stay.[98–101] In addition, a meta-analysis of 2933 participants by Arsenault and colleagues[69] demonstrated a reduction in the incidence of POAF from 32.8% in the control group to 18.7% in the group receiving atrial pacing, a difference that was statistically significant (OR, 0.47; 95% CI, 0.36–0.61; I^2 = 50%). Although these results are encouraging, conflicting reports are also to be found with some studies reporting either no benefit,[102] or indeed an increase in atrial ectopy with pacing.[103] The 2005 American College of Chest Physicians guidelines currently recommend biatrial pacing to help prevent AF after surgery in high-risk patients.[104]

Electrical Cardioversion

The 2006 ACC/AHA guidelines recommend (class IIa) direct-current cardioversion in patients with POAF based on similar indications as nonsurgical patients.[70] Persistent symptoms, hemodynamic instability, and failure of pharmacologic measures comprise the major clinical scenarios in which electrical cardioversion may be considered. In postsurgical patients, cardioversion may be done either externally (transthoracic) or internally, with low-energy, using transvenous electrodes or epicardial wires placed during surgery.

Posterior Pericardiotomy

Posterior pericardiotomy is an intraoperative procedure where a longitudinal incision is made in the posterior pericardium parallel to the left phrenic nerve. The incision usually extends from the left inferior pulmonary vein to the diaphragm.[105] Several studies have demonstrated a benefit of this procedure in preventing postoperative pericardial effusion, tamponade, and AF.[105–107] In a prospective, randomized study of 200 patients undergoing CABG, incidence of AF in the group that underwent pericardiotomy was 6%, compared with 34% in the group that did not undergo pericardiotomy (*P* = .0000007).[105]

Anterior Fat Pad Preservation

An anterior periaortic fat pad (AFP) containing parasympathetic ganglia in the aortopulmonary window has been described in humans. The AFP is usually excised during CABG to fully expose the aortic root. Considering the influence of sympathetic tone on POAF, there has been an interest in studying the effects of AFP preservation on AF after CABG. Despite some early promise,[108]

recent randomized trials have demonstrated no benefit of AFP preservation in decreasing the incidence of POAF.[109,110]

ANTICOAGULATION

Thromboembolic events represent one of the most catastrophic complications of AF. Without anticoagulation the annual stroke risk is estimated to be between 1.9% and 18.2% depending on comorbidities.[111] Consequently, stroke prophylaxis is an aspect of AF management that has been the focus of much attention in recent years. Data related to stroke prophylaxis in postsurgical patients, however, are significantly lacking, and management is often guided by evidence from nonsurgical patients.

Cardiac surgery and cardiopulmonary bypass alter multiple coagulation factors, and enhance the tendency to bleed.[112] While deciding on the optimal anticoagulation strategy, the risk of bleeding in these patients must be weighed against the potential benefit derived from decreasing the stroke risk, and the usually self-limited nature of POAF. The CHADS$_2$[113] and HAS-BLED[114] scores are often used for this purpose; however, their validity in postsurgical patients has not been established.

In patients at low risk for stroke, therapy with aspirin may be adequate.[115] Trials done with warfarin in the immediate post-CABG period for maintenance of graft patency demonstrated only a slightly increased risk of overt bleeding, but a higher incidence of large pericardial effusions and tamponade, compared with patients on aspirin and placebo.[116,117] The ACC/AHA/European Society of Cardiology guidelines recommend anticoagulation with warfarin with a target international normalized ratio (INR) of 2.0 to 3.0 if AF persists for longer than 48 hours, as in nonsurgical patients.[70] There are no data relating to the use of heparin as bridging therapy in this population. The current consensus is that although routine use of heparin for this purpose is generally inadvisable, in patients with high-risk features (age >75 years, hypertension, prior stroke or transient ischemic attack, left ventricular dysfunction) it may be considered after evaluating the individual hemorrhagic risk.[70,115]

The optimal duration for which anticoagulation must be continued after cessation of POAF is also controversial. Impaired atrial contraction and the risk of thrombosis are known to persist for weeks after AF ceases, especially in longstanding AF. In this context, the 2005 American College of Chest Physicians guidelines recommend continuing anticoagulation for 30 days after return to normal rhythm.[115]

RECURRENCE

POAF is a transient, self-limited condition with persistence until discharge being rare. If AF does recur it may be treated as in nonsurgical patients.[95] If the arrhythmia is well tolerated, a rate-control strategy with anticoagulation may be used, with elective cardioversion at 4 to 6 weeks.[118] For patients who are not candidates for rate control, rhythm control by chemical or electrical means may be undertaken.[119] In patients where AF has persisted for longer than 48 hours, or where the time of onset of AF is unclear, it may be prudent to obtain a transesophageal echocardiogram to rule out an atrial thrombus before attempted cardioversion.

SUMMARY

AF is often encountered after cardiac and noncardiac surgical procedures. It is associated with an increased hospital stay and stroke risk, and a reduced in-hospital and long-term survival.[10] Understanding the underlying pathophysiology of POAF remains elusive; however, numerous risk factors predisposing to its development have been identified, including advanced age, structural damage to the heart, left ventricular dysfunction, hypertension, and valve surgery. Further investigation into the mechanisms underlying POAF, and the effects of various therapeutic modalities, will enable a better understanding of this phenomenon. Risk stratification, and targeted interventions for high-risk patients, may hold the key to mitigating the morbidity and financial burden associated with this arrhythmia.

REFERENCES

1. Tamis JE, Steinberg JS. Atrial fibrillation independently prolongs hospital stay after coronary artery bypass surgery. Clin Cardiol 2000;23(3):155–9.
2. Steinberg JS. Postoperative atrial fibrillation: a billion-dollar problem. J Am Coll Cardiol 2004; 43(6):1001–3.
3. Villareal RP, Hariharan R, Liu BC, et al. Postoperative atrial fibrillation and mortality after coronary artery bypass surgery. J Am Coll Cardiol 2004;43(5): 742–8.
4. Lahtinen J, Biancari F, Salmela E, et al. Postoperative atrial fibrillation is a major cause of stroke after on-pump coronary artery bypass surgery. Ann Thorac Surg 2004;77(4):1241–4.
5. Creswell LL, Schuessler RB, Rosenbloom M, et al. Hazards of postoperative atrial arrhythmias. Ann Thorac Surg 1993;56(3):539–49.
6. Aranki SF, Shaw DP, Adams DH, et al. Predictors of atrial fibrillation after coronary artery surgery. Current trends and impact on hospital resources. Circulation 1996;94(3):390–7.
7. Almassi GH, Schowalter T, Nicolosi AC, et al. Atrial fibrillation after cardiac surgery: a major morbid event? Ann Surg 1997;226(4):501–11 [discussion: 511–3].
8. Mathew JP, Fontes ML, Tudor IC, et al. A multicenter risk index for atrial fibrillation after cardiac surgery. JAMA 2004;291(14):1720–9.
9. Banach M, Rysz J, Drozdz JA, et al. Risk factors of atrial fibrillation following coronary artery bypass grafting: a preliminary report. Circ J 2006;70(4): 438–41.
10. Mariscalco G, Engström KG. Postoperative atrial fibrillation is associated with late mortality after coronary surgery, but not after valvular surgery. Ann Thorac Surg 2009;88(6):1871–6.
11. Ahlsson A, Fengsrud E, Bodin L, et al. Postoperative atrial fibrillation in patients undergoing aortocoronary bypass surgery carries an eightfold risk of future atrial fibrillation and a doubled cardiovascular mortality. Eur J Cardiothorac Surg 2010;37(6): 1353–9.
12. Amar D, Roistacher N, Burt M, et al. Clinical and echocardiographic correlates of symptomatic tachydysrhythmias after noncardiac thoracic surgery. Chest 1995;108(2):349–54.
13. Brathwaite D, Weissman C. The new onset of atrial arrhythmias following major noncardiothoracic surgery is associated with increased mortality. Chest 1998;114(2):462–8.
14. Maesen B, Nijs J, Maessen J, et al. Post-operative atrial fibrillation: a maze of mechanisms. Europace 2012;14(2):159–74.
15. Andrews TC, Reimold SC, Berlin JA, et al. Prevention of supraventricular arrhythmias after coronary artery bypass surgery. A meta-analysis of randomized control trials. Circulation 1991;84(Suppl 5): III236–44.
16. Frost L, Mølgaard H, Christiansen EH, et al. Atrial fibrillation and flutter after coronary artery bypass surgery: epidemiology, risk factors and preventive trials. Int J Cardiol 1992;36(3):253–61.
17. Maisel WH, Rawn JD, Stevenson WG. Atrial fibrillation after cardiac surgery. Ann Intern Med 2001; 135(12):1061–73.
18. Auer J, Weber T, Berent R, et al. Risk factors of postoperative atrial fibrillation after cardiac surgery. J Card Surg 2005;20(5):425–31.
19. Leitch JW, Thomson D, Baird DK, et al. The importance of age as a predictor of atrial fibrillation and flutter after coronary artery bypass grafting. J Thorac Cardiovasc Surg 1990;100(3):338–42.
20. Walsh SR, Oates JE, Anderson JA, et al. Postoperative arrhythmias in colorectal surgical patients: incidence and clinical correlates. Colorectal Dis 2006;8(3):212–6.

21. Batra GS, Molyneux J, Scott NA. Colorectal patients and cardiac arrhythmias detected on the surgical high dependency unit. Ann R Coll Surg Engl 2001;83(3):174–6.

22. Christians KK, Wu B, Quebbeman EJ, et al. Postoperative atrial fibrillation in noncardiothoracic surgical patients. Am J Surg 2001;182(6):713–5.

23. Lo B, Fijnheer R, Nierich AP, et al. C-reactive protein is a risk indicator for atrial fibrillation after myocardial revascularization. Ann Thorac Surg 2005;79(5):1530–5.

24. Reed GL III, Singer DE, Picard EH, et al. Stroke following coronary-artery bypass surgery. A case-control estimate of the risk from carotid bruits. N Engl J Med 1988;319(19):1246–50.

25. Hogue CW Jr, Creswell LL, Gutterman DD, et al, American College of Chest Physicians. Epidemiology, mechanisms, and risks: American College of Chest Physicians guidelines for the prevention and management of postoperative atrial fibrillation after cardiac surgery. Chest 2005;128(Suppl 2): 9S–16S.

26. Cox JL. A perspective of postoperative atrial fibrillation in cardiac operations. Ann Thorac Surg 1993; 56(3):405–9.

27. Crosby LH, Pifalo WB, Woll KR, et al. Risk factors for atrial fibrillation after coronary artery bypass grafting. Am J Cardiol 1990;66(20):1520–2.

28. Fuller JA, Adams GG, Buxton B. Atrial fibrillation after coronary artery bypass grafting. Is it a disorder of the elderly? J Thorac Cardiovasc Surg 1989; 97(6):821–5.

29. Tchervenkov CI, Wynands JE, Symes JF, et al. Persistent atrial activity during cardioplegic arrest: a possible factor in the etiology of postoperative supraventricular tachyarrhythmias. Ann Thorac Surg 1983;36(4):437–43.

30. Smith PK, Buhrman WC, Levett JM, et al. Supraventricular conduction abnormalities following cardiac operations. A complication of inadequate atrial preservation. J Thorac Cardiovasc Surg 1983;85(1):105–15.

31. Caretta Q, Mercanti CA, De Nardo D, et al. Ventricular conduction defects and atrial fibrillation after coronary artery bypass grafting. Multivariate analysis of preoperative, intraoperative and postoperative variables. Eur Heart J 1991;12(10):1107–11.

32. Hashimoto K, Ilstrup DM, Schaff HV. Influence of clinical and hemodynamic variables on risk of supraventricular tachycardia after coronary artery bypass. J Thorac Cardiovasc Surg 1991;101(1):56–65.

33. Bruins P, te Velthuis H, Yazdanbakhsh AP, et al. Activation of the complement system during and after cardiopulmonary bypass surgery: postsurgery activation involves C-reactive protein and is associated with postoperative arrhythmia. Circulation 1997;96(10):3542–8.

34. Gaudino M, Andreotti F, Zamparelli R, et al. The -174G/C interleukin-6 polymorphism influences postoperative interleukin-6 levels and postoperative atrial fibrillation. Is atrial fibrillation an inflammatory complication? Circulation 2003;108(Suppl 1): II195–9.

35. Chung MK, Martin DO, Sprecher D, et al. C-reactive protein elevation in patients with atrial arrhythmias: inflammatory mechanisms and persistence of atrial fibrillation. Circulation 2001;104(24): 2886–91.

36. Aviles RJ, Martin DO, Apperson-Hansen C, et al. Inflammation as a risk factor for atrial fibrillation. Circulation 2003;108(24):3006–10.

37. Anselmi A, Possati G, Gaudino M. Postoperative inflammatory reaction and atrial fibrillation: simple correlation or causation? Ann Thorac Surg 2009; 88(1):326–33.

38. Amar D, Zhang H, Heerdt PM, et al. Statin use is associated with a reduction in atrial fibrillation after noncardiac thoracic surgery independent of C-reactive protein. Chest 2005;128(5):3421–7.

39. Kumagai K, Nakashima H, Saku K. The HMG-CoA reductase inhibitor atorvastatin prevents atrial fibrillation by inhibiting inflammation in a canine sterile pericarditis model. Cardiovasc Res 2004;62(1): 105–11.

40. Ho KM, Tan JA. Benefits and risks of corticosteroid prophylaxis in adult cardiac surgery: a dose-response meta-analysis. Circulation 2009;119(14): 1853–66.

41. Bourbon A, Vionnet M, Leprince P, et al. The effect of methylprednisolone treatment on the cardiopulmonary bypass-induced systemic inflammatory response. Eur J Cardiothorac Surg 2004;26(5): 932–8.

42. Kalman JM, Munawar M, Howes LG, et al. Atrial fibrillation after coronary artery bypass grafting is associated with sympathetic activation. Ann Thorac Surg 1995;60(6):1709–15.

43. Hoeldtke RD, Cilmi KM. Effects of aging on catecholamine metabolism. J Clin Endocrinol Metab 1985;60(3):479–84.

44. Dimmer C, Tavernier R, Gjorgov N, et al. Variations of autonomic tone preceding onset of atrial fibrillation after coronary artery bypass grafting. Am J Cardiol 1998;82(1):22–5.

45. Amar D, Zhang H, Miodownik S, et al. Competing autonomic mechanisms precede the onset of postoperative atrial fibrillation. J Am Coll Cardiol 2003; 42(7):1262–8.

46. Lamb RK, Prabhakar G, Thorpe JA, et al. The use of atenolol in the prevention of supraventricular arrhythmias following coronary artery surgery. Eur Heart J 1988;9(1):32–6.

47. White HD, Antman EM, Glynn MA, et al. Efficacy and safety of timolol for prevention of

supraventricular tachyarrhythmias after coronary artery bypass surgery. Circulation 1984;70(3): 479–84.

48. Ali IM, Sanalla AA, Clark V. Beta-blocker effects on postoperative atrial fibrillation. Eur J Cardiothorac Surg 1997;11(6):1154–7.

49. Nazeri A, Razavi M, Elayda MA, et al. Race/ethnicity and the incidence of new-onset atrial fibrillation after isolated coronary artery bypass surgery. Heart Rhythm 2010;7(10):1458–63.

50. Lauer MS, Eagle KA, Buckley MJ, et al. Atrial fibrillation following coronary artery bypass surgery. Prog Cardiovasc Dis 1989;31(5):367–78.

51. Weber UK, Osswald S, Huber M, et al. Selective versus non-selective antiarrhythmic approach for prevention of atrial fibrillation after coronary surgery: is there a need for pre-operative risk stratification? A prospective placebo-controlled study using low-dose sotalol. Eur Heart J 1998;19(5): 794–800.

52. Furberg CD, Psaty BM, Manolio TA, et al. Prevalence of atrial fibrillation in elderly subjects (the Cardiovascular Health Study). Am J Cardiol 1994; 74(3):236–41.

53. Vaporciyan AA, Correa AM, Rice DC, et al. Risk factors associated with atrial fibrillation after noncardiac thoracic surgery: analysis of 2588 patients. J Thorac Cardiovasc Surg 2004;127(3): 779–86.

54. Spach MS, Dolber PC. Relating extracellular potentials and their derivatives to anisotropic propagation at a microscopic level in human cardiac muscle. Evidence for electrical uncoupling of side-to-side fiber connections with increasing age. Circ Res 1986;58(3):356–71.

55. Mariscalco G, Engström KG, Ferrarese S, et al. Relationship between atrial histopathology and atrial fibrillation after coronary bypass surgery. J Thorac Cardiovasc Surg 2006;131(6):1364–72.

56. Kannel WB, Abbott RD, Savage DD, et al. Epidemiologic features of chronic atrial fibrillation: the Framingham Study. N Engl J Med 1982;306(17): 1018–22.

57. Zacharias A, Schwann TA, Riordan CJ, et al. Obesity and risk of new-onset atrial fibrillation after cardiac surgery. Circulation 2005;112(21): 3247–55.

58. Chua SK, Shyu KG, Lu MJ, et al. Clinical utility of CHADS2 and CHA2DS2-VASc scoring systems for predicting postoperative atrial fibrillation after cardiac surgery. J Thorac Cardiovasc Surg 2013; 146(4):919–26.e1.

59. Chandy J, Nakai T, Lee RJ, et al. Increases in P-wave dispersion predict postoperative atrial fibrillation after coronary artery bypass graft surgery. Anesth Analg 2004;98(2):303–10. table of contents.

60. Steinberg JS, Zelenkofske S, Wong SC, et al. Value of the P-wave signal-averaged ECG for predicting atrial fibrillation after cardiac surgery. Circulation 1993;88(6):2618–22.

61. Mathew JP, Parks R, Savino JS, et al. Atrial fibrillation following coronary artery bypass graft surgery: predictors, outcomes, and resource utilization. MultiCenter Study of Perioperative Ischemia Research Group. JAMA 1996;276(4):300–6.

62. Ducceschi V, D'Andrea A, Liccardo B, et al. Perioperative clinical predictors of atrial fibrillation occurrence following coronary artery surgery. Eur J Cardiothorac Surg 1999;16(4):435–9.

63. Cochrane AD, Siddins M, Rosenfeldt FL, et al. A comparison of amiodarone and digoxin for treatment of supraventricular arrhythmias after cardiac surgery. Eur J Cardiothorac Surg 1994;8(4):194–8.

64. Campbell TJ, Morgan JJ. Treatment of atrial arrhythmias after cardiac surgery with intravenous disopyramide. Aust N Z J Med 1980;10(6):644–9.

65. Soucier RJ, Mirza S, Abordo MG, et al. Predictors of conversion of atrial fibrillation after cardiac operation in the absence of class I or III antiarrhythmic medications. Ann Thorac Surg 2001;72(3):694–7 [discussion: 697–8].

66. Solomon AJ, Kouretas PC, Hopkins RA, et al. Early discharge of patients with new-onset atrial fibrillation after cardiovascular surgery. Am Heart J 1998;135(4):557–63.

67. Mendes LA, Connelly GP, McKenney PA, et al. Right coronary artery stenosis: an independent predictor of atrial fibrillation after coronary artery bypass surgery. J Am Coll Cardiol 1995;25(1): 198–202.

68. Rubin DA, Nieminski KE, Reed GE, et al. Predictors, prevention, and long-term prognosis of atrial fibrillation after coronary artery bypass graft operations. J Thorac Cardiovasc Surg 1987;94(3):331–5.

69. Arsenault KA, Yusuf AM, Crystal E, et al. Interventions for preventing post-operative atrial fibrillation in patients undergoing heart surgery. Cochrane Database Syst Rev 2013;(1):CD003611.

70. Fuster V, Rydén LE, Cannom DS, et al. ACC/AHA/ESC 2006 guidelines for the management of patients with atrial fibrillation: full text: a report of the American College of Cardiology/American Heart Association Task Force on practice guidelines and the European Society of Cardiology Committee for Practice Guidelines (Writing Committee to Revise the 2001 guidelines for the management of patients with atrial fibrillation) developed in collaboration with the European Heart Rhythm Association and the Heart Rhythm Society. Europace 2006;8(9):651–745.

71. Dunning J, Treasure T, Versteegh M, et al, EACTS Audit and Guidelines Committee. Guidelines on the prevention and management of de novo atrial

fibrillation after cardiac and thoracic surgery. Eur J Cardiothorac Surg 2006;30(6):852–72.

72. Akbarzadeh F, Kazemi-Arbat B, Golmohammadi A, et al. Biatrial pacing vs. intravenous amiodarone in prevention of atrial fibrillation after coronary artery bypass surgery. Pak J Biol Sci 2009;12(19):1325–9.

73. Aasbo JD, Lawrence AT, Krishnan K, et al. Amiodarone prophylaxis reduces major cardiovascular morbidity and length of stay after cardiac surgery: a meta-analysis. Ann Intern Med 2005;143(5):327–36.

74. Mitchell LB, Exner DV, Wyse DG, et al. Prophylactic oral amiodarone for the prevention of arrhythmias that begin early after revascularization, valve replacement, or repair: PAPABEAR: a randomized controlled trial. JAMA 2005;294(24):3093–100.

75. Hohnloser SH, Meinertz T, Dammbacher T, et al. Electrocardiographic and antiarrhythmic effects of intravenous amiodarone: results of a prospective, placebo-controlled study. Am Heart J 1991; 121(1 Pt 1):89–95.

76. Butler J, Harriss DR, Sinclair M, et al. Amiodarone prophylaxis for tachycardias after coronary artery surgery: a randomised, double blind, placebo controlled trial. Br Heart J 1993;70(1):56–60.

77. Daoud EG, Strickberger SA, Man KC, et al. Preoperative amiodarone as prophylaxis against atrial fibrillation after heart surgery. N Engl J Med 1997; 337(25):1785–91.

78. Guarnieri T, Nolan S, Gottlieb SO, et al. Intravenous amiodarone for the prevention of atrial fibrillation after open heart surgery: the Amiodarone Reduction in Coronary Heart (ARCH) trial. J Am Coll Cardiol 1999;34(2):343–7.

79. Suttorp MJ, Kingma JH, Peels HO, et al. Effectiveness of sotalol in preventing supraventricular tachyarrhythmias shortly after coronary artery bypass grafting. Am J Cardiol 1991;68(11):1163–9.

80. Pfisterer ME, Klöter-Weber UC, Huber M, et al. Prevention of supraventricular tachyarrhythmias after open heart operation by low-dose sotalol: a prospective, double-blind, randomized, placebo-controlled study. Ann Thorac Surg 1997;64(4):1113–9.

81. Gomes JA, Ip J, Santoni-Rugiu F, et al. Oral d,l sotalol reduces the incidence of postoperative atrial fibrillation in coronary artery bypass surgery patients: a randomized, double-blind, placebo-controlled study. J Am Coll Cardiol 1999;34(2):334–9.

82. Serafimovski N, Burke P, Khawaja O, et al. Usefulness of dofetilide for the prevention of atrial tachyarrhythmias (atrial fibrillation or flutter) after coronary artery bypass grafting. Am J Cardiol 2008;101(11):1574–9.

83. Nichol G, McAlister F, Pham B, et al. Meta-analysis of randomised controlled trials of the effectiveness of antiarrhythmic agents at promoting sinus rhythm in patients with atrial fibrillation. Heart 2002;87(6): 535–43.

84. Frost L, Mortensen PE, Tingleff J, et al. Efficacy and safety of dofetilide, a new class III antiarrhythmic agent, in acute termination of atrial fibrillation or flutter after coronary artery bypass surgery. Dofetilide Post-CABG Study Group. Int J Cardiol 1997; 58(2):135–40.

85. Torp-Pedersen C, Møller M, Bloch-Thomsen PE, et al. Dofetilide in patients with congestive heart failure and left ventricular dysfunction. Danish Investigations of Arrhythmia and Mortality on Dofetilide Study Group. N Engl J Med 1999;341(12): 857–65.

86. Yilmaz AT, Demírkiliç U, Arslan M, et al. Long-term prevention of atrial fibrillation after coronary artery bypass surgery: comparison of quinidine, verapamil, and amiodarone in maintaining sinus rhythm. J Card Surg 1996;11(1):61–4.

87. Gold MR, O'Gara PT, Buckley MJ, et al. Efficacy and safety of procainamide in preventing arrhythmias after coronary artery bypass surgery. Am J Cardiol 1996;78(9):975–9.

88. Laub GW, Janeira L, Muralidharan S, et al. Prophylactic procainamide for prevention of atrial fibrillation after coronary artery bypass grafting: a prospective, double-blind, randomized, placebo-controlled pilot study. Crit Care Med 1993;21(10): 1474–8.

89. Merrick AF, Odom NJ, Keenan DJ, et al. Comparison of propafenone to atenolol for the prophylaxis of postcardiotomy supraventricular tachyarrhythmias: a prospective trial. Eur J Cardiothorac Surg 1995;9(3):146–9.

90. Smith EE, Shore DF, Monro JL, et al. Oral verapamil fails to prevent supraventricular tachycardia following coronary artery surgery. Int J Cardiol 1985;9(1):37–44.

91. Fanning WJ, Thomas CS Jr, Roach A, et al. Prophylaxis of atrial fibrillation with magnesium sulfate after coronary artery bypass grafting. Ann Thorac Surg 1991;52(3):529–33.

92. Wistbacka JO, Koistinen J, Karlqvist KE, et al. Magnesium substitution in elective coronary artery surgery: a double-blind clinical study. J Cardiothorac Vasc Anesth 1995;9(2):140–6.

93. Zangrillo A, Landoni G, Sparicio D, et al. Perioperative magnesium supplementation to prevent atrial fibrillation after off-pump coronary artery surgery: a randomized controlled study. J Cardiothorac Vasc Anesth 2005;19(6):723–8.

94. Ozaydin M, Peker O, Erdogan D, et al. N-acetylcysteine for the prevention of postoperative atrial fibrillation: a prospective, randomized, placebo-controlled pilot study. Eur Heart J 2008;29(5):625–31.

95. Peretto G, Durante A, Limite LR, et al. Postoperative arrhythmias after cardiac surgery: incidence, risk factors, and therapeutic management. Cardiol Res Pract 2014;2014:615987.

96. Fan K, Lee KL, Chiu CS, et al. Effects of biatrial pacing in prevention of postoperative atrial fibrillation after coronary artery bypass surgery. Circulation 2000;102(7):755–60.

97. Daoud EG, Dabir R, Archambeau M, et al. Randomized, double-blind trial of simultaneous right and left atrial epicardial pacing for prevention of post-open heart surgery atrial fibrillation. Circulation 2000;102(7):761–5.

98. Levy T, Fotopoulos G, Walker S, et al. Randomized controlled study investigating the effect of biatrial pacing in prevention of atrial fibrillation after coronary artery bypass grafting. Circulation 2000; 102(12):1382–7.

99. Blommaert D, Gonzalez M, Mucumbitsi J, et al. Effective prevention of atrial fibrillation by continuous atrial overdrive pacing after coronary artery bypass surgery. J Am Coll Cardiol 2000;35(6): 1411–5.

100. Greenberg MD, Katz NM, Iuliano S, et al. Atrial pacing for the prevention of atrial fibrillation after cardiovascular surgery. J Am Coll Cardiol 2000; 35(6):1416–22.

101. Gerstenfeld EP, Khoo M, Martin RC, et al. Effectiveness of bi-atrial pacing for reducing atrial fibrillation after coronary artery bypass graft surgery. J Interv Card Electrophysiol 2001;5(3):275–83.

102. Gerstenfeld EP, Hill MR, French SN, et al. Evaluation of right atrial and biatrial temporary pacing for the prevention of atrial fibrillation after coronary artery bypass surgery. J Am Coll Cardiol 1999; 33(7):1981–8.

103. Chung MK, Augostini RS, Asher CR, et al. Ineffectiveness and potential proarrhythmia of atrial pacing for atrial fibrillation prevention after coronary artery bypass grafting. Ann Thorac Surg 2000; 69(4):1057–63.

104. Maisel WH, Epstein AE, American College of Chest Physicians. The role of cardiac pacing: American College of Chest Physicians guidelines for the prevention and management of postoperative atrial fibrillation after cardiac surgery. Chest 2005; 128(Suppl 2):36S–8S.

105. Kuralay E, Ozal E, Demirkili U, et al. Effect of posterior pericardiotomy on postoperative supraventricular arrhythmias and late pericardial effusion (posterior pericardiotomy). J Thorac Cardiovasc Surg 1999;118(3):492–5.

106. Kaygin MA, Dag O, Güneş M, et al. Posterior pericardiotomy reduces the incidence of atrial fibrillation, pericardial effusion, and length of stay in hospital after coronary artery bypasses surgery. Tohoku J Exp Med 2011;225(2):103–8.

107. Cakalagaoglu C, Koksal C, Baysal A, et al. The use of posterior pericardiotomy technique to prevent postoperative pericardial effusion in cardiac surgery. Heart Surg Forum 2012;15(2):E84–9.

108. Cummings JE, Gill I, Akhrass R, et al. Preservation of the anterior fat pad paradoxically decreases the incidence of postoperative atrial fibrillation in humans. J Am Coll Cardiol 2004;43(6):994–1000.

109. White CM, Sander S, Coleman CI, et al. Impact of epicardial anterior fat pad retention on postcardiothoracic surgery atrial fibrillation incidence: the AFIST-III Study. J Am Coll Cardiol 2007;49(3): 298–303.

110. Kazemi B, Ahmadzadeh A, Safaei N, et al. Influence of anterior periaortic fat pad excision on incidence of postoperative atrial fibrillation. Eur J Cardiothorac Surg 2011;40(5):1191–6.

111. Gage BF, Waterman AD, Shannon W, et al. Validation of clinical classification schemes for predicting stroke: results from the National Registry of Atrial Fibrillation. JAMA 2001;285(22):2864–70.

112. McKeown P, Epstein AE, American College of Chest Physicians. Future directions: American College of Chest Physicians guidelines for the prevention and management of postoperative atrial fibrillation after cardiac surgery. Chest 2005; 128(Suppl 2):61S–4S.

113. Lip GY, Nieuwlaat R, Pisters R, et al. Refining clinical risk stratification for predicting stroke and thromboembolism in atrial fibrillation using a novel risk factor-based approach: the euro heart survey on atrial fibrillation. Chest 2010;137(2):263–72.

114. Pisters R, Lane DA, Nieuwlaat R, et al. A novel user-friendly score (HAS-BLED) to assess 1-year risk of major bleeding in patients with atrial fibrillation: the Euro Heart Survey. Chest 2010;138(5):1093–100.

115. Epstein AE, Alexander JC, Gutterman DD, et al. Anticoagulation: American College of Chest Physicians guidelines for the prevention and management of postoperative atrial fibrillation after cardiac surgery. Chest 2005;128(Suppl 2):24S–7S.

116. Weber MA, Hasford J, Taillens C, et al. Low-dose aspirin versus anticoagulants for prevention of coronary graft occlusion. Am J Cardiol 1990;66(20): 1464–8.

117. Malouf JF, Alam S, Gharzeddine W, et al. The role of anticoagulation in the development of pericardial effusion and late tamponade after cardiac surgery. Eur Heart J 1993;14(11):1451–7.

118. Martinez EA, Epstein AE, Bass EB, American College of Chest Physicians. Pharmacologic control of ventricular rate: American College of Chest Physicians guidelines for the prevention and management of postoperative atrial fibrillation after cardiac surgery. Chest 2005;128(Suppl 2):56S–60S.

119. Martinez EA, Bass EB, Zimetbaum P, American College of Chest Physicians. Pharmacologic control of rhythm: American College of Chest Physicians guidelines for the prevention and management of postoperative atrial fibrillation after cardiac surgery. Chest 2005;128(Suppl 2):48S–55S.

Novel Upstream Approaches to Prevent Atrial Fibrillation Perpetuation

José Jalife, MD

KEYWORDS

- Atrial fibrillation • Myofibroblast • Fibrosis • Myocytes

KEY POINTS

- The mechanisms underlying atrial fibrillation (AF) in humans are poorly understood. In particular, it is unknown how sustained high-frequency excitation leads to electrical remodeling and fibrosis of the atria and results in AF perpetuation.
- Sustained high-frequency atrial excitation results in intracellular accumulation of reactive oxygen species, also known as "oxidative stress", which likely plays important roles in the pathogenesis of AF, triggering both electrical and structural remodeling.
- Inflammation is known to play an important pathogenic role leading to cardiac fibrosis in several cardiovascular diseases, including AF; activated inflammatory cells, such as polymorphonucleated neutrophils, lymphocytes, monocytes, resident macrophages, and activated platelets are all important players in this picture.
- The role of the renin-angiotensin-aldosterone system (RAAS) in AF is a new area of investigation. Both structural and electrical remodeling produced by sustained AF may share common pathways in which the main fibrogenic cell type in the heart, the myofibroblast, plays a central role through its activation by RAAS.
- Through its effects promoting gene transcription via cytokine-mediated signaling pathways, galectin-3 might represent a common upstream link for both structural and electrical remodeling and a mediator in the transition to persistent AF.

THE EPIDEMIC OF ATRIAL FIBRILLATION

Atrial fibrillation (AF) is the most common sustained arrhythmia seen by physicians in their practice. It affects about 1.5% of the population in the developed world.[1] In the United States and Europe, overall prevalence of AF is 0.9%. These numbers are projected to grow dramatically and to more than double over the next 2 decades as the elderly proportion of the population increases.[2–4] Thus, in the Western world AF has already reached epidemic proportions.

AF is a major cause of hospitalization and is associated with an increased risk of stroke, heart failure, dementia, and death.[5–7] Yet despite its epidemiologic importance and more than 100 years of basic and clinical research, physicians still do not fully understand its fundamental mechanisms and have not learned how to treat it effectively. When AF lasts continuously for more than 7 days it is designated as persistent AF; shorted episodes are termed paroxysmal.[8] Spontaneous, pharmacologic or ablative resumption of sinus rhythm is infrequent in persistent AF, with prompt recurrences or commonly failed cardioversions. Episodes lasting for more than 1 year are termed "long-term persistent AF". Many drugs have been tried in persistent AF and permanent AF with very limited success. On the other hand, the demonstration of AF triggers in the atrial sleeves

This article originally appeared in Cardiology Clinics, Volume 32, Issue 4, November 2014.
Center for Arrhythmia Research, Cardiovascular Research Center, University of Michigan, 2800 Plymouth Road, Ann Arbor, MI 48109, USA
E-mail address: jjalife@umich.edu

of the pulmonary veins[9] (PVs) has led to a significant improvement in therapy, and today PV isolation using radiofrequency (RF) ablation is curative in about ~70% to 80% of patients with paroxysmal AF.[10] However, the success rate of RF ablation in the more prevalent and highly heterogeneous persistent and long-term persistent AF population has been inadequate. Arguably only a profound and complete understanding of the mechanisms involved in the maintenance and perpetuation of AF will allow us to generate more specific prevention and/or treatment of this dangerous and debilitating disease.

Persistent AF leads to electrical remodeling and fibrosis of the atria but the mechanism remains poorly understood. The objective of this article is to address the most important factors involved in the mechanism of AF stabilization in the long term, paying particular attention to possible molecular mechanisms leading to both structural remodeling in the form of fibrosis and electrical remodeling secondary to ion channel expression changes, which might contribute to persistent AF. Although excellent reviews have appeared on the subject on AF-related atrial remodeling,[11–13] the tantalizing possibility that both fibrosis and electrical remodeling might in fact be prevented when intervening early enough before the remodeling process reaches a point of no return has seldom been addressed. The idea is based on the repeated demonstration in the literature that during sustained AF the renin-angiotensin-aldosterone (RAAS) system activates common signaling pathways involving galectin-3 (Gal-3), transforming growth factor β1 (TGF-β1), and platelet-derived growth factor (PDGF) that contribute to structural and electrophysiologic remodeling leading to AF stabilization and perpetuation. In this regard, it seems reasonable to postulate that the early use of such agents as mineralocorticoid blockers or Gal-3 inhibitors in hypertensive patients who are at risk of developing AF, or in patients showing the initial symptoms of paroxysmal AF, may be efficacious in preventing sustained AF and adverse cardiac remodeling.

A NEW ANIMAL MODEL OF PERSISTENT AF

Multiple profibrotic conditions, including heart failure, hypertension, a history of myocardial infarction, diabetes mellitus, or obesity, predispose to AF.[14] In addition, AF itself somehow leads to electrical remodeling and fibrosis of the atria but the mechanism remains poorly understood. Atrial electrical remodeling and functional changes in subcellular atrial myocyte function in the short term lead to abbreviation of atrial action potential duration (APD) and refractory period,[15–17] which would help to promote the stabilization of reentry. However, whether and how these changes contribute to AF perpetuation in the long term has not been fully determined. In humans, chronic AF decreases the L-type calcium current in atrial myocytes.[18] In addition, chronic AF increases the inward rectifier potassium current,[19] but decreases the transient outward current and the ultrarapid component of the delayed rectifier current differentially on each atria and increases the slow component of the delayed rectifier current in both.[20] However, the time course of these changes mentioned earlier has not been established. In a recent study in a sheep model of persistent AF induced by intermittent atrial tachypacing, there was a progressive spontaneous increase in the dominant frequency (DF) of AF activation during a 2-week period after the first detected AF episode (**Fig. 1**).[21] The results suggested that, unlike the tachypacing-induced electrical remodeling that can occur over minutes or hours,[15] there existed a protracted, slowly progressing electrical remodeling, which occurred secondary to an AF that sustained for days or weeks.[21] In addition, a consistent left versus right atrial DF difference lasting greater than 22 weeks in most animals (see **Fig. 1**) correlated with the presence of rotors, DF gradients, and outward propagation from the posterior left atrium (PLA) during sustained AF in the explanted, Langendorff-perfused sheep hearts.[21] Similar to other animal models, long-term atrial tachypacing in the sheep resulted in atrial fibrosis,[22] with concomitant release of cytokines that are known to modify atrial electrical function.[23] Also in the sheep model, atrial structural changes leading to PLA enlargement and stretch likely made rotors less likely to drift or to collide with anatomic boundaries, thus contributing to their stabilization and AF persistence.[21,24]

The changes in DF discussed earlier reflect a progressive decrease in the atrial APD, refractory period, and purported stabilization of rotor activity over a 22-day period. They also reflect long-term tachycardia-induced reduction in the gene expression, protein levels, and transmembrane currents of the inward sodium and L-type calcium channels, but increase the expression and transmembrane currents of the inward rectifier potassium current.[25] In addition, there were concomitant increases in serum markers of fibrosis as well as atrial tissue collagen gene transcription and fiber deposition. Moreover, although structural and electrical remodeling are both thought to promote AF persistence, it is unknown whether it is the high-frequency excitation itself that provides the insult that results in the molecular changes

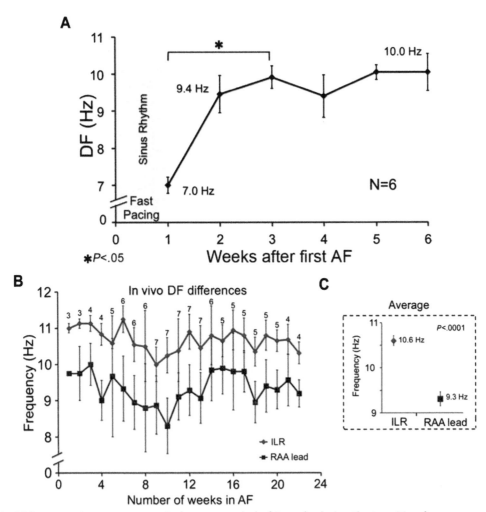

Fig. 1. AF frequency increases progressively over a period of 6 weeks during the transition from paroxysmal to persistent AF. (*A*) DF values from the implantable loop recorder traces show an increase in DF during a 2-week period after the first tachypacing-induced AF episode. (*B, C*) DF values obtained from the left atrium (*red symbols*) are significantly higher than those obtained from the right atrial appendage. Twenty-two weeks of follow-up are shown. (*Adapted from* Filgueiras-Rama D, Price NF, Martins RP, et al. Long-term frequency gradients during persistent atrial fibrillation in sheep are associated with stable sources in the left atrium. Circ Arrhythm Electrophysiol 2012;5:1160–7; with permission.)

leading to rotor stabilization or whether it is the atrial dilatation, the inflammatory response, or the oxidative stress that has been associated with AF. Arguably, activated myofibroblasts are likely to be important cellular effectors in atrial fibrosis, although monocytes/macrophages and other cell types may also contribute to the fibrotic response and even to the eventual remodeling of the atrial myocytes. As shown in **Fig. 2** and discussed later in this article, reactive oxygen species (ROS), inflammatory cytokines, chemokines, the RAAS, and growth factors such as TGF-β1 and PDGF are some of the best-studied mediators implicated in cardiac fibrosis and electrical remodeling.[23,26,27]

SUSTAINED HIGH-FREQUENCY ATRIAL EXCITATION RESULTS IN OXIDATIVE STRESS

Strong evidence continues to accumulate suggesting that intracellular accumulation of ROS, also known as "oxidative stress", likely plays important roles in the pathogenesis of AF (see **Fig. 2**).[11,28,29] Although there is increasing evidence for a physiologic ROS regulation of cardiac Na^+ and Ca^{2+} handling in healthy cardiac myocytes, ROS are known to be generated in increased amounts in failing hearts,[11] as well as the fibrillating atria. Moreover, they appear to be causally linked to the impairment in Ca^{2+} and Na^+ handling in diseased myocytes.[30] The most relevant intracellular sources

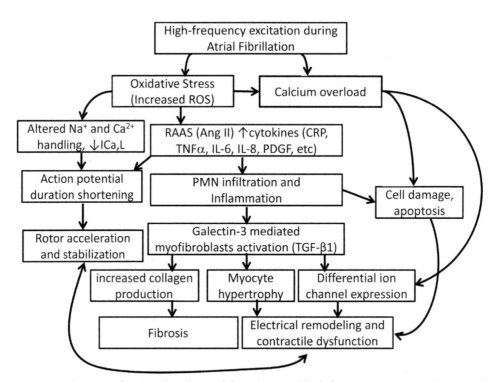

Fig. 2. Hypothetical scenario for AF-induced remodeling. Sustained high-frequency excitation during AF leads to the activation of multiple signaling pathways leading to structural and electrical remodeling with consequent rotor stabilization. Increased reactive oxygen species (ROS) alters Na^+ and Ca^{2+} handling leading to $[Ca^{2+}]_i$ overload and reduction of L-type Ca^{2+} current (I_{CaL}); this shortens the action potential duration and refractory period with consequent acceleration and stabilization of AF sources (rotors). Continuation of AF and elevated ROS also activates the RAAS leading to release of multiple proinflammatory cytokines, which results in inflammatory infiltration of the atrial tissue. Polymorphonucleated macrophages release profibrotic proteins like Gal-3 and activate the myofibroblasts to secrete cytokines TGF-β1 and PDGF, which together with calcium overload increase collagen production, produce myocyte hypertrophy, and lead to differential transcriptional changes in ion channel expression. The resulting fibrosis, contractile dysfunction, and electrical remodeling contribute to rotor stabilization and AF perpetuation.

of elevated ROS in the cardiac myocyte include a gp91-containing nicotinamide adenine dinucleotide phosphate (NADPH) oxidase (NOX2), xanthine oxidoreductase, uncoupled nitric oxide synthase, and the electron transport chain in the mitochondria. However, the molecular mechanisms responsible for increased ROS production in AF including the enzymatic sources and their regulation and the downstream pathways as to how ion channel handling is altered to result in electrical remodeling have not been determined in any detail. The exceedingly high-frequency excitation of the atria that prevails during AF is likely to result in dysfunctional intracellular Na^+ and Ca^{2+} handling in the atrial myocytes, which might be mediated by 2 kinds of redox-dependent modifications: (1) direct redox modifications of central Na^+- and Ca^{2+}-handling proteins such as oxidation of free sulfhydril groups in functionally relevant parts of these proteins; (2) ROS-dependent oxidation of kinases or phosphatases that are known to regulate the function of the

proteins mentioned earlier, including cyclic adenosine monophosphate–dependent protein kinase A, protein kinase C, and Ca/calmodulin-dependent protein kinase II, as well as on redox-regulated downstream targets such as Na^+ and Ca^{2+} transporters and channels.[30]

Increased levels of ROS in myocardial tissues[31–34] and markers of oxidative stress in blood samples have been found in patients with AF.[35] In addition, the occurrence of AF in the post-operative period has been independently associated with NOX2-dependent generation of ROS in right atrial samples in patients undergoing cardiac surgery.[36] Increased ROS levels damage proteins, lipids, and DNA and increase inflammation by promoting cytokine production from activated macrophages, which in turn further induces tissue damage.[28] Further, ROS are also involved in cardiac structural and electrical remodeling, all of which increase susceptibility to AF.

The notion that sustained AF promotes oxidative stress was derived in part from studies demonstrating that chronic human AF is associated with increased peroxynitrite formation.[37] Thereafter, long-term rapid atrial pacing experiments in dogs demonstrated pacing-induced shortening of the atrial effective refractory period, which was associated with decreased tissue ascorbate levels and increased protein nitration. The latter is a biomarker of peroxynitrite formation.[38] Oral ascorbate supplementation attenuated all changes. In a parallel study, supplemental ascorbate was given to 43 patients before and for 5 days after cardiac bypass graft surgery.[38] Patients receiving ascorbate had a 16.3% incidence of post-operative AF compared with 34.9% in control subjects. On the other hand, antioxidant treatment with Vitamin C or N-acetylcysteine has been shown to prevent post-operative AF.[38–40] Oral Vitamin C treatment was reported to reduce early recurrence and inflammation after electrical cardioversion of persistent AF.[41] However, although antioxidant treatment appears to have some preventive effects on post-operative AF, the overall clinical impact of antioxidant therapy in the treatment of long-term persistent AF remains to be determined. Further research is necessary to elucidate detailed ROS-dependent mechanisms involved in AF pathogenesis and to stimulate the development of novel therapeutic strategies for the prevention and treatment of AF.

ROLE OF INFLAMMATION

Inflammation is known to play an important pathogenic role leading to cardiac fibrosis in several cardiovascular diseases, including AF.[42] Cardiac inflammatory disorders such as myocarditis, pericarditis, and cardiac surgery frequently are accompanied by AF.[43] Inflammation has been shown to be involved both before the first occurrence[44] and in the risk of recurrence of AF.[45] In addition, inflammation plays an important role in post-operative AF as shown by intracardiac expression of specific markers.[42] Activated inflammatory cells, such as polymorphonucleated neutrophils, lymphocytes, monocytes, resident macrophages, and activated platelets, are all important players in this picture (see **Fig. 2**).

Substantial clinical and experimental evidence supports a role for C-reactive protein (CRP) as a strong and independent marker of risk of primary and secondary adverse cardiovascular events.[46] CRP has also been reported as a risk factor for recurrences of lone AF, and elevated CRP levels have been related to AF recurrences after successful cardioversion.[47] However, clinical data on the relationship of CRP levels and clinical presentation/duration of AF remain debated.[48–50]

Fig. 2 illustrates a hypothetical scenario linking inflammation produced by sustained high-frequency atrial excitation with subsequent fibrosis, electrical remodeling, and AF perpetuation. Whether spontaneous or pacing-induced, sustained AF would result in the release of proinflammatory cytokines and hormones, such as angiotensin II (Ang II), tumor necrosis factor α, interleukin (IL)-6, and IL-8, related to cardiovascular disease and tissue injury.[46] Injury promotes activation of leukocytes with subsequent release of inflammatory stimuli such as NADPH-oxidase–derived ROS, growth factors, and other hormones, as well as mechanical stretch. Multiple studies have demonstrated a role for NADPH oxidases in Ang II function. Although many downstream targets have been identified, the temporal sequence of events that lead to the proper activation and function of NADPH oxidase is not completely understood, and the compartmentalization of signaling remains to be fully investigated. In addition, more work is necessary to identify the precise molecular modifications of the putative signaling targets of ROS after Ang II stimulation. Understanding which NADPH oxidases are activated by Ang II in the atria, in normal physiology, and in development is also important and may help us to define better interventions aimed at preventing the profibrillatory effects of Ang II activation. These are well-known triggers of fibroblast differentiation into myofibroblasts, which are critical players in the development of fibrosis.[42] Inflammatory cascades also lead to ion channel dysfunction, which along with myocyte apoptosis and matrix generation and turnover, likely contributes to both electrical and structural remodeling and predisposes individuals to AF (see **Fig. 2**).[42]

Whether the antiinflammatory and antioxidant effects of statin therapy will benefit the patient with paroxysmal or persistent AF awaits demonstration in large clinical trials. As recently reviewed by Pinho-Gomes and colleagues,[11] studies in relatively small numbers of patients showed that statins can prevent post-operative AF. On the other hand, statins appear to be of little benefit in the primary prevention of AF, although the efficacy for secondary prevention might be significant when used early in patients at risk before significant remodeling has taken place, but not later when atrial fibrosis has already matured, or after ablation. To date, the antiarrhythmic effect of statins does not support them solely to prevent incident AF or its recurrence. Large-scale randomized clinical trials are necessary to better establish the benefit of statins for the management of AF in specific patients' subgroups, such as younger patients who are at risk but have not yet developed the arrhythmia or those in whom the arrhythmia has just become manifest.

THE RAAS AND ATRIAL FIBROSIS

The role of the RAAS is well established in many cardiovascular disorders, including hypertension, cardiac hypertrophy, and atherosclerosis.[51] Yet, its relationship to cardiac arrhythmias, particularly AF, is a new area of investigation.[52] RAAS has a multitude of electrophysiologic effects and can potentially cause arrhythmia through a variety of mechanisms, including atrial structural and electrical remodeling. Therefore, AF and malignant ventricular tachyarrhythmias, especially in the setting of cardiac hypertrophy or failure, may be considered examples of RAAS-related arrhythmias because treatment with RAAS modulators, including angiotensin-converting enzyme inhibitors, angiotensin receptor blockers, and mineralocorticoid receptor blockers, reduces the incidence of these arrhythmias.[53]

The RAAS has long been suggested by experimental models to be involved in the pathophysiology of AF.[54] RAAS is involved in atrial electroanatomic remodeling and is likely to play an important role in the development of atrial fibrosis and the perpetuation of AF.[55–57] Furthermore, several clinical studies have reported a lower prevalence of AF in selected patient populations treated with RAAS inhibitors compared with controls.[58] AF is also less likely to recur after cardioversion in patients treated with RAAS inhibitors than controls. Recently, rapid atrial pacing in a porcine model increased the activity of the profibrotic enzymes matrix metalloproteinase 2 (MMP2) and MMP9 in the atrial interstitium, increased MMP9 messenger RNA (mRNA) expression, and increased the activity of tissue inhibitor of metalloproteinase 1 (TIMP1) and TIMP3.[59]

Hence, it is tempting to speculate that both structural and electrical remodeling produced by sustained AF may share common pathways in which the main fibrogenic cell type in the heart, the myofibroblast, plays a central role through its activation by RAAS. Ang II activates various profibrotic pathways via the Ang II receptor type 1 (AT1 receptor) in the myofibroblast not only in the lung, liver, and kidney but also in heart tissue.[22] Stimulation of the AT1 receptor promotes the transformation of the quiescent atrial fibroblast into myofibroblast and the synthesis of TGF-β1 (see Fig. 2), the major profibrotic cytokine in the heart,[60] which has been shown to preferentially induce fibrosis in the atria over the ventricles.[61,62]

In addition, aldosterone has been shown to induce fibrosis in chronic lung, liver, and heart diseases.[54] Moreover, the significance of investigating the role played by specific signaling pathways of RAAS in the molecular mechanisms that lead to the transition from paroxysmal to persistent AF is highlighted by the fact that myofibroblasts are the primary mediators of fibrosis in the damaged heart through activation of TGF-β/SMAD signaling.[63–65] They also contribute to cardiac fibrosis through their relatively greater ability to produce fibrillar and nonfibrillar collagens[66,67] and to induce extracellular matrix remodeling through production of focal adhesion–associated proteins.[64,68,69] The importance of these studies is enhanced also by knowledge that paracrine factors released from myofibroblasts lead to myocyte hypertrophy and diastolic dysfunction.[70,71] The best-studied factors include TGF-β, PDGF, fibroblast growth factor 2 and members of the IL-6 family of proteins.[70–72] Whether and how such factors affect myocyte electrical function in the atria or ventricles has only recently been addressed. For example, TGF-β1 released by myofibroblasts differentially regulates transcription and function of the main cardiac sodium channel and of the channel responsible for the transient outward current.[23] Those results provided new mechanistic insight into the molecular mechanisms of electrical remodeling associated with myocardial injury.[23]

Recently published in-vitro experiments[27] strongly suggest that, in addition to leading to fibrosis, atrial myofibroblasts contribute to electromechanical remodeling of myocytes via direct physical contact and release of PDGF, which may be a factor in persistent AF-induced remodeling. The PDGF family is composed of 4 different isoforms, PDGF-A, -B, -C, and -D.[73] These isotypes dimerize to form active proteins creating 4 homodimers and one heterodimer (PDGF-AB). To identify the predominant isoform of PDGF in unpaced ovine atria, the author performed Western blot analysis using primary antibodies directed at PDGF-AB, PDGF-BB, and PDGF-AA. Isoforms C and D are primarily found in the ventricle. PDGF-AB was the predominant isoform detected in atrial homogenates. PDGF isotype expression was normalized to glyceraldehyde 3-phosphate dehydrogenase (GAPDH) (Fig. 3A, B). To determine if atrial myofibroblasts are a potential source of PDGF-AB, conditioned medium collected from primary fibroblast cultures, transformed myofibroblast cultures, and myocyte culture were collected and analyzed for the presence of PDGF-AB by enzyme-linked immunosorbent assay. Atrial myofibroblasts secrete significantly higher amounts of PDGF-AB than atrial myocytes and trend higher

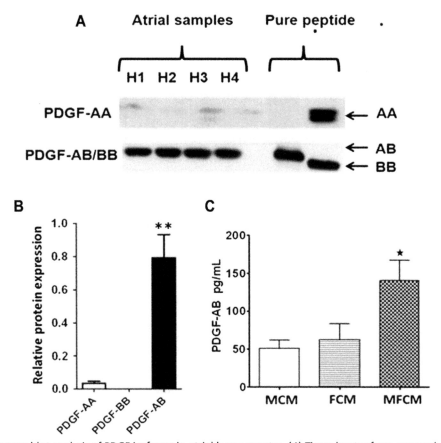

Fig. 3. Western blot analysis of PDGF isoforms in atrial homogenates. (*A*) Tissue lysates from unpaced sheep atria were probed with a PDGF antibody known to recognize 2 major isoforms, PDGF-AB and PDGF-BB, and a separate antibody recognizing the PDGF-AA isoform. Lanes H1 through H4 represent homogenate samples from 4 separate ovine atrial preparations and the final 3 lanes represent 3 recombinant PDGF dimers: PDGF-AA, PDGF-AB, and PDGF-BB. (*B*) Expression levels of 3 PDGF isoforms relative to GAPDH (N = 4). (*C*) Proteomic analysis of conditioned media demonstrates that ovine atrial myofibroblasts (myofibroblast-conditioned medium [MFCM]) secrete significantly higher amounts of PDGF-AB than atrial myocytes (myocyte-conditioned medium [MCM]) and primary atrial fibroblasts (FCM) (*P<.05; **P≤.01). (*Adapted from* Musa H, Kaur K, O'Connell R, et al. Inhibition of platelet-derived growth factor-ab signaling prevents electromechanical remodeling of adult atrial myocytes that contact myofibroblasts. Heart Rhythm 2013;10:1044–51; with permission.)

compared with primary atrial fibroblasts (see **Fig. 3**C). These data support the idea that an increased presence of myofibroblasts in the atrial parenchyma would likely enhance the levels of PDGF-AB in the ovine atria. Next, we determined the effects of PDGF-AB on the APD of normal unpaced ovine atrial myocytes. Cells were incubated with 1 ng/mL recombinant PDGF-AB peptide for 24 hours in culture. This PDGF-AB concentration is somewhat higher than that released by atrial myofibroblasts (see **Fig. 3**B) but well within the range reported by other investigators.[74] As shown in **Fig. 4**A–C, PDGF-AB causes significant reductions in both APD_{50} and APD_{80}. Similar to what has been demonstrated in the co-cultures, PDGF Neuntralizing antibody (N-ab) prevented this effect. **Fig. 4**E, F illustrates that both atrial myocytes

isolated from a persistent AF animal (see below) and atrial myocytes isolated from an unpaced heart but incubated with PDGF-AB can be stimulated rapidly, up to 10 Hz. In contrast, myocytes from unpaced atria, and myocytes treated with PDGF in the presence of N-ab were unable to respond in a 1:1 manner to pacing frequencies of 3 Hz or higher (see **Fig. 4**D, G).

One hallmark of electrophysiological remodeling in both chronically paced atria in animals and PAF in humans is a reduction of I_{CaL}.[18] Thus, to directly assess the effects of heterocellular contact on I_{CaL} we performed whole-cell patch clamp recordings in atrial myocytes isolated from unpaced ovine atria that were in direct contact with myofibroblasts and compared them to ($I_{Ca,L}$) recordings from isolated myocytes in the same dish (**Fig. 5**A–C). The

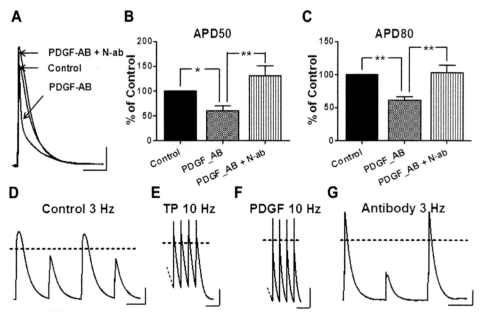

Fig. 4. (*A–C*) PDGF-AB (PDGF-AB; 1 ng/mL) shortens sheep atrial myocyte APD50 and APD80 (*$P<.05$; **$P<.01$). Neutralizing antibody (N-ab) blocks the effect (all conditions; $n \geq 9$). (*D–G*) After 24-h incubation with PDGF-AB, atrial myocytes could be stimulated up to 10 Hz (panel *F*) similar to cells from a tachypaced (TP) animal (panel *E*). In contrast, atrial cells from an unpaced animal (panel *D*) as well as those exposed to PDGF-AB+N-ab (panel *G*) could not be paced higher than 3 Hz. Scale bars = 20 mV, 100 ms (panel *A*), 200 ms (panels *D–F*). (*From* Musa H, Kaur K, O'Connell R, et al. Inhibition of platelet-derived growth factor-ab signaling prevents electromechanical remodeling of adult atrial myocytes that contact myofibroblasts. Heart Rhythm 2013;10:1044–51; with permission.)

$I_{Ca,L}$ current-voltage (I-V) profile of myocytes in direct contact with myofibroblasts demonstrates a significant attenuation of inward currents at several tested voltages. Furthermore, the I-V relationship of myocytes in contact with myofibroblasts and also in the presence of N-ab retained a profile similar to isolated myocytes. The voltage-dependent inactivation and time-dependent recovery of $I_{Ca,L}$ were unaffected, as shown in **Fig. 5**B, C, respectively. In addition, representative traces of calcium transients elicited at 0.5 Hz pacing demonstrate reduced calcium transient amplitudes in atrial myocytes, isolated from unpaced hearts, in direct contact with myofibroblasts (see **Fig. 5**D). A quantitative analysis of the results is shown in **Fig. 5**E. Peak calcium transient amplitudes were reduced from a control mean value of 5.20 ± 0.61% to a value of 2.34 ± 0.30% in the presence of heterocellular contact (*$P<.01$). Preincubation with a neutralizing PDGF-AB antibody partially restored the transient with a value of 3.47 ± 0.74%. Values were calculated as a percentage increase of fluorescence relative to baseline values. These data allow us to suggest that PDGF-AB released by myofibroblasts residing in close proximity to atrial myocytes can lead to calcium channel remodeling compromising the balance of inward

currents and contributing to the observed heterogeneous shortening of APD previously demonstrated in atrial myocytes obtained from sheep and human atria undergoing persistent AF.[75,76]

IS GAL-3 A NEW PLAYER IN AF REMODELING?

Gal-3 is a β-galactoside–binding lectin[77] that is highly expressed in fibrotic tissues.[78] Gal-3 plays a key role in hepatic,[79] renal,[80] and pulmonary fibrosis[81] following pro-fibrotic insults. Upregulation of Gal-3 has been demonstrated in different human inflammatory and fibrotic conditions, such as cirrhosis,[82] idiopathic lung fibrosis,[83] and chronic pancreatitis.[84] In the latter study, Gal-3 mRNA expression correlated significantly with the extent of fibrosis. Similarly, animal models of hepatic,[82] renal,[85] and cardiac fibrosis[86] have demonstrated the upregulation of Gal-3. Moreover, Gal-3 expression has been shown to be temporarily and spatially associated with fibrosis,[79] being minimal in normal liver, maximal at peak fibrosis, and virtually absent after recovery from fibrosis.[79] Further, it has been shown that Gal-3 infusion causes myocardial fibrosis, which may be neutralized by the antifibrotic tetrapeptide N-acetyl-seryl-aspartyl-lysyl-proline (Ac-SDKP).[86] Moreover, Gal-3 is

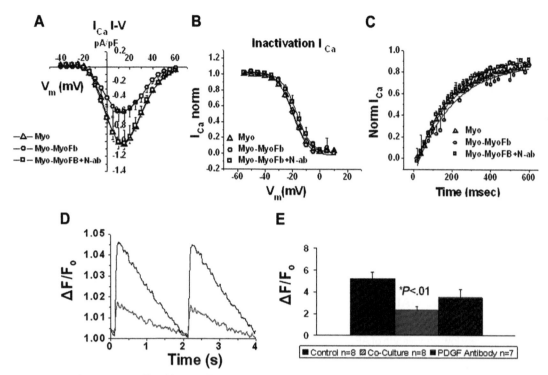

Fig. 5. Contact between myofibroblasts and unpaced atrial myocytes remodels L-type calcium current (ICa,L). (*A*) ICa,L was reduced at several voltages (*P*≤.05) when myocytes were in direct contact with a myofibroblast (circles; n = 4) relative to isolated myocytes (triangles; n = 5) and myocytes preincubated with PGDF antibody (PDGF N-ab; squares; n = 4) (n = 2 for all subsets). (*B, C*) ICa,L voltage-dependent inactivation and time dependence of recovery remain unaltered. (*D*) Representative calcium transients at 0.5 Hz from atrial cells in coculture. (*E*) Calcium transient amplitude (0.5 Hz) of atrial cells experiencing heterocellular contact (*red*) was reduced to 2.34% ± 0.30% from a control value (*black*) of 5.20% ± 0.61% (*P*≤.01). Preincubation with PDGF-AB N-ab partially restored the transient amplitudes to 3.47% ± 0.74% (*blue*) (n = 8, 8, 7, respectively). All values reflect a percentage increase over baseline fluorescence set to 1. Myo, myocyte; MyoFB, myofibroblast. (*From* Musa H, Kaur K, O'Connell R, et al. Inhibition of platelet-derived growth factor-ab signaling prevents electromechanical remodeling of adult atrial myocytes that contact myofibroblasts. Heart Rhythm 2013;10:1044–51; with permission.)

associated with age and risk factors of cardiovascular disease and predicts all-cause mortality in the general population.[78,87] Therefore, in addition to its diagnostic merit in heart failure patients, it has been proved that Gal-3 influences cardiac fibrosis to a high extent.[78]

The carboxyl-terminal domain of Gal-3 contains a carbohydrate-binding region linked by an amino-terminal domain consisting primarily of tandem repeats of 9 amino acids[88] to cross-link carbohydrate and noncarbohydrate ligands. It is a pleiotropic molecule found in the nucleus, cytoplasm, and at the cell surface, where Gal-3 pentamers bind to poly N-acetyllactosamine residues on TGF-β receptors of fibroblasts causing cell surface retention and promoting its signaling through SMADs and Akt.[81,89] To my knowledge, a possible role of Gal-3 in AF-induced atrial remodeling has never been explored, yet it is tempting to speculate that similar to what has been demonstrated in pulmonary fibrosis,[81] Gal-3 may regulate the effects of

TGF-β1 and other cytokines by promoting the retention of their receptors on the surface membrane of the atrial myofibroblast, thus acting to increase transcription of profibrotic molecules via stimulation of phosphorylation and nuclear translocation of the SMAD2/3 complex. Alternatively, Gal-3 may act by promoting Akt-mediated nuclear translocation of β-catenin via inhibition of GSK-3β phosphorylation and activity, which has been shown to be important in lung fibrosis.[81] Atrial fibrosis causes intra- and interatrial inhomogeneity in conduction, creating a substrate for reentry and contributing to the progressive nature of AF.[90] Among many other profibrotic factors, both Gal-3 and TGF-β1 have been implicated in the development of cardiac remodeling during heart failure, and TGF-β1 is of importance in tachypacing-induced fibrosis,[22] but the role of either TGF-β1 or Gal-3 in AF-induced electrical remodeling is unknown. Recently, Yu and colleagues[91] demonstrated that genetic disruption and pharmacologic inhibition of Gal-3 attenuates cardiac fibrosis, left ventricular dysfunction, and subsequent heart failure development. More recently, Sonmez and colleagues[92] showed that Gal-3, MMP9, and N-terminal propeptide of type III procollagen levels were significantly higher in the serum of AF patients compared with patients in sinus rhythm. However, Ho and colleagues[93] who examined the association of Gal-3 and incident AF in 3306 participants of a Framingham Offspring reported that higher circulating Gal-3 concentrations were associated with increased risk of developing AF but not after accounting for other traditional clinical AF risk factors. Altogether, the evidence discussed earlier indicates that although Gal-3 is a potential mediator of cardiac fibrosis in AF, additional preclinical and clinical studies are needed to evaluate its role in AF-related remodeling.

OUTLOOK ON PREVENTATIVE AF THERAPY

A study conducted in Geneva, Switzerland, in 2010 described a very low prevalence of AF in a survey of the general population of the elderly.[94] It was suggested that a high density of primary care physicians and cardiologist in Geneva may have resulted in better and broader screening and treatment of risk factors of AF. In addition, the Genevan population has a low exposure to the classical cardiovascular risk factors. Although needing confirmation in larger trials, the natural conclusion of that study is that a healthy population with a low exposure to the classical cardiovascular risk factors, with sufficient medical professionals who cautiously consider the guidelines, will have a lower percentage of AF than could be expected from previous studies.[95] Unfortunately, the characteristics of the Geneva population do not seem to repeat in the population of Europe and the United States at large, where the prevalence of AF is large and where an emphasis on health and risk factor prevention has not been comprehensively applied. Therefore, the accelerated growth in the incident AF rates in the Western world, together with the rising prevalence of AF in emerging Asian economies, is driving the growth of this market. According to a report by Transparency Market Research *(Atrial Fibrillation Market [Pharmacological and Non-Pharmacological Treatment, Electric Cardioversion, Radiofrequency, Cryo, Laser and Microwave Catheter Ablation, Maze Surgery, Anti-Coagulant and Anti-Arrhythmic Drugs]* - Global Industry Analysis, Size, Share, Growth, Trends and Forecast, 2013–2019), the AF market is valued at USD 6.1 billion in 2012 and is expected to reach an estimated value of USD 14.8 billion in 2019. Pharmacologic treatment procedures are more frequently administered to the patients suffering from AF and are a cheaper alternative to nonpharmacologic procedures. Therefore, pharmacologic procedures held most of the market share in 2012. In addition, favorable results exhibited by clinical trials promoting combined pharmacologic therapy and rising prevalence of disorders causing AF such as hypertension, obesity, and heart failure will also serve the market as drivers. Moreover, the future growth of this market and the rising prevalence of AF in emerging Asian economies will ensure the success of introducing novel advanced prevention therapies with the use of nonantiarrhythmic drugs that target specific mechanisms and signaling pathways involved in atrial remodeling to prevent the perpetuation or recurrence of the arrhythmia. Such agents include angiotensin-converting enzyme inhibitors, angiotensin receptor blockers, statins, mineralocorticoid blockers, and Gal-3 inhibitors. Through its effects promoting gene transcription via cytokine-mediated signaling pathways, Gal-3 might represent a common upstream link for both structural and electrical remodeling and a mediator in the transition to persistent AF. Should that prove to be true, then demonstration that one of several types of Gal-3 inhibitors that have been described recently[96] prevents the tachypacing-induced increase in DF[21] and halts AF progression might lead the way to the first generation of disease-modifying therapies to inhibit atrial remodeling and prevent AF perpetuation.

ACKNOWLEDGMENTS

I thank Drs S. Pandit and K. Kaur for excellent comments and recommendations in the preparation of the manuscript. This work was supported in part by the Leducq Foundation.

REFERENCES

1. Savelieva I, Camm J. Update on atrial fibrillation: part I. Clin Cardiol 2008;31:55–62.
2. Majeed A, Moser K, Carroll K. Trends in the prevalence and management of atrial fibrillation in general practice in England and Wales, 1994-1998: analysis of data from the general practice research database. Heart 2001;86:284–8.
3. Wolf PA, Abbott RD, Kannel WB. Atrial fibrillation as an independent risk factor for stroke: the Framingham study. Stroke 1991;22:983–8.
4. Feinberg WM, Blackshear JL, Laupacis A, et al. Prevalence, age distribution, and gender of patients with atrial fibrillation. Analysis and implications. Arch Intern Med 1995;155:469–73.
5. Stewart S, Hart CL, Hole DJ, et al. A population-based study of the long-term risks associated

with atrial fibrillation: 20-year follow-up of the Ren-frew/Paisley study. Am J Med 2002;113:359–64.

6. Bunch TJ, Weiss JP, Crandall BG, et al. Atrial fibrillation is independently associated with senile, vascular, and alzheimer's dementia. Heart Rhythm 2010;7:433–7.

7. Magnani JW, Rienstra M, Lin H, et al. Atrial fibrillation: current knowledge and future directions in epidemiology and genomics. Circulation 2011; 124:1982–93.

8. Calkins H, Kuck KH, Cappato R, et al. 2012 HRS/EHRA/ECAS expert consensus statement on catheter and surgical ablation of atrial fibrillation: recommendations for patient selection, procedural techniques, patient management and follow-up, definitions, endpoints, and research trial design. Europace 2012;14: 528–606.

9. Haissaguerre M, Jais P, Shah DC, et al. Spontaneous initiation of atrial fibrillation by ectopic beats originating in the pulmonary veins. N Engl J Med 1998;339:659–66.

10. Cappato R, Calkins H, Chen SA, et al. Updated worldwide survey on the methods, efficacy, and safety of catheter ablation for human atrial fibrillation. Circ Arrhythm Electrophysiol 2010;3:32–8.

11. Pinho-Gomes AC, Reilly S, Brandes RP, et al. Targeting inflammation and oxidative stress in atrial fibrillation: role of 3-hydroxy-3-methylglutaryl-coenzyme a reductase inhibition with statins. Antioxid Redox Signal 2014;20:1268–85.

12. Corradi D. Atrial fibrillation from the pathologist's perspective. Cardiovasc Pathol 2014;23:71–84.

13. Nattel S, Harada M. Atrial remodeling and atrial fibrillation: recent advances and translational perspectives. J Am Coll Cardiol 2014;63:2335–45.

14. Menezes AR, Lavie CJ, DiNicolantonio JJ, et al. Atrial fibrillation in the 21st century: a current understanding of risk factors and primary prevention strategies. Mayo Clin Proc 2013;88:394–409.

15. Wijffels MC, Kirchhof CJ, Dorland R, et al. Atrial fibrillation begets atrial fibrillation. A study in awake chronically instrumented goats. Circulation 1995; 92:1954–68.

16. Workman AJ, Kane KA, Rankin AC. The contribution of ionic currents to changes in refractoriness of human atrial myocytes associated with chronic atrial fibrillation. Cardiovasc Res 2001;52:226–35.

17. Ausma J, Wijffels M, Thone F, et al. Structural changes of atrial myocardium due to sustained atrial fibrillation in the goat. Circulation 1997;96:3157–63.

18. Van Wagoner DR, Pond AL, Lamorgese M, et al. Atrial l-type Ca2+ currents and human atrial fibrillation. Circ Res 1999;85:428–36.

19. Voigt N, Trausch A, Knaut M, et al. Left-to-right atrial inward rectifier potassium current gradients in patients with paroxysmal versus chronic atrial fibrillation. Circ Arrhythm Electrophysiol 2010;3: 472–80.

20. Caballero R, de la Fuente MG, Gomez R, et al. In humans, chronic atrial fibrillation decreases the transient outward current and ultrarapid component of the delayed rectifier current differentially on each atria and increases the slow component of the delayed rectifier current in both. J Am Coll Cardiol 2010;55: 2346–54.

21. Filgueiras-Rama D, Price NF, Martins RP, et al. Long-term frequency gradients during persistent atrial fibrillation in sheep are associated with stable sources in the left atrium. Circ Arrhythm Electrophysiol 2012;5:1160–7.

22. He X, Gao X, Peng L, et al. Atrial fibrillation induces myocardial fibrosis through angiotensin II type 1 receptor-specific arkadia-mediated downregulation of SMAD7. Circ Res 2011;108:164–75.

23. Kaur K, Zarzoso M, Ponce-Balbuena D, et al. TGF-beta1, released by myofibroblasts, differentially regulates transcription and function of sodium and potassium channels in adult rat ventricular myocytes. PLoS One 2013;8:e55391.

24. Yamazaki M, Mironov S, Taravant C, et al. Heterogeneous atrial wall thickness and stretch promote scroll waves anchoring during atrial fibrillation. Cardiovasc Res 2012;94:48–57.

25. Martins RP, Kaur K, Hwang E, et al. Dominant frequency increase rate predicts transition from paroxysmal to long-term persistent atrial fibrillation. Circulation 2014;129:1472–82.

26. Kong P, Christia P, Frangogiannis NG. The pathogenesis of cardiac fibrosis. Cell Mol Life Sci 2014; 71:549–74.

27. Musa H, Kaur K, O'Connell R, et al. Inhibition of platelet-derived growth factor-AB signaling prevents electromechanical remodeling of adult atrial myocytes that contact myofibroblasts. Heart Rhythm 2013;10:1044–51.

28. Youn JY, Zhang J, Zhang Y, et al. Oxidative stress in atrial fibrillation: an emerging role of nadph oxidase. J Mol Cell Cardiol 2013;62:72–9.

29. Elahi MM, Flatman S, Matata BM. Tracing the origins of postoperative atrial fibrillation: the concept of oxidative stress-mediated myocardial injury phenomenon. Eur J Cardiovasc Prev Rehabil 2008;15:735–41.

30. Sag CM, Wagner S, Maier LS. Role of oxidants on calcium and sodium movement in healthy and diseased cardiac myocytes. Free Radic Biol Med 2013;63:338–49.

31. Chang JP, Chen MC, Liu WH, et al. Atrial myocardial NOX2 containing nadph oxidase activity contribution to oxidative stress in mitral regurgitation: potential mechanism for atrial remodeling. Cardiovasc Pathol 2011;20:99–106.

32. Kim YM, Guzik TJ, Zhang YH, et al. A myocardial NOX2 containing NAD(P)H oxidase contributes to oxidative stress in human atrial fibrillation. Circ Res 2005;97:629–36.

33. Kim YM, Kattach H, Ratnatunga C, et al. Association of atrial nicotinamide adenine dinucleotide phosphate oxidase activity with the development of atrial fibrillation after cardiac surgery. J Am Coll Cardiol 2008;51:68–74.

34. Zhang J, Youn JY, Kim AY, et al. Nox4-dependent hydrogen peroxide overproduction in human atrial fibrillation and hl-1 atrial cells: relationship to hypertension. Front Physiol 2012;3:140.

35. Neuman RB, Bloom HL, Shukrullah I, et al. Oxidative stress markers are associated with persistent atrial fibrillation. Clin Chem 2007;53:1652–7.

36. Antoniades C, Bakogiannis C, Tousoulis D, et al. Preoperative atorvastatin treatment in cabg patients rapidly improves vein graft redox state by inhibition of Rac1 and NADPH-oxidase activity. Circulation 2010;122:S66–73.

37. Mihm MJ, Yu F, Carnes CA, et al. Impaired myofibrillar energetics and oxidative injury during human atrial fibrillation. Circulation 2001;104:174–80.

38. Carnes CA, Chung MK, Nakayama T, et al. Ascorbate attenuates atrial pacing-induced peroxynitrite formation and electrical remodeling and decreases the incidence of postoperative atrial fibrillation. Circ Res 2001;89:E32–8.

39. Ozaydin M, Peker O, Erdogan D, et al. N-acetylcysteine for the prevention of postoperative atrial fibrillation: a prospective, randomized, placebo-controlled pilot study. Eur Heart J 2008;29:625–31.

40. Rodrigo R, Vinay J, Castillo R, et al. Use of vitamins C and E as a prophylactic therapy to prevent postoperative atrial fibrillation. Int J Cardiol 2010;138:221–8.

41. Korantzopoulos P, Kolettis TM, Kountouris E, et al. Oral vitamin c administration reduces early recurrence rates after electrical cardioversion of persistent atrial fibrillation and attenuates associated inflammation. Int J Cardiol 2005;102:321–6.

42. Friedrichs K, Klinke A, Baldus S. Inflammatory pathways underlying atrial fibrillation. Trends Mol Med 2011;17:556–63.

43. Klein WW. Arrhythmias in inflammatory heart disease (author's transl). Wien Klin Wochenschr 1975;87:465–8 [in German].

44. Aviles RJ, Martin DO, Apperson-Hansen C, et al. Inflammation as a risk factor for atrial fibrillation. Circulation 2003;108:3006–10.

45. Loricchio ML, Cianfrocca C, Pasceri V, et al. Relation of C-reactive protein to long-term risk of recurrence of atrial fibrillation after electrical cardioversion. Am J Cardiol 2007;99:1421–4.

46. Guo Y, Lip GY, Apostolakis S. Inflammation in atrial fibrillation. J Am Coll Cardiol 2012;60:2263–70.

47. Rizos I, Rigopoulos AG, Kalogeropoulos AS, et al. Hypertension and paroxysmal atrial fibrillation: a novel predictive role of high sensitivity C-reactive protein in cardioversion and long-term recurrence. J Hum Hypertens 2010;24:447–57.

48. Chung MK, Martin DO, Sprecher D, et al. C-reactive protein elevation in patients with atrial arrhythmias: inflammatory mechanisms and persistence of atrial fibrillation. Circulation 2001;104:2886–91.

49. Pellegrino PL, Brunetti ND, De Gennaro L, et al. Inflammatory activation in an unselected population of subjects with atrial fibrillation: links with structural heart disease, atrial remodeling and recent onset. Intern Emerg Med 2013;8:123–8.

50. Marcus GM, Smith LM, Ordovas K, et al. Intracardiac and extracardiac markers of inflammation during atrial fibrillation. Heart Rhythm 2010;7:149–54.

51. Mentz RJ, Bakris GL, Waeber B, et al. The past, present and future of renin-angiotensin aldosterone system inhibition. Int J Cardiol 2013;167:1677–87.

52. Iravanian S, Dudley SC Jr. The renin-angiotensin-aldosterone system (RAAS) and cardiac arrhythmias. Heart Rhythm 2008;5:S12–7.

53. Ito Y, Yamasaki H, Naruse Y, et al. Effect of eplerenone on maintenance of sinus rhythm after catheter ablation in patients with long-standing persistent atrial fibrillation. Am J Cardiol 2013;111:1012–8.

54. Kimura S, Ito M, Tomita M, et al. Role of mineralocorticoid receptor on atrial structural remodeling and inducibility of atrial fibrillation in hypertensive rats. Hypertens Res 2011;34:584–91.

55. Iraqi W, Rossignol P, Angioi M, et al. Extracellular cardiac matrix biomarkers in patients with acute myocardial infarction complicated by left ventricular dysfunction and heart failure: insights from the eplerenone post-acute myocardial infarction heart failure efficacy and survival study (EPHESUS) study. Circulation 2009;119:2471–9.

56. Pitt B, Stier CT Jr, Rajagopalan S. Mineralocorticoid receptor blockade: new insights into the mechanism of action in patients with cardiovascular disease. J Renin Angiotensin Aldosterone Syst 2003;4:164–8.

57. Burstein B, Nattel S. Atrial fibrosis: mechanisms and clinical relevance in atrial fibrillation. J Am Coll Cardiol 2008;51:802–9.

58. Ehrlich JR, Hohnloser SH, Nattel S. Role of angiotensin system and effects of its inhibition in atrial fibrillation: clinical and experimental evidence. Eur Heart J 2006;27:512–8.

59. Chen CL, Huang SK, Lin JL, et al. Upregulation of matrix metalloproteinase-9 and tissue inhibitors of metalloproteinases in rapid atrial pacing-induced atrial fibrillation. J Mol Cell Cardiol 2008;45:742–53.

60. Frangogiannis NG, Michael LH, Entman ML. Myofibroblasts in reperfused myocardial infarcts express the embryonic form of smooth muscle myosin heavy chain (smemb). Cardiovasc Res 2000;48:89–100.

61. Verheule S, Sato T, Everett T, et al. Increased vulnerability to atrial fibrillation in transgenic mice with selective atrial fibrosis caused by overexpression of TGF-beta1. Circ Res 2004;94:1458–65.

62. Rahmutula D, Marcus GM, Wilson EE, et al. Molecular basis of selective atrial fibrosis due to overexpression of transforming growth factor-beta1. Cardiovasc Res 2013;99:769–79.

63. Dixon IM. The soluble interleukin 6 receptor takes its place in the pantheon of interleukin 6 signaling proteins: phenoconversion of cardiac fibroblasts to myofibroblasts. Hypertension 2010;56:193–5.

64. Santiago JJ, Dangerfield AL, Rattan SG, et al. Cardiac fibroblast to myofibroblast differentiation in vivo and in vitro: expression of focal adhesion components in neonatal and adult rat ventricular myofibroblasts. Dev Dyn 2010;239:1573–84.

65. Dobaczewski M, Bujak M, Zymek P, et al. Extracellular matrix remodeling in canine and mouse myocardial infarcts. Cell Tissue Res 2006;324:475–88.

66. Espira L, Czubryt MP. Emerging concepts in cardiac matrix biology. Can J Physiol Pharmacol 2009;87:996–1008.

67. Dobaczewski M, Bujak M, Li N, et al. SMAD3 signaling critically regulates fibroblast phenotype and function in healing myocardial infarction. Circ Res 2010;107:418–28.

68. Thum T, Gross C, Fiedler J, et al. Microrna-21 contributes to myocardial disease by stimulating MAP kinase signalling in fibroblasts. Nature 2008;456:980–4.

69. Cleutjens JP, Verluyten MJ, Smiths JF, et al. Collagen remodeling after myocardial infarction in the rat heart. Am J Pathol 1995;147:325–38.

70. Kakkar R, Lee RT. Intramyocardial fibroblast myocyte communication. Circ Res 2010;106:47–57.

71. Souders CA, Bowers SL, Baudino TA. Cardiac fibroblast: the renaissance cell. Circ Res 2009; 105:1164–76.

72. Banerjee I, Fuseler J, Souders CA, et al. The role of interleukin-6 in the formation of the coronary vasculature. Microsc Microanal 2009;15:415–21.

73. Zhao W, Zhao T, Huang V, et al. Platelet-derived growth factor involvement in myocardial remodeling following infarction. J Mol Cell Cardiol 2011;51:830–8.

74. Ivarsson M, McWhirter A, Borg TK, et al. Type i collagen synthesis in cultured human fibroblasts: regulation by cell spreading, platelet-derived growth factor and interactions with collagen fibers. Matrix Biol 1998;16:409–25.

75. Gaborit N, Steenman M, Lamirault G, et al. Human atrial ion channel and transporter subunit gene-expression remodeling associated with valvular heart disease and atrial fibrillation. Circulation 2005;112: 471–81.

76. Lau DH, Psaltis PJ, Mackenzie L, et al. Atrial remodeling in an ovine model of anthracycline-induced non-ischemic cardiomyopathy: remodeling of the same sort. J Cardiovasc Electrophysiol 2011;22:175–82.

77. Barondes SH, Castronovo V, Cooper DN, et al. Galectins: a family of animal beta-galactoside-binding lectins. Cell 1994;76:597–8.

78. de Boer RA, Yu L, van Veldhuisen DJ. Galectin-3 in cardiac remodeling and heart failure. Curr Heart Fail Rep 2010;7:1–8.

79. Henderson NC, Mackinnon AC, Farnworth SL, et al. Galectin-3 regulates myofibroblast activation and hepatic fibrosis. Proc Natl Acad Sci U S A 2006; 103:5060–5.

80. Henderson NC, Mackinnon AC, Farnworth SL, et al. Galectin-3 expression and secretion links macrophages to the promotion of renal fibrosis. Am J Pathol 2008;172:288–98.

81. Mackinnon AC, Gibbons MA, Farnworth SL, et al. Regulation of tgf-beta1 driven lung fibrosis by galectin-3. Am J Respir Crit Care Med 2012;185:537–46.

82. Hsu DK, Dowling CA, Jeng KC, et al. Galectin-3 expression is induced in cirrhotic liver and hepatocellular carcinoma. Int J Cancer 1999;81:519–26.

83. Nishi Y, Sano H, Kawashima T, et al. Role of galectin-3 in human pulmonary fibrosis. Allergol Int 2007;56: 57–65.

84. Wang L, Friess H, Zhu Z, et al. Galectin-1 and galectin-3 in chronic pancreatitis. Lab Invest 2000;80:1233–41.

85. Sasaki S, Bao Q, Hughes RC. Galectin-3 modulates rat mesangial cell proliferation and matrix synthesis during experimental glomerulonephritis induced by anti-thy1.1 antibodies. J Pathol 1999; 187:481–9.

86. Liu YH, D'Ambrosio M, Liao TD, et al. N-acetyl-seryl-aspartyl-lysyl-proline prevents cardiac remodeling and dysfunction induced by galectin-3, a mammalian adhesion/growth-regulatory lectin. Am J Physiol Heart Circ Physiol 2009;296:H404–12.

87. Lopez-Andres N, Rossignol P, Iraqi W, et al. Association of galectin-3 and fibrosis markers with long-term cardiovascular outcomes in patients with heart failure, left ventricular dysfunction, and dyssynchrony: insights from the care-hf (cardiac resynchronization in heart failure) trial. Eur J Heart Fail 2012;14:74–81.

88. Liu FT. Molecular biology of ige-binding protein, ige-binding factors, and ige receptors. Crit Rev Immunol 1990;10:289–306.

89. Bonniaud P, Margetts PJ, Ask K, et al. Tgf-beta and smad3 signaling link inflammation to chronic fibrogenesis. J Immunol 2005;175:5390–5.

90. Li D, Fareh S, Leung TK, et al. Promotion of atrial fibrillation by heart failure in dogs: atrial remodeling of a different sort. Circulation 1999;100:87–95.

91. Yu L, Ruifrok WP, Meissner M, et al. Genetic and pharmacological inhibition of galectin-3 prevents cardiac remodeling by interfering with myocardial fibrogenesis. Circ Heart Fail 2013;6:107–17.

92. Sonmez O, Ertem FU, Vatankulu MA, et al. Novel fibro-inflammation markers in assessing left atrial remodeling in non-valvular atrial fibrillation. Med Sci Monit 2014;20:463–70.

93. Ho JE, Yin X, Levy D, et al. Galectin 3 and incident atrial fibrillation in the community. Am Heart J 2014; 167:729–34.e1.

94. Schmutz M, Beer-Borst S, Meiltz A, et al. Low prevalence of atrial fibrillation in asymptomatic adults in geneva, switzerland. Europace 2010;12:475–81.

95. Heeringa J. Atrial fibrillation: is the prevalence rising? Europace 2010;12:451–2.

96. Tellez-Sanz R, Garcia-Fuentes L, Vargas-Berenguel A. Human galectin-3 selective and high affinity inhibitors. Present state and future perspectives. Curr Med Chem 2013;20:2979–90.

Moving?

Make sure your subscription moves with you!

To notify us of your new address, find your **Clinics Account Number** (located on your mailing label above your name), and contact customer service at:

Email: journalscustomerservice-usa@elsevier.com

800-654-2452 (subscribers in the U.S. & Canada)
314-447-8871 (subscribers outside of the U.S. & Canada)

Fax number: 314-447-8029

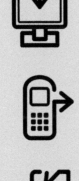

Elsevier Health Sciences Division
Subscription Customer Service
3251 Riverport Lane
Maryland Heights, MO 63043

ELSEVIER

Printed and bound by CPI Group (UK) Ltd, Croydon, CR0 4YY

03/10/2024

01040304-0010